Biodegradation
of Pesticides

Biodegradation of Pesticides

Edited by

Fumio Matsumura
Michigan State University
East Lansing, Michigan

and

C. R. Krishna Murti
Industrial Toxicology Research Centre
Lucknow, India

SPRINGER SCIENCE+BUSINESS MEDIA, LLC

Library of Congress Cataloging in Publication Data

Main entry under title:

Biodegradation of pesticides.

Includes bibliographical references and index.
1. Pesticides—Biodegradation. I. Matsumura, Fumio. II. Krishna Murti, C. R.
SB951.145.B54B56   628.9′6   82-7570
ISBN 978-1-4684-4090-4   ISBN 978-1-4684-4088-1 (eBook)   AACR2
DOI 10.1007/ 978-1-4684-4088-1

© 1982 Springer Science+Business Media New York
Originally published by Plenum Press, New York in 1982
Softcover reprint of the hardcover 1st edition 1982

Contributors

T. K. Adhya, Laboratory of Soil Microbiology, Central Rice Research Institute, Cuttack 753006, India

Floyd M. Ashton, Department of Botany, University of California, Davis, California 95616

Sue K. Ballard, Department of Entomology and Graduate Center for Toxicology, University of Kentucky, Lexington, Kentucky 40546

Carl E. Crisp, Pacific Southwest Forest and Range Experiment Station, Forest Service, U.S. Department of Agriculture, Berkeley, California 94701

Gene R. DeFoliart, Department of Entomology, University of Wisconsin, Madison, Wisconsin 53706

T. S. S. Dikshith, Industrial Toxicology Research Centre, Lucknow 226001, India

H. Wyman Dorough, Department of Entomology and Graduate Center for Toxicology, University of Kentucky, Lexington, Kentucky 40546

D. Stuart Frear, U.S. Department of Agriculture, Science and Education Administration, Agricultural Research, Metabolism and Radiation Research Laboratory, Fargo, North Dakota 58105

C. R. Krishna Murti, Industrial Toxicology Research Centre, Lucknow 226001, India

Gerald L. Lamoureux, U.S. Department of Agriculture, Science and Education Administration, Agricultural Research, Metabolism and Radiation Research Laboratory, Fargo, North Dakota 58105

Fumio Matsumura, Pesticide Research Center, Michigan State University, East Lansing, Michigan 48824

J. R. Plimmer, Organic Chemical Synthesis Laboratory, Agricultural Research Services, U.S. Department of Agriculture, Beltsville, Maryland 20705

K. Raghu, Biology and Agriculture Division, Bhabha Atomic Research Centre, Bombay 400085, India

N. Sethunathan, Laboratory of Soil Microbiology, Central Rice Research Institute, Cuttack 753006, India

Richard H. Shimabukuro, U.S. Department of Agriculture, Science and Education Administration, Agricultural Research, Metabolism and Radiation Research Laboratory, Fargo, North Dakota 58105

Hugh D. Sisler, Department of Botany, University of Maryland, College Park, Maryland 20742

Preface

When first developed, chlorinated pesticides such as DDT, dieldrin, and mirex were received with open arms, quickly becoming popular as effective, economic agents against pests. But evidence began to mount that residues of these chemicals remained in the environment, not breaking down, often appearing in plants and animals. By the late seventies many pesticides had achieved a terrible notoriety and were subsequently banned in a number of countries. Of tremendous concern, then, is the persistence of pesticides in the environment.

The major thrust of research and development in the area of pesticides has properly been the creation of substances that are both effective and degradable. Yet in order to successfully promote the use of biodegradable pesticides, one must fully understand the mechanism of degradation, and it is to this vital subject that we address ourselves in the present volume.

According to the Biodegradation Task Force, Safety of Chemicals Committee, Brussels (1978), *biodegradation* may be defined as

> the molecular degradation of an organic substance resulting from the complex action of living organisms. A substance is said to be biodegraded to an environmentally acceptable extent when environmentally undesirable properties are lost. Loss of some characteristic function or property of substance by biodegradation may be referred to as biological transformation.

Since the subject of pesticide degradation is complex, often involving sophisticated knowledge of the mutual interaction between chemical and environment, we have attempted to summarize current knowledge of, and thinking on, pesticide degradation, presenting scientific principles as well as describing their practical applications. Our intended audience comprises those who develop new pesticides, who assess their environmental hazards, or who regulate their use.

The idea for this book originated from productive sessions at the United States–India Workshop on Biodegradable Pesticides, held in Lucknow, India, under the auspices of the National Science Foundation's International Programs

Division and Department of Science and Technology, India. We would like to thank Ms. Alice Ellis and Ms. Sharon Puchalski for assisting us in editing the manuscripts.

Fumio Matsumura
C. R. Krishna Murti

Contents

Chapter 2

Pesticide Metabolism in Plants: Reactions and Mechanisms

Richard H. Shimabukuro, Gerald L. Lamoureux, and
D. Stuart Frear

Chapter 3

Degradation of Pesticides in the Environment by Microorganisms and Sunlight

Fumio Matsumura

PART II • APPLICATION OF THE PRINCIPLES OF BIODEGRADATION OF PESTICIDES

Chapter 4
Microbial Degradation of Pesticides in Tropical Soils
N. Sethunathan, T. K. Adhya, and K. Raghu

Chapter 5
Persistence and Biodegradation of Herbicides
Floyd M. Ashton

Chapter 6
Biodegradation of Agricultural Fungicides
Hugh D. Sisler

Chapter 7
Biodegradable Insecticides: Their Application in Forestry
Carl E. Crisp

Chapter 8
The Use of Biodegradable Pesticides in Public Health Entomology
Gene R. DeFoliart

Chapter 9
Pesticides for Stored Products
J. R. Plimmer

Chapter 10

Application of Biodegradable Pesticides in India
C. R. Krishna Murti and T. S. S. Dikshith

PART I

Biodegradation of Pesticides
Principles and Mechanisms

1

Degradation of Pesticides by Animals

H. Wyman Dorough and Sue K. Ballard

1.1. INTRODUCTION

Once a pesticide enters the animal body through ingestion, inhalation, or dermal absorption, it is subject to metabolism by a variety of mechanisms. The types of chemical or biochemical transformations a pesticide may undergo in the animal are varied, and knowledge of the fate of these toxicants in animals contributes to a better understanding of their advantages and limitations for specific use situations. This is an important consideration since the almost universal usage of wide varieties of pesticides may result in the exposure of man and other nontarget organisms on a regular basis. The effect of this exposure on animals depends upon many factors such as the concentration and chemical composition of the pesticide, the species of animal, and the sex and age of the animal. While complete coverage of the fate of pesticides in animals exceeds the intent of the present presentation, a general discussion of the biochemistry of pesticides in animals is necessary if one is to gain even the slightest appreciation of the complexity of the many factors involved.

Basically, the various types of pesticides (e.g., herbicides, insecticides, fungicides) may be considered essentially as lipophilic compounds containing certain functional groups that may undergo well-recognized biochemical reactions. For the most part, these reactions lead to compounds that are more polar than the parent molecule and more easily excreted from the body. Therefore, most metabolic transformations of pesticides are detoxification processes. It is well-established, however, that metabolism often leads to more active com-

H. Wyman Dorough and Sue K. Ballard • Department of Entomology and Graduate Center for Toxicology, University of Kentucky, Lexington, Kentucky 40546.

pounds, as in the case with the conversion of parathion to paraoxon. Fortunately, the more active compounds are usually further metabolized to nontoxic forms and eventually eliminated from the body.

Most data available indicate that the ability of different animal species to metabolize a pesticide vary quantitatively rather than qualitatively. For this reason the present discussion will center around the metabolism of parent pesticide molecules that occur within animal systems generally. The term *metabolite* will be used here to denote any derivative of the parent molecule, and bioalteration reactions that lead to metabolites will be divided into two broad categories: *phase I (primary) metabolism* and *phase II metabolism*, referred to as *secondary* or *conjugation metabolism*.

Phase I metabolism involves the production of a free metabolite through biotransformation reactions such as dehydrohalogenation, dehalogenation, desulfuration, epoxidation, hydrolysis, hydroxylation–isomerization, oxidation, reduction, and nitrosation (Menn and Still, 1977). The term *free metabolite* refers to metabolites which are derived from the parent pesticide and have not reacted further with natural components of a biological system. These can normally be extracted from the substrate and partitioned from water into an organic solvent. Thus, free metabolites are often referred to as *organosolubles*.

Phase II metabolism involves the formation of conjugates through glycoside formation, sulfoconjugation, glutathione conjugation, amino acid conjugation, acetylation, and methylation (Dorough, 1979a). Thus, conjugated metabolites are derivatives of the pesticide that have reacted with a natural component of the organism to form a new material. Generally, this type of reaction involves the formation of a free metabolite, followed by a second step converting the metabolite to a conjugate. These conjugates are usually extractable from the substrate with polar solvents but do not partition from water into organic solvents. Components of the pesticide that cannot be removed from the substrate by thorough extraction are called *bound residues*. In this case, conjugation may have occurred with endogenous portions of the organisms such as proteins or cell membranes. However, little is actually known about the chemical nature of the bound residues.

Further information on general pesticide degradation can be found in the works of Wilkinson (1976), Matsumura (1975), and Melnikov (1971). A more detailed review of conjugation metabolism of pesticides was recently reported by Dorough (1979a).

1.2. PHASE I METABOLISM

1.2.1. Dehydrohalogenation and Dehalogenation

One of the more familiar dehydrocholorination reactions in animals is the enzymatic conversion of DDT to DDE (Fig. 1.1). DDT also undergoes reductive

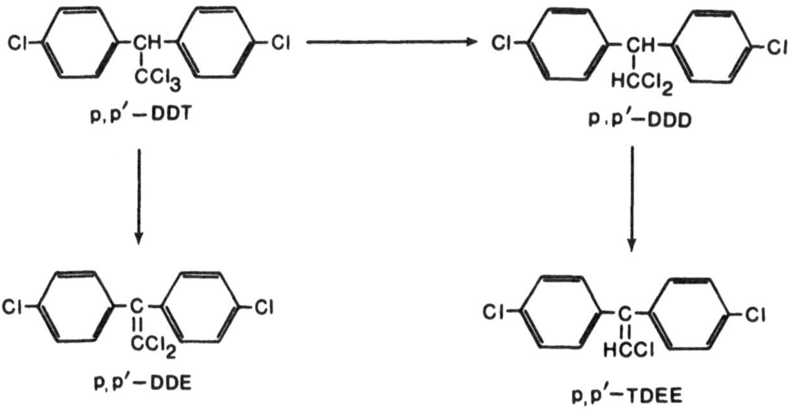

Figure 1.1. Metabolic dechlorination of DDT.

dechlorination to DDD. The metabolic conversion of p,p'-DDT in the pig has been shown to follow two major routes (Sundroik *et al.*, 1977). One of these routes involves the conversion of p,p'-DDT to p,p'-DDE, which is then excreted in the urine as such, or after enzymatic hydroxylation. The other route involves the oxidation of the aliphatic portion of p,p'-DDT to p,p'-DDA, which is a major excretory product in most animals.

White-tail deer metabolized 20% of administered DDT to DDE, most of which was eliminated in the feces (Kurtz and George, 1977). In general, vertebrates produce both p,p'-DDE and p,p'-DDD from p,p'-DDT, and the former product is often the major tissue residue (Addison and Willis, 1978).

The main product of dehydrohalogenation of the insecticide BHC is 1,2,4-trichlorobenzene (Benson, 1969). Once the first chlorine molecule is eliminated, the other two are lost so rapidly that metabolites containing 4 and 5 chlorines have not been isolated. Dogs, rabbits, and rats are among those animal species which metabolize BHC to 1,2,4-trichlorobenzene (Menzie, 1969).

In vitro work by Tashiro and Matsumura (1978) indicates that dechlorination is an important detoxification step in the metabolism of *trans*-nonachlor. It was demonstrated that metabolism of the compound was extremely slow in the human liver in comparison to the rat liver. The low metabolism of *trans*-nonachlor by human liver was thought to result from an inability of the liver preparations to form *trans*-chlordane. When *trans*-chlordane was added to the same preparations, the interspecies difference in metabolism rates diminished. Apparently, there is an efficient mechanism to dechlorinate *trans*-nonachlor to *trans*-chlordane in the rat.

Reductive debromination of the herbicide 3,4,5-tribromo-N,N-α-trimethyl-$1H$-pyrazole-1-acetamide has been shown to be a metabolic pathway in the rat (Hornish and Nappier, 1978). The reductive debromination of the tribromo acid

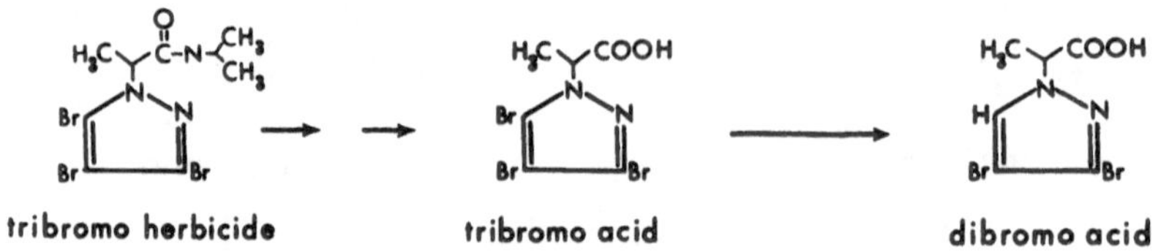

Figure 1.2.   Rats debrominate this compound selectively at the number 5 carbon.

that is first formed is apparently compound-specific and position-selective. The debromination occurred selectively at the C-5 position to produce the second most abundant metabolite (Fig. 1.2). Debromination at the other sites was not detected, and this selectivity is probably controlled by the electronic effects in the pyrazole ring. Reductive debromination is thought to be very unusual in the mammalian system.

1.2.2.   Desulfuration

Desulfuration is a well-known metabolic pathway for organophosphorus pesticides that contain a phosphorothioic moiety. This reaction is often an activation step in animals, since the resulting metabolite can be more toxic than the parent molecule. The desulfuration of malathion to malaoxon (Fig. 1.3) is a good example of this type of metabolic reaction (Eto, 1974). The parent compound has an acute oral LD_{50} in rats of approximately 2500 mg/kg while for the oxon derivative, the LD_{50} is about 300 mg/kg.

The formation of the more potent anticholinesterase compounds by desulfuration of thiophosphates has been demonstrated with many other common insecticides, including parathion (O,O-diethyl-O-p-nitrophenyl phosphorothioate), dimethoate [O,O-dimethyl S-(N-methyl-carbamoyl-methyl) phosphorothioate], and sumithion (O,O-dimethyl O-3-methyl-4-nitrophenyl phosphorothioate) (Fukuto and Metcalf, 1969).

1.2.3.   Epoxidation

It has been well established that microsomal enzymes are responsible for the epoxidation of the double bond that occurs in many cyclodiene insecticides

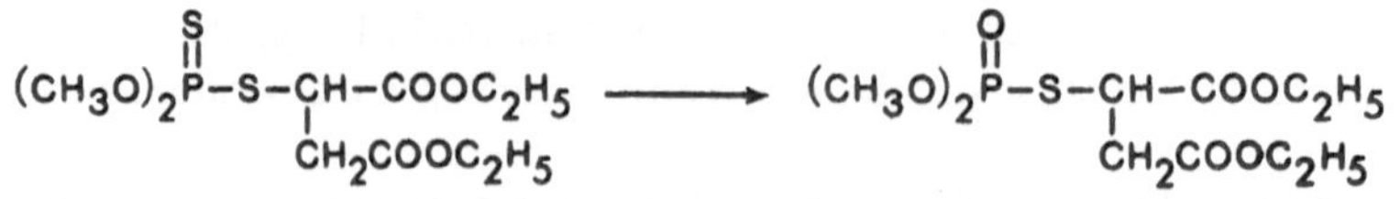

Figure 1.3.   Metabolic activation of malathion via desulfuration.

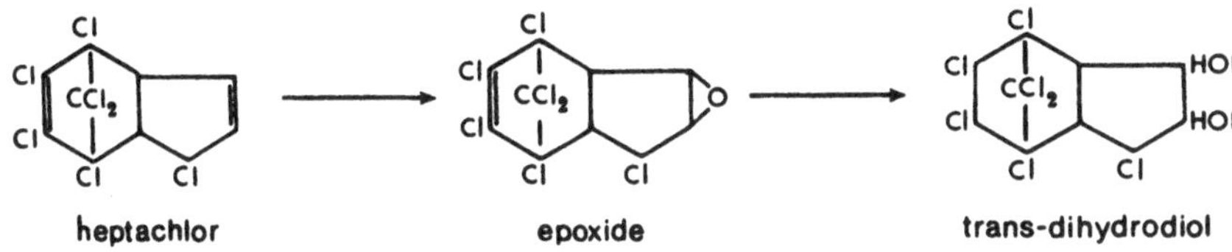

heptachlor   epoxide   trans-dihydrodiol

Figure 1.4. Metabolic epoxidation and subsequent hydration of heptachlor.

such as heptachlor, aldrin, isodrin, and chlordane (Brooks, 1974). Exampies of epoxidation have been shown to occur *in vivo* in dogs (Davidow and Radomski, 1953) and rats (Tashiro and Matsumura, 1978). Although epoxides can be very stable compounds, most are subject to hydration (Brooks and Harrison, 1969) and the resulting dihydrols are further metabolized and excreted from the body (Fig. 1.4).

Heptachlor epoxide is a major metabolite of heptachlor and is more toxic to animals than heptachlor (Melnikov, 1971). Aldrin and isodrin are epoxidized to dieldrin and endrin, respectively, and are as toxic or more toxic to animals than the parent compound (Casida and Lykken, 1969).

1.2.4. Hydrolysis

Pesticides with ester groups can be degraded by enzymatic or chemical hydrolysis. The result is the cleaving of the molecule by the addition of water, usually forming nontoxic products or products that can be detoxified by conjugation.

Carbamate insecticides are hydrolyzed by esterases to form carbamic acid, which instantaneously decomposes to carbon dioxide and methyl- or dimethylamine (Kuhr and Dorough, 1976). The carbamate ester bond is usually relatively stable in plants and insects but is hydrolyzed fairly readily in most animal species. For example, carbaryl (1-naphthyl-*N*-methylcarbamate) is readily hydrolyzed in rats, sheep, guinea pigs, and dogs. However, carbaryl is fairly resistant to hydrolysis in monkeys and pigs (Kuhr, 1971).

Organophosphorus insecticides undergo hydrolysis by a number of different enzymatic processes (Dauterman, 1971). The generalized reactions are shown in Fig. 1.5, where R is an alkyl group and X is either a halide, another substituted phosphorus group attached by an anhydride bond, or an alkoxy or aryloxy group. Hydrolysis may occur at the ester or acid anhydride bond.

The first reaction yields a dialkylphosphorothioic acid (or dialkyl phosphoric acid), while the second reaction yields a desalkyl derivative. The enzymes involved may be phosphotriester hydrolases, mixed-function oxidases, or glutathione transferases (Dauterman, 1971).

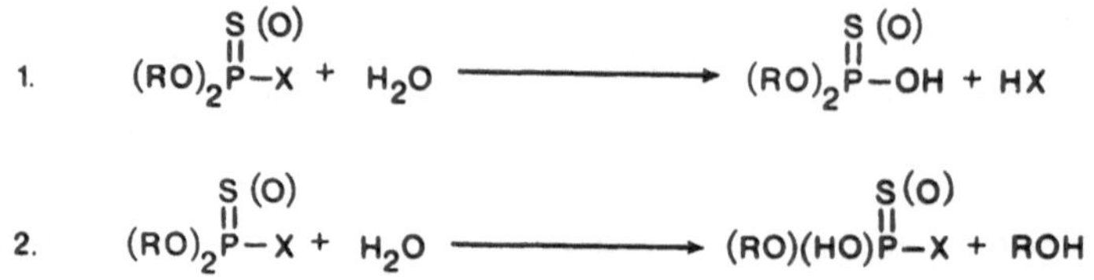

$$1. \quad (RO)_2 \overset{S\ (O)}{\overset{\|}{P}} - X + H_2O \longrightarrow (RO)_2 \overset{S\ (O)}{\overset{\|}{P}} - OH + HX$$

$$2. \quad (RO)_2 \overset{S\ (O)}{\overset{\|}{P}} - X + H_2O \longrightarrow (RO)(HO) \overset{S\ (O)}{\overset{\|}{P}} - X + ROH$$

Figure 1.5. Hydrolytic pathways common to most organophosphorus insecticides.

Although the alkyl phosphates are major metabolites of many organophosphorus pesticides, some of these compounds are subject to hydrolysis at other sites. For instance, several products can occur from malathion by hydrolytic cleavage at five different sites (Bradway and Shafik, 1977), as indicated by the position of the arrows in the structure of this insecticide shown in Fig. 1.6.

The metabolites occurred in the urine of a man who attempted suicide by drinking 200 ml of a 50% malathion preparation. Malathion monoacid was the most abundant metabolite, followed by dimethylphosphorothioate, and dimethylphosphate. Only small amounts of the dicarboxylic acid and monomethyl phosphate were detected.

1.2.5. Hydroxylation

Hydroxylation reactions are common in the formation of numerous pesticide metabolites in animals. The hydroxylation reaction can lead to further oxidation to form a carbonyl compound, or may serve as a site for further detoxification by O-conjugate formation. The proposed pathway for metabolism of the herbicide flamprop-isopropyl in rats and dogs (Fig. 1.7) shows hydroxylations on the isopropyl group of the molecule, which in one case leads to deesterification while in the other case leads to oxidation of the alcohol moiety to the acid derivative (Bedford et al., 1978). Quantitation of these metabolites showed that side chain hydroxylation was twice as great in dogs as in rats.

Aromatic hydroxylation reactions also occur readily in mammals. For example, several investigations have revealed that carbaryl is metabolized by hepatic enzymes to 1-naphthyl-N-hydroxymethylcarbamate, 4-hydroxy-1-naphthyl-N-methylcarbamate, and 5-hydroxy-1-naphthyl-N-methylcarbamate. Maximum

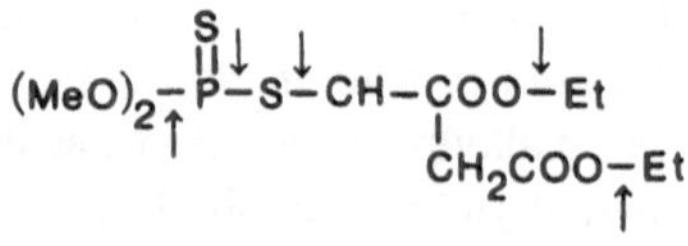

Figure 1.6. Points of hydrolytic cleavage on the malathion molecule.

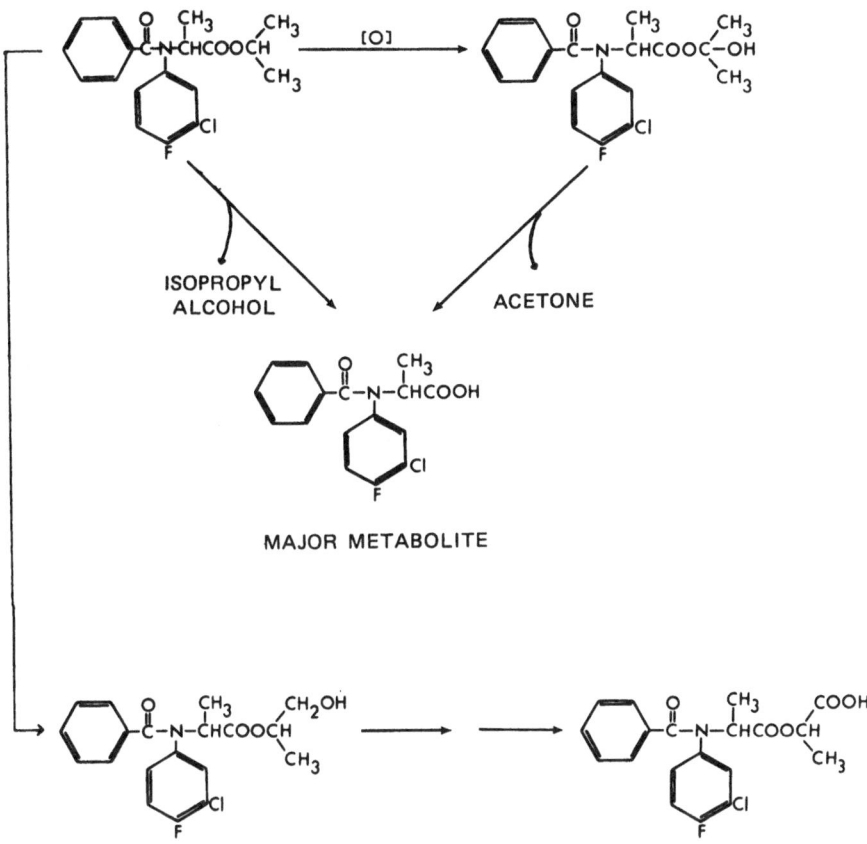

Figure 1.7. Hydroxylation reactions involved in the mammalian metabolism of the herbicide flamprop-isopropyl.

rates of formation *in vitro* were achieved with the microsome plus some fractions of rat liver in the presence of NADPH (Kuhr and Dorough, 1976). Most animals excrete about 70% of an administered dose of [^{14}C]-ring-labeled carbaryl in the urine within 24 hr after treatment. Much of the excreted radioactivity consists of metabolites formed by the hydroxylation of the naphthyl ring.

O-, S-, and N-alkyl hydroxylation are other possible features of microsomal hydroxylation. The electronegativity of the adjacent hetero-atom often leads to dealkylation. Many pesticides contain alkoxy groups in ester or ether structures that can be degraded by dealkylation of the O-alkyl group.

The reaction involves the formation of an unstable α-hydroxy intermediate (Fig. 1.8), which spontaneously produces an aldehyde or ketone depending on

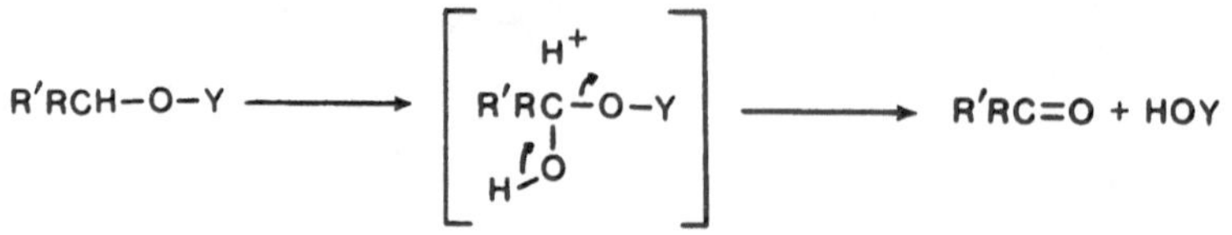

$$R'RCH-O-Y \longrightarrow \left[R'RC \overset{H^+}{\underset{H\overset{\prime}{\nearrow}O}{\cdot}} O-Y \right] \longrightarrow R'RC=O + HOY$$

Figure 1.8. Role of hydroxylation in O-dealkylation.

whether the carbonyl carbon is primary or secondary. With the organophosphates, it is known that glutathione S-alkyltransferase plays a role in demethylation and that the reaction varies considerably according to substrate and species (Nakatsugawa and Morelli, 1976).

N-alkyl hydroxylation and dealkylation occur in a manner that is chemically analogous to O-dealkylation. The N-hydroxylalkyl intermediate (Fig. 1.9) is more stable than the O-hydroxylalkyl intermediate, probably because of the lower electronegativity of nitrogen. Nonetheless, the intermediate does degrade to yield the dealkylated compound and an aldehyde (Nakatsugawa and Morelli, 1976).

1.2.6. Oxidation–Reduction Reactions

Some oxidation reactions such as epoxidation and hydroxylation have already been discussed. The fact that many thiophosphorus compounds are desulfurated by microsomal oxidases to their corresponding oxygen analogs also has been pointed out. Some of these esters are also hydrolyzed to phosphoric acids by the oxidase system, and may be an important degradation step in animals (Dauterman, 1971). The work of Nakatsugawa et al. (1969) indicates that diazinon undergoes oxidative metabolism which results in the formation of diazoxon and subsequent degradation to diethylphosphorothioic acid.

Oxidation of thioether compounds has long been recognized as a very significant reaction in the metabolism of pesticides containing an R-S-R group. Compounds such as demeton (Fig. 1.10) are oxidized to the sulfoxide and sulfone (March et al., 1955), and these metabolites may contribute markedly to the biological activity exhibited by these pesticides.

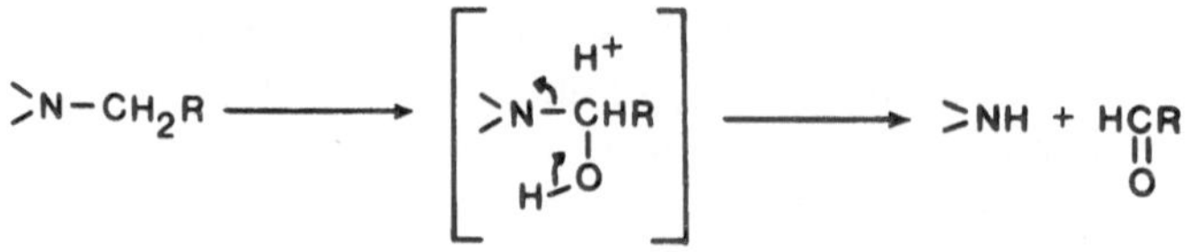

$$>N-CH_2R \longrightarrow \left[>N \overset{H^+}{\underset{H\overset{\prime}{\nearrow}O}{\cdot}} CHR \right] \longrightarrow >NH + H\underset{O}{\overset{\parallel}{C}}R$$

Figure 1.9. Role of hydroxylation in N-dealkylation.

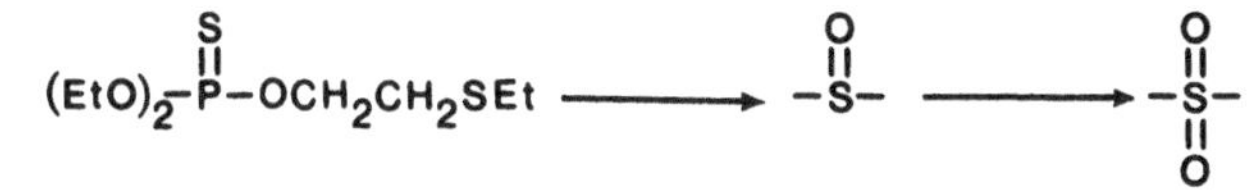

$$(EtO)_2-\overset{\overset{S}{\|}}{P}-OCH_2CH_2SEt \longrightarrow -\overset{\overset{O}{\|}}{S}- \longrightarrow -\overset{\overset{O}{\|}}{\underset{\underset{O}{\|}}{S}}-$$

Figure 1.10. Thioether oxidation of demeton.

Sulfoxidation is a major metabolic route for carbamates such as aldicarb (Kuhr and Dorough, 1976) and Croneton® (Nye *et al.*, 1976). In rats, the principal urinary metabolites of Croneton® (2-ethylthiomethylphenyl-*N*-methylcarbamate) were Croneton® sulfoxide, Croneton® sulfone, phenol sulfoxide, and phenol sulfone after both a single oral dose and in long-term feeding studies.

Probably the most common type of reduction reaction of pesticides in animals is the reduction of a nitro group to an amino group. Diphenyl ethers such as the herbicide nitrofen serve as excellent examples of pesticides having nitro substituents which can be reduced (Hunt *et al.*, 1977).

1.2.7. Isomerization

Reports of isomerization reactions in pesticide metabolism in animals are rare. However, it has been shown that *in vivo* isomerization and Beckmann rearrangement reactions are important in the metabolism of the insecticide methomyl in rats (Huhtanen and Dorough, 1976). The mechanism may also apply to other thiohydroximate esters. Methomyl may exist in two geometric configurations, *syn* and *anti*, but the more stable *syn* isomer is the form applied as an insecticide. *Syn* methomyl radiolabeled as indicated in Fig. 1.11 was shown to be metabolized to CO_2 and acetonitrile. It was proposed that *syn* methomyl was metabolized to CO_2 and isomerized, in part, to *anti* methomyl, which was then hydrolyzed and degraded to acetonitrile. The proposed mechanism is shown in Fig. 1.11 along with the percentages of the dose voided in the urine and expired as carbon dioxide and acetonitrile.

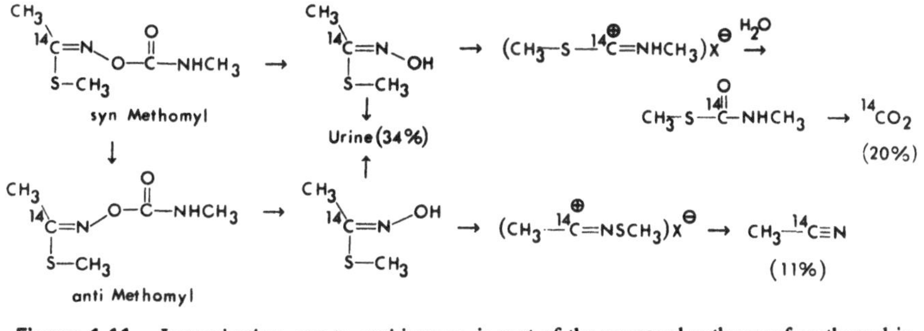

Figure 1.11. Isomerization, *syn* to *anti* isomer, is part of the proposed pathway of methomyl in rats.

1.2.8.   Nitrosation

There are many examples where nitrogen-containing pesticides react with nitrite to form *N*-nitroso compounds (Elespuru and Lijinsky, 1973). Many of these are potent mutagens. The reaction is a nonenzymatic synthesis which is highly pH-dependent, and relatively strong acid conditions are generally required to convert the nitrite into nitrous acid. Nitrous acid is further converted to active nitrosating agents such as nitrous anhydride or nitrous acidium ion (Mirvish, 1975). Pesticides nitrosated under these conditions include those compounds that contain an amine or amide moiety. Atrazine, a triazine herbicide, was converted to a nitrosamine derivative when reacted with nitrite under acid conditions (Wolfe *et al.*, 1976). Nitrosamines also have been formed from dithiocarbamate fungicides such as ziram, ferbam, and thiram (Eisenbrand *et al.*, 1974; Sen *et al.*, 1975). However, nitroso derivatives of the parent fungicide were not produced. It was necessary for these compounds to be degraded under acid conditions to release dimethylnitrosamine (Fig. 1.12).

Carbamates and ureas are the major classes of pesticides which react with nitrite to form nitrosamides. Many *N*-methylcarbamates have been nitrosated (Fig. 1.12) and the derivatives tested for mutagenicity and carcinogenicity (Lijinsky and Schmahl, 1978; Seiler, 1977; Uchiyama *et al.*, 1975). Thus far, the compounds tested have proven to be potent mutagens and animal carcinogens. *In vivo* nitrosation has been demonstrated in rats (Eisenbrand *et al.*, 1974) and guinea pigs (Rickard and Dorough, 1978).

1.3.   PHASE II METABOLISM

Conjugation metabolism of insecticides has been reviewed by Dorough (1979a), and the material generally applies to all groups of pesticides. In animal

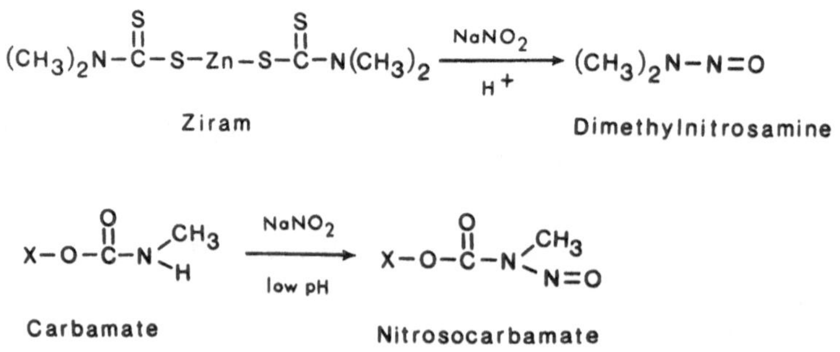

Figure 1.12.   Examples of *N*-nitroso formation from pesticides.

species the endogenous substrates are commonly glucuronic acid, sulfate, and amino acids. Glucose instead of glucuronic acid, is the most common endogenous substrate in insects and plants (Parke, 1968).

Pesticides usually require some type of phase I metabolism to produce an -OH, -COOH, $-NH_2$, -NHOH, or -SH site for subsequent conjugation with an endogenous compound (Smith, 1968; Jenner and Testa, 1978). If the endogenous compound is glucose, the conjugate is called a glucoside, and when it is glucuronic acid, it is referred to as a glucuronide. The terms that differentiate between the exogenous and endogenous moieties of the sugar conjugate or glycoside are *glycone* (sugar moiety) and *aglycone* (exogenous portion). The other types of conjugates do not have comparable terms to distinguish between the exogenous and endogenous portions of any conjugate, so the term *exocon* has been used to indicate the exogenous portion, and endocon to note the endogenous moiety (Dorough, 1976).

1.3.1. Glycoside Formation

While glucoside conjugation of xenobiotics is rare in mammals, some exceptions are reported in the literature. An example of this is the conjugation of a xanthine oxidase inhibitor with glucose in dogs, rats, and monkeys (Duggan *et al.*, 1974). Conclusive evidence that pesticides undergo glucose conjugation in mammals has yet to be presented.

In vertebrate species, many pesticides or their metabolites are conjugated as glucuronides. Glucuronic acid does not react directly, but is present in an active form (uridine diphosphate glucuronic acid, UDPGA), which is synthesized enzymatically from α-glucose-6-phosphate and glucuronic acid. Conjugation with a pesticide or its metabolite is mediated by glucuronyltransferase enzymes. This type of conjugation is one of the most important conjugation mechanisms in animals (Miettinen and Leskinen, 1970; Williams, 1967). Some examples of these glucuronide conjugates are shown in Fig. 1.13. Two animal groups which appear to have only minimal capacity for glucuronidation are cats and fishes. The reasons may be a reduced transferase activity in the cat, and a deficiency in the endogenous glucuronic acid donor in the fish (Parke, 1968).

1.3.2. Sulfoconjugation

Sulfotransferases are enzymes that catalyze sulfate conjugation in various organisms (Florkin and Stotz, 1973). The conjugation of compounds with sulfate is common in microorganisms, plants, and animals; the subject has been reviewed by Dodgson and Rose (1970).

The endogenous donor of the sulfate group is 3'-phosphoadenosine-5'-phosphosulfate (PAPS), which is an activated form of sulfate. *O*-sulfate conjugates

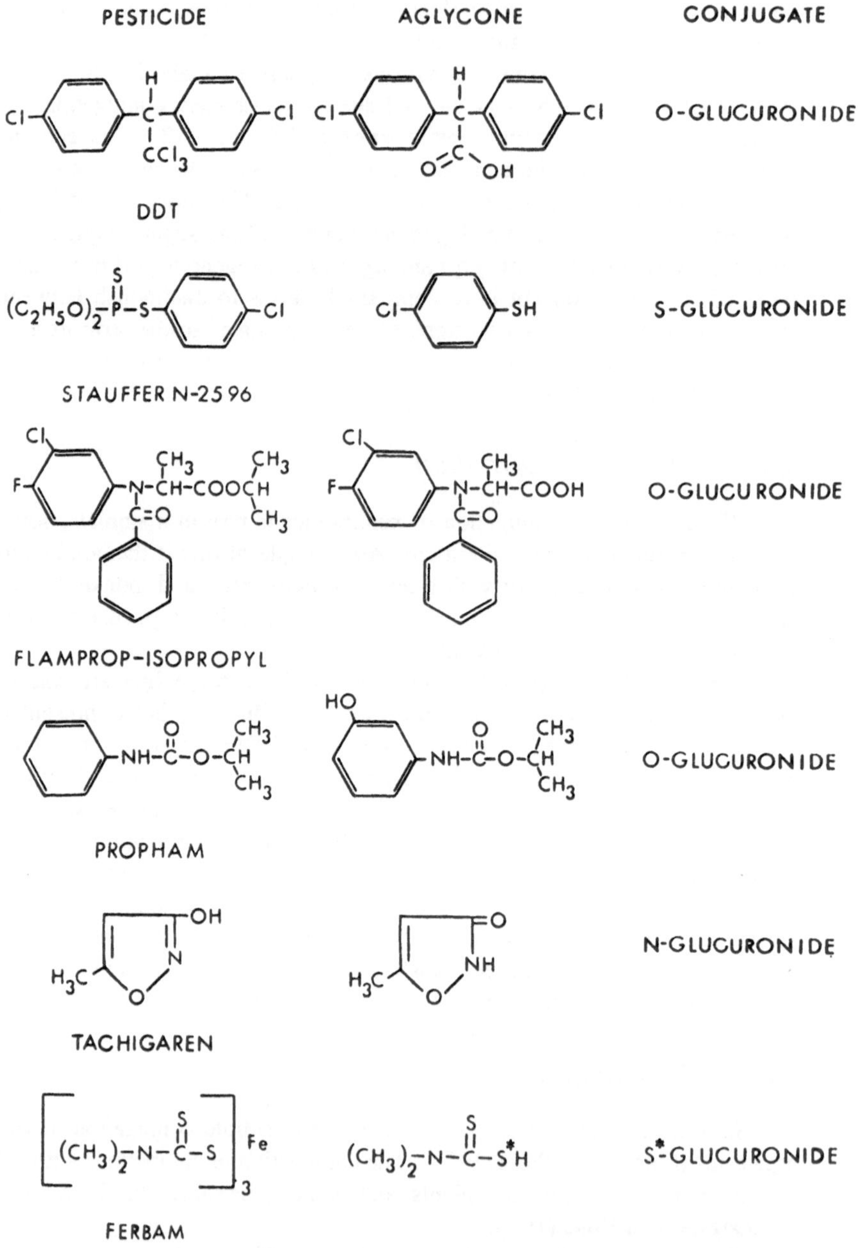

PESTICIDE	AGLYCONE	CONJUGATE

DDT   O-GLUCURONIDE

STAUFFER N-2596   S-GLUCURONIDE

FLAMPROP-ISOPROPYL   O-GLUCURONIDE

PROPHAM   O-GLUCURONIDE

TACHIGAREN   N-GLUCURONIDE

FERBAM   S*-GLUCURONIDE

Figure 1.13. Examples of pesticides which undergo glucuronide metabolism in animals.

are frequently formed from aromatic and aliphatic compounds containing a hydroxyl group. In other instances, sulfate conjugates are formed with amino groups. The resulting conjugates of hydroxyl and amino groups are referred to as sulfate ester conjugates or ethereal sulfates. Ethereal sulfate conjugation occurs in all mammals, and in birds, reptiles, mollusks, and insects. It does not occur in some microorganisms or in plants due to a lack of sulfotransferase enzymes (Dodgson and Rose, 1970). Most animal species conjugate phenolic compounds as both sulfates and glucuronides, and the ratio of the conjugates will vary according to the substrate and species involved (Berenbom and Young, 1951; Capel *et al.*, 1974; Usui *et al.*, 1977).

1.3.3. Other Conjugation Reactions

Glutathione (GSH) conjugation or mercapturic acid formation is an important metabolic pathway for some pesticides in plants and animals. GSH conjugation of pesticides was reviewed by Hutson with an emphasis on herbicides (1976).

GSH is a tripeptide containing glutamic acid, cysteine, and glycine. GSH conjugation is catalyzed by enzymes called GSH-S-transferases, which are located in the soluble fraction of tissue homogenates. The general reaction is outlined in Fig. 1.14.

Many types of chemicals undergo GSH conjugation because of the various types of substrate-specific GSH-S-transferases that mediate this reaction (Boyland and Chasseaud, 1969). These include GSH-S-aryl, -aralkyl, and -alkenetransferases. Organophosphorous triesters, S-triazines, diphenyl ethers, organothiocyanates, and thiocarbamates (sulfoxide) are among the pesticides known to be substrates of GSH-S-transferases (Usui *et al.*, 1977). Mercapturic acid formation

$$1. \quad RX + GSH \xrightarrow{\text{GSH}-S-\text{transferase}} RSG + HX$$

$$2. \quad RSG \xrightarrow{\gamma\text{-glutamyl transferase}} R-Cys-Gly + \text{glutamate}$$

$$3. \quad R-Cys-Gly \xrightarrow{\text{peptidase}} R-SCH_2\underset{\underset{NH_2}{|}}{CH}COOH + \text{glycine}$$

$$4. \quad R-SCH_2\underset{\underset{NH_2}{|}}{CH}COOH + \text{acetyl}-CoA \xrightarrow[\text{transferase}]{\text{acetyl}-} R-SCH_2\underset{\underset{NHCOCH_3}{|}}{CH}COOH + CoA$$

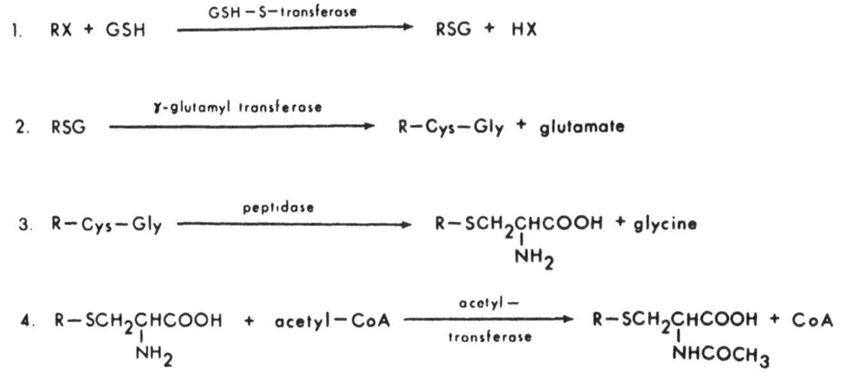

Figure 1.14. General reaction scheme for glutathione conjugation.

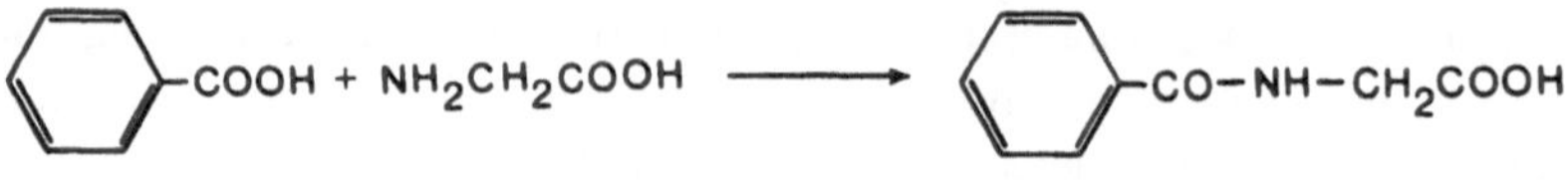

Figure 1.15. Conjugation of benzoic acid with glycine.

occurs when further metabolism results in the removal of glutamic acid, followed by acetylation of the cysteine amino group to form the mercapturic acid shown in step 4 of Fig. 1.14.

Conjugation of exocons with GSH is possible in a wide variety of animals (Boyland and Chasseaud, 1969), but the ability of animals to form mercapturic acids has not been as widely indicated (Williams, 1971). Kurihara et al. (1977) presented evidence for the presence of several previously unreported chloro-phenyl-mercapturic acids as urinary metabolites of lindane in rats. They reported that the 4-Cl, 3,4-Cl$_2$, 2,5-Cl$_2$, 2,3,5-Cl$_3$, and 2,4,5-Cl$_3$ phenyl mercapturic acids were formed, as well as the previously reported 2,4-dichlorophenyl-mer-capturic acid. Hutson et al. (1970) reported the isolation of a triazin mercapturic acid that was formed from 2-chloro-4-ethylamino-6-(1-methyl-1-cyanoethylam-ino)-S-triazine in the rat.

Pesticides containing aromatic carboxylic acid groups may be conjugated with amino acids, especially glycine (Fig. 1.15). As early as 1842, Keller showed the conversion of benzoic acid to hippuric acid in the animal body by reacting with glycine (Williams, 1967). The insecticide isoxathion is an example of a pesticide that undergoes this type of metabolism (Ando et al., 1975). Isoxathion is a phenylphosphorothioate which is hydrolyzed in the rat to yield a phenyl moiety which is oxidized to benzoic acid. The acid then conjugates with glycine to yield hippuric acid. Many other amino acids have been shown to be involved in conjugation metabolism, and the amino acids vary considerably depending upon the species in question (Mandel, 1971; Tashiro and Matsumura, 1978; Williams, 1967).

Metabolism studies of the miticide cyclopropate in the dog revealed that about half of the administered radiolabel was retained in the muscle as a unique conjugated pesticide metabolite, O-(cyclopropylcarbonyl) carnitine (Quistad et al., 1978). It was suggested that this was the first evidence of carnitine's role in pesticide metabolism. While carnitine (α-amino-β-hydroxybutyric acid tri-methylbetaine) is not an amino acid, it is mentioned here as an example of a novel conjugation reaction.

1.4. CONCLUSION

The degradation of pesticides by animals will remain an important facet of pesticide chemistry for many years to come. Regulatory requirements and the scientific obligation to assess the safety of xenobiotics will provide the impetus for these studies. Moreover, novel reactions and unusual biological activities will continue to serve as stimuli for studying the fate of pesticides in animals and other organisms.

One thing that must not happen is that we become complacent about the status of the science of pesticide degradation. While many pesticides undergo biochemical reactions that are now highly predictable, the toxicological significance of these reactions and their products is not always so apparent. It is essential that greater emphasis be placed on the significance of specified bioalteration mechanisms in allowing man to cope successfully with toxic substances, and on the susceptibility of these mechanisms to the physical, chemical, and emotional stresses to which man is exposed.

ACKNOWLEDGMENTS.   The assistance of Robert Rickard and Mary Dorough in the preparation of this manuscript is gratefully acknowledged. Appreciation also is extended to the U.S. Environmental Protection Agency (Grant No. R805143) for support that has enabled the author and his students to investigate insecticide metabolism in animals and other organisms. Similarly, acknowledgment is given for support received from Regional Research Project S-73.

REFERENCES

Addison, R. F., and Willis, D. E., 1978, The metabolism by rainbow trout *(Slamo gairdnerii)* of *p,p'*-(^{14}C) DDT and some of its possible degradation products labeled with ^{14}C, *Toxicol. Appl. Pharmacol.* **43**(2):303.

Ando, M., Nakagawa, M., Nakamura, T., and Tomita, K., 1975, Metabolism of Isoxathion, *O,O*-diethyl *O*-(5-phenyl-3-isoxazolyl)phosphorothioate in the rats, *Agric. Biol. Chem.* **30**(4):803.

Bedford, C. T., Crayford, J. V., Hutson, D. H. and Wiggins, D. E., 1978, An example of the oxidative de-esterification of an isopropyl ester. Its role in the metabolism of the herbicide flamprop-iso-propyl, *Xenobiotica* **8**(6):383.

Benson, W. R., 1969, The chemistry of pesticides, *Ann. N.Y. Acad. Sci.* **160**:7.

Berenbom, M., and Young, L., 1951, Biochemical studies of toxic agents. 3. The isolation of 1- and 2-naphthylsulphuric acid and 1- and 2-naphthylglucuronide from the urine of rats dosed with 1- and 2-naphthol, *Biochem. J.* **49**:165.

Boyland, E., and Chasseaud, L. F., 1969, The rate of glutathione and glutathine-*S*-transferase in mercapturic acid biosynthesis, *Adv. Enzymol.* **32**:173.

Bradway, D. E., and Shafik, T. M., 1977, Malathion exposure studies. Determination of mono- and dicarboxylic acids and alkyl phosphates in urine, *J. Agric. Food Chem.* **25**(6):1342.

Brooks, G. T., 1974, *Chlorinated Insecticides,* Vol. II, CRC Press, Cleveland.

Brooks, G. T., and Harrison, A., 1969, Hydration of HEOD (dieldrin) and the heptachlor epoxides by microsomes from the livers of pigs and rabbits, *Bull. Env:ron. Contam. Toxicol.* **4**:352.

Capel, I. D., Millburn, P. and Williams, R. T., 1974, The conjugation of 1- and 2-naphthols and other phenols in the cat and pig, *Xenobiotica* **4**:601.

Casida, J. E., and Lykken, L., 1969, Metabolism of organic pesticide chemicals in higher plants, *Annu. Rev. Plant Physiol.* **20**:606.

Dauterman, W. C., 1971, Biological and non-biological modifications of organophosphorus compounds, *Bull. W.H.O.* **44**:133.

Davidow, B., and Radomski, J. L., 1953, Isolation of an epoxide metabolite from fat tissues of dogs fed heptachlor, *J. Pharmacol. Exp. Ther.* **107**:259.

Dodgson, K. S., and Rose, F. A., 1970, Sulfoconjugation and sulfohydrolysis, in: *Metabolic Conjugation and Metabolic Hydrolysis*, Vol. I (W. Fishman, ed.), pp. 239–325, Academic Press, New York.

Dorough, H. W., 1976, Biological activity of pesticide conjugates, in: *Bound and Conjugated Pesticide Residues* (D. Kaufman, G. Still, G. Paulson and S. Bandal, eds.), pp. 11–35, ACS American Chemical Society, Washington, D.C. Symposium Series 29.

Dorough, H. W., 1979*a*, Metabolism of insecticides by conjugation mechanisms, *Pharmacol. Ther.* **4**:433.

Dorough, H. W., 1979*b*, Conjugation reactions of pesticides and their metabolites with sugars, in: *Advances in Pesticide Science*, Part 3 (H. Geissbuhler, ed.), pp. 526–536, Pergamon Press, New York.

Duggan, D. E., Baldwin, J. J., Arison, B. H., and Rhodes, R. E., 1974, *N*-glucoside formation as a detoxification mechanism in mammals, *J. Pharmacol. Exp. Ther.* **190**:563.

Eisenbrand, G., Ungerer, O., and Preussmann, R., 1974, Rapid formation of carcinogenic *N*-nitrosamine by interaction of nitrite with fungicides derived from dithiocarbamic acid *in vitro* under simulated gastric conditions and *in vivo* in the rat stomach, *Food Cosmet. Toxicol.* **12**:229.

Elespuru, R. K., and Lijinsky, W., 1973, The formation of carcinogenic nitroso compounds from nitrite and some types of agricultural chemicals, *Food Cosmet. Toxicol.* **11**:807.

Eto, M., 1974, *Organophosphorus Pesticides: Organic and Biological Chemistry*, CRC Press, Cleveland.

Florkin, M., and Stotz, E. H., 1973, *Comprehensive Biochemistry*, Vol. 13, Elsevier, New York.

Fukuto, T. R., and Metcalf, R. L., 1969, Metabolism of insecticides in plants and animals, *Ann. N.Y. Acad. Sci.* **160**:97.

Hornish, R. E., and Nappier, J. L., 1978, Excretion and metabolism of 3,4,5-tribromo-*N*,*N*-α-trimethyl-1*H*-pyrazole-1-acetamide in the rat, *J. Agric. Food Chem.* **26**(5):1083.

Huhtanen, K., and Dorough, H. W., 1976, Isomerization and Beckmann rearrangement reactions in the metabolism of methomyl in rats, *Pest. Biochem. Phys.* **6**:571.

Hunt, L. M., Chamberlain, W. F., Gilbert, B. N., Hopkins, D. E., and Gingrich, Q. R., 1977, Absorption, excretion, and metabolism of nitrogen by a sheep, *J. Agric. Food Chem.* **24**(5):1062.

Hutson, P. H., 1976, Glutathione conjugates, in: *Bound and Conjugated Pesticide Residues* (D. Kaufman, G. Still, G. Paulson and S. Bandal, eds.), pp. 103–131, ACS Symposium Series 29, American Chemical Society, Washington D.C.

Hutson, D. H., Hoadley, E. C., Griffiths, M. H., and Donninger, C., 1970, Mercapturic acid formation in the metabolism of 2-chloro-4-ethylamino-6-(1-methyl-1-cyanothylamino)-*S*-triazine in the rat, *J. Agric. Food. Chem.* **78**(3):507.

Jenner, P., and Testa, B., 1978, Novel pathways in drug metabolism, *Xenobiotica* **8**(1):1.

Kuhr, R. J., 1971, The formation and importance of carbamate insecticide metabolites as terminal residues, *Pure Appl. Chem. Suppl.* **1**:199.

Kuhr, R. J., and Dorough, H. W., 1976, *Carbamate Insecticides: Chemistry, Biochemistry, and Toxicology*, CRC Press, Cleveland.

Kurihara, N., Tanaka, K., and Nakajima, M., 1977, Pathways of chlorophenyl-mercapturic acids formation in biodegradation of lindane, *Agric. Biol. Chem.* **41**(7):1317.

Kurtz, D. A., and George, J. L., 1977, DDT metabolism in Pennsylvania white-tail deer, in: *Fate of Pesticides in Large Animals* (G. Ivie and H. Dorough, eds.), pp. 193–215, Academic Press, New York.

Lijinsky, W., and Schmahl, D., 1978, Carcinogenesis by nitroso derivatives of methylcarbamate insecticides and other nitrosamides in rats and mice, *Int. Agency Res. Cancer Sci. Publ. No.* 19, pp. 495–501.

Mandel, H. W., 1971, Pathways of drug biotransformation: Biochemical conjugations, in: *Fundamentals of Drug Metabolism and Drug Disposition* (B. LaDu, H. Mandel and E. Way, eds.), pp. 149–186, Williams and Wilkins, Baltimore.

March, R. B., Metcalf, R. L., Fukuto, T. R., and Maxon, M. G., 1955, Metabolism of Systox in the white mouse and American cockroach, *J. Econ. Entomol.* **48**:355.

Matsumura, F., 1975, *Toxicology of Insecticides*, Plenum Press, New York.

Melnikov, N. N., 1971, *Chemistry of Pesticides*, p. 59, Springer-Verlag, New York.

Menn, J. J., and Still, G. G., 1977, Metabolism of insecticides and herbicides in higher plants, *Crit. Rev. Toxicol.* **5**:3.

Menzie, C. M., 1969, *Metabolism of Pesticides*, U. S. Department of the Interior, Fish and Wildlife Service.

Miettinen, T. A., and Leskinen, E., 1970, Glucuronic acid pathway, in: *Metabolic Conjugation and Metabolic Hydrolysis*, Vol. I (W. Fishman, ed.), pp. 157–237, Academic Press, New York.

Mirvish, S. S., 1975, Formation of *N*-nitroso compounds: Chemistry, kinetics, and *in vivo* occurrances, *Toxicol. Appl. Pharmacol.* **31**:325.

Nakatsugawa, T., and Morelli, M. A., 1976, Microsomal oxidation and insecticide metabolism, in: *Insecticide Biochemistry and Physiology* (C. F. Wilkinson, ed.), pp. 80–100, Plenum Press, New York.

Nakatsugawa, T., Tolman, N. M., and Dahm, P. A., 1969, Oxidative degradation of diazinon by rat liver microsomes, *Biochem. Pharmacol.* **18**:685.

Nye, D. E., Hurst, H. E., and Dorough, H. W., 1976, Fate of Croneton (2-ethylthiomethylphenyl *N*-methylcarbamate) in rats, *J. Agric. Food Chem.* **24**(2):371.

Parke, D. V., 1968, *The Biochemistry of Foreign Compounds*, Pergamon Press, Oxford.

Quistad, G. B., Staiger, L. E., and Schooley, D. A., 1978, Environmental degradation of the miticide cyclopropate (hexadecyl cyclopropane carboxylate). Beagle dog metabolism, *J. Agric. Food Chem.* **26**(1):76.

Rickard, R., and Dorough, H. W., 1978, *In vivo* synthesis of 1-naphthyl *N*-methylnitrosocarbamate (nitrosocarbaryl) in the rat and guinea pig, *Pharmacologist* **20**(3):146.

Seiler, J. P., 1977, Nitrosation *in vitro* and *in vivo* by sodium nitrite, and mutagenicity of nitrogenous pesticides, *Mutat. Res.* **48**:225.

Sen, N. P., Donaldson, B. A., and Charbonneau, C., 1975, Formation of nitrosodimethylamine from the interaction of certain pesticides and nitrite, International Agency for Research on Cancer. IARC Scientific Publication No. 9, pp. 75–79.

Smith, J. N., 1968, The comparative metabolism of xenobiotics, *Adv. Comp. Physiol. Biochem.* **3**:173.

Sundroik, G., Hutzinger, O., Safe, S. and Platonow, N., 1977, The metabolism of *p,p'*-DDT and *p,p'*-DDE in the pig, in: *Fate of Pesticides in Large Animals* (G. Ivie and H. Dorough, eds.), pp. 175–182, Academic Press, New York.

Tashiro, S., and Matsumura, F., 1978, Metabolism of *trans*-nonachlor and related chlordane components in rat and man, *Arch. Environ. Contam. Toxicol.* **7**:113.

Uchiyama, M., Takeda, M., Suzuki, T., and Yoshikawa, K., 1975, Mutagenicity of nitroso derivatives of *N*-methylcarbamate insecticides in microbiological method, *Bull. Environ. Contam. Toxicol.* **14**:389.

Usui, K., Shishido, T., and Fukami, J., 1977, Glutathione *S*-transferases of rat liver active on organophosphorus triesters, *Agric. Biol. Chem.* **41**(12):2491.

Wilkinson, C. F. (ed.), 1976, *Insecticide Biochemistry and Physiology*, Plenum Press, New York.

Williams, R. T., 1967, The biogenesis of conjugation and detoxification products, in: *Biogenesis of Natural Compounds* (P. Bernfeld, ed.), pp. 427–474, Pergamon Press, Oxford.

Williams, R. T., 1971, Species variation in drug biotransformations, in: *Fundamentals of Drug Metabolism and Drug Disposition* (B. LaDu, H. Mandel and E. Way, eds.), pp. 187–205, Williams and Wilkins, Baltimore.

Wolfe, N. L., Fepp, R. D., Gordon, J. A., and Fincher, R. C., 1976, *N*-Nitrosamine formation from atrazine, *Bull. Environ. Contam. Toxicol.* **15**:342.

2

Pesticide Metabolism in Plants
Reactions and Mechanisms

Richard H. Shimabukuro, Gerald L. Lamoureux, and D. Stuart Frear

2.1. INTRODUCTION

The use of pesticides to protect crop plants from weeds, insects, and other pests has increased steadily. In 1975 the total production of organic pesticides in the United States was 1609 million pounds (USDA, 1977). A great variety of pesticides, including herbicides, insecticides, and fungicides is applied to crop plants. Pesticides are inherently toxic and may be degraded to either toxic or nontoxic forms. Therefore, it is important to know the intermediate degradation products and the ultimate fate of pesticides in plants.

Much is known about the degradation and dissipation of pesticides in plants, but detailed knowledge of biotransformation reaction mechanisms is often lacking (Baldwin, 1977). Pesticide metabolism in plants has been reviewed extensively (Baldwin, 1977; Bull, 1972; Casida and Lykken, 1969; Kearney and Kaufman, 1975; Lamoureux and Frear, 1979; Menzer, 1973; Sandermann et al., 1977). It is not the intent of this review to present an exhaustive coverage of pesticide

Richard H. Shimabukuro, Gerald L. Lamoureux, and D. Stuart Frear ● U.S. Department of Agriculture, Science and Education Administration, Agricultural Research, Metabolism and Radiation Research Laboratory, Fargo, North Dakota 58105.

metabolism in plants, but rather to illustrate selected degradation reactions known to occur in plants. The biological significance of these degradation reactions will be discussed primarily with respect to their importance in plants.

2.2. PESTICIDE METABOLISM IN PLANTS

Plants metabolize pesticides through a series of intermediates ultimately to insoluble residues (Baldwin, 1977; Frear *et al.*, 1972*a*). The complete course of metabolism in a plant is not understood for any pesticide in use today. The chemical nature and the quantity of intermediate metabolites and insoluble residues in a plant are influenced by the site of absorption of the pesticide, translocation, and time of residence in the plant (Baldwin, 1977; Shimabukuro and Walsh, 1979). Several important differences between plants and animals that are relevant to the metabolism of pesticides in plants have been established recently.

2.2.1. Absorption

Regardless of how a pesticide is applied to a plant, it must ultimately penetrate the cells where phytotoxic and biotransformation reactions occur. In animals, oral administration or dosing by injection minimizes exposure of the pesticides to external microbial and environmental factors. Root or foliar treatment is common in plants. Long-term treatments of plants by soil or leaf application of pesticides increase the probability that plants may absorb a mixture of degradation products formed by microbial and/or photochemical activity (Crosby, 1973). These problems may be circumvented to a large extent by short-term treatments with excised leaves, roots, leaf disks, and isolated mesophyll cells (Shimabukuro and Walsh, 1979).

The absorption of pesticides by the gastrointestinal tract of animals poses similar barriers to all ingested pesticides. The root tips and leaf surfaces are the major sites of penetration into plants (Bukovac, 1976; Hay, 1976). These two sites present distinctly different barriers to penetration by the same pesticides. The cuticle, a thin, lipoidal membrane that covers the entire above-ground parts of a plant, is the primary barrier to penetration by foliar application. In roots, the primary barrier appears to be the endodermis, an internal root structure that must be traversed by an active mechanism before transport to the shoots can occur.

2.2.2. Translocation and Distribution

Absorbed pesticides are distributed throughout the animal body in a well-defined circulatory system. In plants, translocation and distribution occur in two distinct vascular systems (Crafts and Crisp, 1971). Generally, pesticides are translocated apoplastically in the xylem (passive transport) from roots to all transpiring leaves. Symplastic translocation in the phloem (active transport) occurs selectively from mature leaves to centers of high metabolic activity associated with the young growing points of the shoot and root (Zimmerman and Milburn, 1975). Therefore, the distribution of pesticides in plants may not be uniform and may vary according to the pesticide and the site of penetration into the plant. Redistribution of pesticides or their metabolites is often limited in plants, and translocation does not appear to be related to the hydrophilic properties of the pesticide or its metabolites (Hussain *et al.*, 1974; Shimabukuro and Walsh, 1979).

2.2.3. Metabolism

Metabolism of pesticides in plants may be slower than in animals (Casida and Lykken, 1969). Plants do not have a specific organ as highly active in pesticide degradation as the mammalian liver. In contrast to animals, senescence is a hormonally controlled phenomenon in plants that may be induced, retarded, or reversed by different environmental factors (Thiman, 1977; Woolhouse, 1974). The same organs may be in various stages of senescence on the same plant. The leaves and roots, which are the likely centers of pesticide metabolism in plants, range in physiological age from senescent organs to young, developing primordia. Therefore, a pesticide may be subjected to a wide range of metabolic or degradation activities that vary according to the site of penetration into the plant and its translocation.

In plants, the metabolism of organic pesticides to more hydrophilic forms by oxidation and conjugation does not result primarily in secretion of the pesticides as it does in mammals. Plants lack an excretory mechanism comparable to the enterohepatic and renal excretory systems in mammals. Therefore, plants metabolize pesticides to water-soluble conjugates and insoluble "terminal" residues that remain in the plant during its life (Baldwin, 1977; Kaufman *et al.*, 1976) or until the organ containing the residue is detached from the plant. Complete oxidation of organic pesticides in plants to CO_2 and H_2O is generally not a significant reaction (Frear *et al.*, 1972a).

2.3. DEGRADATION REACTIONS OF PESTICIDES IN PLANTS

Much is known about the metabolic fate of pesticides in plants (Casida and Lykken, 1969; Kearney and Kaufman, 1975). However, our understanding of biotransformation mechanisms based on the plant enzyme systems involved is very limited. Only a few of the plant enzymes involved in pesticide metabolism have been investigated in any detail (Lamoureux and Frear, 1979).

2.3.1. Oxidation

Oxidative reactions of pesticides in plants are frequently primary reactions that result in either detoxication or activation. Comparative biochemistry indicates that several reactions known to occur in both plants and animals are possibly mixed function oxidase-catalyzed reactions (mfo). These reactions include *N*-dealkylation, *O*-dealkylation, aromatic hydroxylation, alkyl oxidation, epoxidation, desulfuration, sulfur oxidation, ester hydrolysis, and nitrogen oxidation (Lamoureux and Frear, 1979). However, direct evidence for the involvement of cytochrome P-450 exists for only a few of the reactions demonstrated in plants (Sandermann *et al.*, 1977). In plants some of the oxidation reactions presumed to be due to mixed function oxidases may be catalyzed by peroxidases or other oxygenases (Lamoureux and Frear, 1979).

Aldrin epoxidation to dieldrin was reported to occur in excised plant tissues (Table 2.1) (Fig. 2.1) (Oloff and Lichtenstein, 1969), but it is still not certain whether aldrin epoxidase is an mfo system (Earl and Kennedy, 1975; Yu *et al.*, 1971). Cytochrome P-450 was not detected in pea aldrin epoxidase, and its activity was stimulated by deoxycholate, Triton X-100, and other solubilizing and chelating agents that inhibit cytochrome P-450 systems (Earl and Kennedy, 1975).

In plants, dieldrin does not appear to be the precursor to aldrin *trans*-diol as it is in mammals (Brooks, 1974) and soil microorganisms (Matsumura *et al.*, 1968; Matsumura and Boush, 1967). Dieldrin was not metabolized to aldrin *trans*-diol in cell-free preparations of pea and bean roots (McKinney and Mehendale, 1973; Yu *et al.*, 1971). Aldrin *trans*-diol was formed in bean and potato cell suspension cultures only when aldrin but not dieldrin was a substrate (Fig. 2.1) (Brain and Lines, 1977). Cell suspension cultures of bean shoots but not bean roots converted small amounts of dieldrin to photodieldrin by a nonphotochemical pathway (Brain and Lines, 1977) similar to that in microorganisms (Brooks, 1974). Plant enzymes that oxidize cyclodiene insecticides appear to exhibit greater substrate specificity but are less widely distributed than corresponding animal enzymes. Aldrin, isodrin, and heptachlor were not metabolized in corn root homogenates, whereas aldrin and isodrin but not heptachlor were epoxidized in bean and pea root homogenates (Yu *et al.*, 1971).

Stable epoxide metabolites of herbicides have not been isolated in plants. However, the hydroxylation of 2,4-D in bean plants to 2,5-dichloro-4-hydroxyphenoxyacetic acid (Hamilton *et al.*, 1971; Montgomery *et al.*, 1971) implicated the formation of an epoxide intermediate (Fig. 2.2). Chlorine migration or the NIH shift (Guroff *et al.*, 1967) occurred in 2,4-D metabolism. The NIH shift

Table 2.1. Common and Chemical Names of Pesticides Mentioned in Text[a]

Pesticide	Chemical name
Aldicarb (Temik®)	2-Methyl-2-(methylthio)propionaldehyde-O-(methylcarbamoyl)oxime
Aldrin	1,2,3,4,10,10-Hexachloro-1,4,4a,5,8,8a-hexahydro-$endo$-exo-1,4:5,8-dimethanonaphthalene
Atrazine	2-Chloro-4-(ethylamino)-6-(isopropylamino)-s-triazine
Banol® (carbanolate)	2-Chloro-4,5-dimethylphenyl methylcarbamate
Barban	4-Chloro-2-butynyl m-chlorocarbanilate
Baygon® (propoxur)	2-(1-Methylethoxy)phenyl methylcarbamate
BAY NTN 9306® (Sulprofos)	O-Ethyl O-[4-(methylthio)phenyl] S-propyl phosphorodithioate
Benzoylprop-ethyl	Ethyl($\pm$)-2-(N-benzoyl-3,4-dichloroanilino)propionate
Carbaryl	1-Naphthyl methylcarbamate
Carbofuran	2,3-Dihydro-2,2-dimethyl-7-benzofuranyl methylcarbamate
CDAA	N,N-Diallyl-2-chloroacetamide
Chloramben	3-Amino-2,5-dichlorobenzoic acid
Chlorfenprop-methyl	Methyl 2-chloro-3-(4-chlorophenyl)propanoate
Chlorpropham	Isopropyl m-chlorocarbanilate
Cisanilide	cis-2,5-Dimethyl-N-phenyl-1-pyrrolidine carboxamide
Croneton®	2-Ethylthiomethylphenyl-N-methylcarbamate
Cyanazine	2-[(4-Chloro-6-(ethylamino)-s-triazin-2-yl)amino]-2-methylpropionitrile
Cyprazine	2-Chloro-4-(cyclopropylamino)-6-(isopropyl amino)-s-triazine
2,4-D	2,4-Dichlorophenoxyacetic acid
DCPB	4,4'-Dichlorobenzophenone
DDD (TDE)	2,2-bis(p-Chlorophenyl)-1,1-dichloroethane
DDE	2,2-bis(p-Chlorophenyl)-1,1-dichloroethylene
DDT	2,2-bis(p-Chlorophenyl)-1,1,1-trichloroethane
Diazinon	O,O-Diethyl O-(2-isopropyl-6-methyl-4-pyrimidinyl) phosphorothioate
Dichlobenil	2,6-Dichlorobenzonitrile
Diclofop-methyl	Methyl 2-[4-(2',4'-dichlorophenoxy)phenoxy]propanoate
Dicrotophos (Bidrin®)	3-(Dimethylamino)-1-methyl-3-oxo-1-propenyl dimethyl phosphate
Dieldrin	1,2,3,4,10,10-Hexachloro-6,7-epoxy-1,4,4a,5,6,7,8,8a-octahydro-1,4-$endo$-exo-5,8-dimethanonaphthalene, 85% minimum
Dimethoate	O,O-Dimethyl S-(N-methylcarbamoyl-methyl)phosphorodithioate
Dinoben®	2,5-Dichloro-3-nitrobenzoic acid

(Continued)

Table 2.1. *(Continued)*

Pesticide	Chemical name
Diphenamid	*N,N*-Dimethyl-2,2-diphenylacetamide
Diuron	3-(3,4-Dichlorophenyl)-1,1-dimethylurea
Dyfonate® (fonofos)	*O*-Ethyl *S*-phenyl ethylphosphonodithioate
EPTC	*S*-Ethyl dipropylthiocarbamate
Etrimfos	*O,O*-Dimethyl *O*-(6-ethoxy-2-ethyl-4-pyrimidinyl) phosphorothioate
Fenitrothion	*O,O*-Dimethyl *O*-(4-nitro-*m*-tolyl) phosphorothioate
Fensulfothion	*O,O*-Diethyl *O*-[*p*-(methylsulfinyl)-phenyl] phosphorothioate
Flamprop-methyl	Methyl(±)-2-[*N*-(3-chloro-4-fluorophenyl)benzamido]propionate
Fluorodifen	*p*-Nitrophenyl α,α,α-trifluoro-2-nitro-*p*-toly lether
Heptachlor	1,4,5,6,7,8,8-Heptachloro-3a,4,7,7a-tetrahydro-4,7-methanoindene
IAA	Indole-3-acetic acid
Isodrin	1,2,3,4,10,10-Hexachloro-1,4,4a,5,8,8a-hexahydro-1,4-*endo-endo*-5,8-dimethanonapthalene
Kelthane® (dicofol)	2,2-bis(*p*-Chlorophenyl)-1,1,1-trichloroethanol
Malathion	*S*-[1,2-bis(ethoxycarbonyl)ethyl]*O,O*-dimethyl phosphorodithioate
Methazole	2-(3,4-Dichlorophenyl)-4-methyl-1,2,4-oxadiazolidine-3,5-dione
Monuron	3-(*p*-Chlorophenyl)-1,1-dimethylurea
Oxamyl	Methyl *N',N'*-dimethyl-*N*-[(methylcarbamyl)oxy]-1-thiooxamidate
Parathion	*O,O*-Diethyl *O-p*-nitrophenyl phosphorothioate
PCNB	Pentachloronitrobenzene
Perfluidone	1,1,1-Trifluoro-*N*-[2-methyl-4-(phenylsulfonyl)phenyl]methanesulfonamide
Phorate	*O,O*-Diethyl *S*-[(ethylthio)methyl] phosphorodithioate
Prometryne	2,4-bis(Isopropylamino)-6-(methylthio)-*s*-triazine
Propachlor	2-Chloro-*N*-isopropylacetanilide
Propanil	3',4'-Dichloropropionanilide
Propham	Isopropyl carbanilate
R-25788	*N,N*-Diallyl-2,2-dichloroacetamide
SAN 6706	4-Chloro-5-(dimethylamino)-2-(α,α,α-trifluoro-*m*-tolyl)-3(2H)-pyridazinone
SAN 9789® (norflurazon)	4-Chloro-5-(methylamino)-2-(α,α,α-trifluoro-*m*-tolyl)-3(2H)-pyridazinone
Simazine	2-Chloro-4,6-bis(ethylamino)-*s*-triazine
2,4,5-T	2,4,5-Trichlorophenoxyacetic acid
Tetrachlorvinphos	2-Chloro-1-(2,4,5-trichlorophenyl)vinyl dimethyl phosphate

[a] The trademarked (®) names of some pesticides with their common names in parentheses are listed in the table and given as used in the listed references.

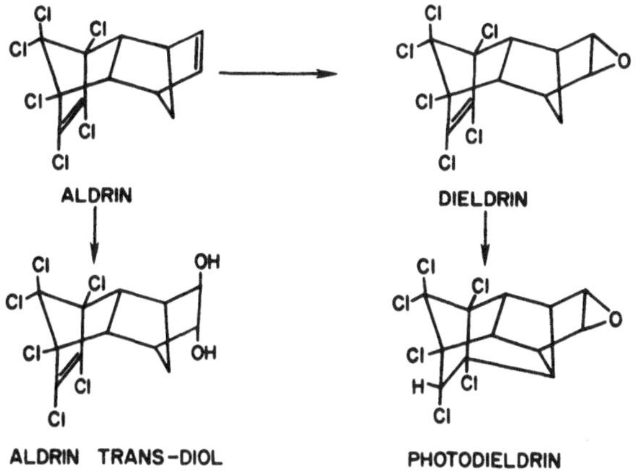

ALDRIN

DIELDRIN

ALDRIN TRANS-DIOL

PHOTODIELDRIN

Figure 2.1. Oxidation of aldrin in plants.

is considered as probable evidence for an epoxide intermediate (Guroff et al., 1967; Jerina and Daley, 1974) and is characteristic of liver mfo hydroxylations (Jerina and Daley, 1974). An mfo system for 2,4-D hydroxylation was isolated from cucumber leaves (Makeev et al., 1977). This enzyme also hydroxylated cinnamic acid, a reaction that was demonstrated to be an mfo-catalyzed reaction in preparations from pea apexes (Russell and Conn, 1967; Russell, 1971).

Aryl hydroxylations of other pesticides in plants may also be mfo-catalyzed reactions (Fig. 2.2). The herbicide, 2,4,5-T, was hydroxylated in the 4-position with chlorine replacement instead of migration (Hamilton et al., 1971). Cisanilide was hydroxylated in either the pyrrolidine or phenyl rings in carrot and cotton leaves (Frear and Swanson, 1975). Both hydroxylated metabolites were subsequently glycosylated (Frear and Swanson, 1975). In soybean, aryl hydroxylation of chlorpropham occurred in either the 2- or 4-positions in shoots but only in the 2-position in roots (Still and Mansager, 1973). Diclofop-methyl was hydroxylated rapidly and predominantly in the 5-position of the 2,4-dichlorophenoxy moiety in resistant wheat (Gorbach et al., 1977; Shimabukuro et al., 1979). However, this was not the predominant reaction in susceptible wild oat (Shimabukuro et al., 1979).

Carbamate insecticides are metabolized readily in plants by oxidation and conjugation (Casida and Lykken, 1969; Kuhr and Casida, 1967). The carbamate ester group of carbaryl and several phenyl-N-methyl carbamates remained largely intact in bean plants (Fig. 2.3), but very little unchanged carbaryl was detected. Within 6 days, most of the insecticide was metabolized to water-soluble glycosides and insoluble residue (Kuhr and Casida, 1967). The aglycones were predominantly in the 4-hydroxy-, 5-hydroxy-, N-hydroxymethyl, and 5,6-dihydro-5,6-dihydroxycarbaryl (Kuhr and Casida, 1967; Mumma et al., 1971).

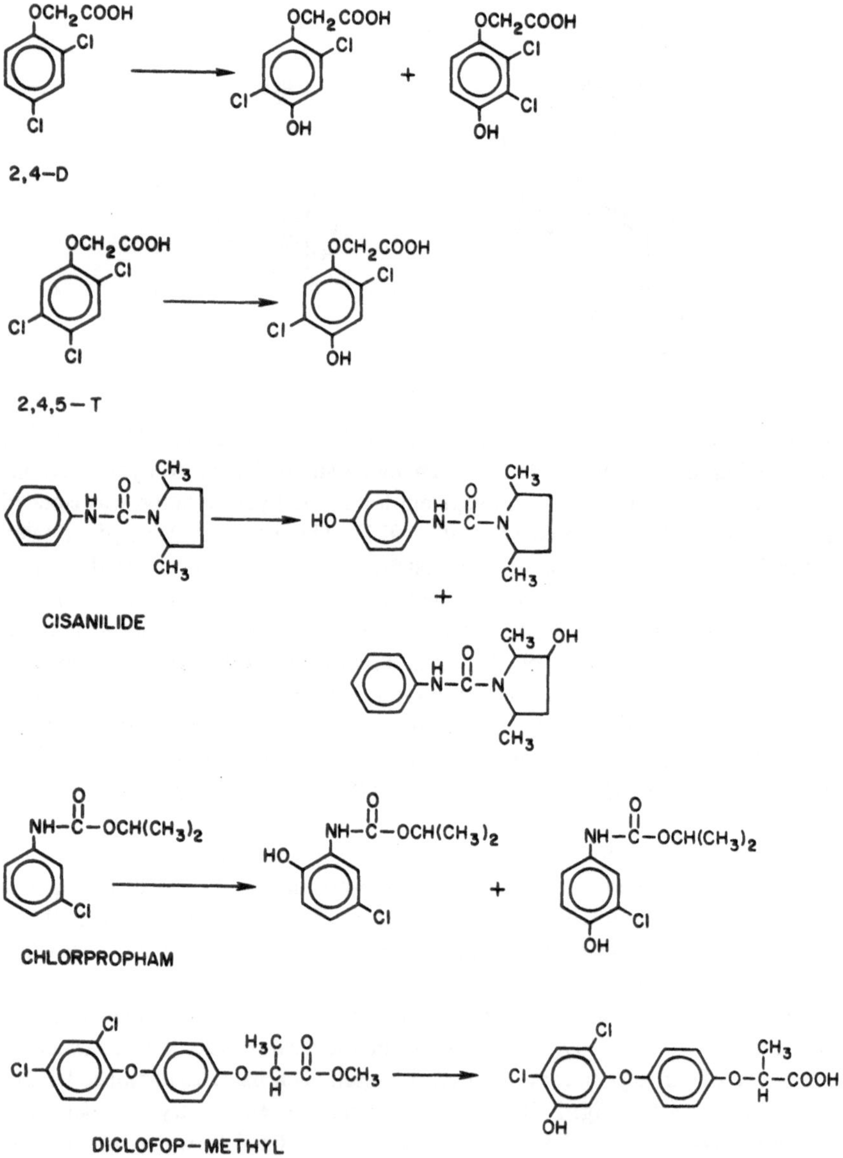

Figure 2.2. Aryl hydroxylation of the herbicides 2,4-D, 2,4,5-T, cisanilide, chlorpropham, and diclofop-methyl.

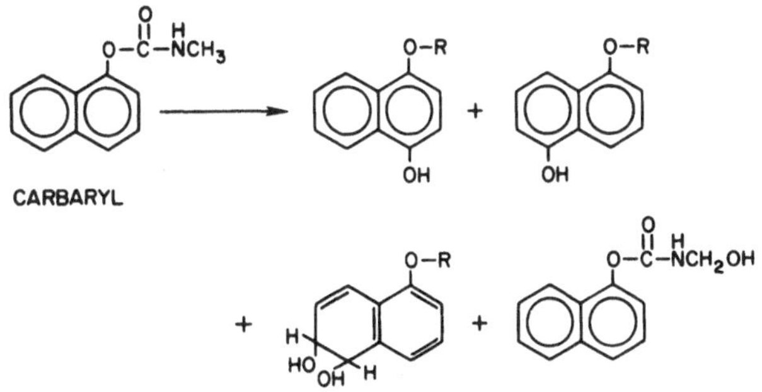

Figure 2.3. Oxidation of carbaryl in beans.

The rate of metabolism of carbamate insecticides differed greatly among plant species. Carbofuran metabolism ranged from 68% of the injected carbofuran within 3 days in beans (Dorough *et al.*, 1973*a*) to 80% of the translocated carbofuran in mugho pine needles after 70 days (Pree and Saunders, 1974). Within a species such as bean, carbaryl and carbofuran were metabolized much faster than aldicarb and Croneton® (Marshall and Dorough, 1977). After 20 days, only 15–19% of the injected carbofuran and carbaryl remained in the organosoluble fractions as compared to 46% and 58% for Croneton® and aldicarb (Marshall and Dorough, 1977). The carbamate ester linkage of Croneton® and aldicarb was hydrolyzed in contrast to that of carbofuran and carbaryl. Many of the glycosides of hydroxylated carbamate insecticides yielded aglycones that were potent anticholinesterase agents after cleavage with β-glucosidase (Kuhr and Casida, 1967).

Organophosphate insecticides are activated by oxidative reactions such as desulfuration, sulfur oxidation, and *N*-dealkylation and inactivated by *O*-dealkylation and hydrolysis of the acid anhydride bond. The activation and inactivation reactions above occur in plants, but studies on their reaction mechanisms with *in vitro* preparations from plants are lacking (Bull, 1972; Casida and Lykken, 1969). In plants, the desulfuration of the thiono sulfur apparently does not occur as readily as the oxidation of thioether sulfur (Bull, 1972; Bull *et al.*, 1976; Eto, 1974). Very little of the *O*-analogs of BAY NTN 9306® (sulprofos) (Fig. 2.4) (Bull *et al.*, 1976), Dyfonate® (fonofos) (McBain *et al.*, 1970) or dimethoate (Narayan and Lichtenstein, 1973) were detected in plants. Generally, the alkyl sulfur in pesticides is rapidly oxidized to the sulfoxide and more slowly to the sulfone (Bull, 1972; Bull *et al.*, 1976). The concentration of BAY NTN 9306® sulfoxide in cotton leaves was much higher than its sulfone or its *O*-analog over a 16-day treatment period (Bull *et al.*, 1976). However, cleavage of the thiophenyl group of Dyfonate® followed by *S*-methylation and oxidation gave methylphenyl sulfone as a major metabolite in potatoes (McBain *et al.*, 1970).

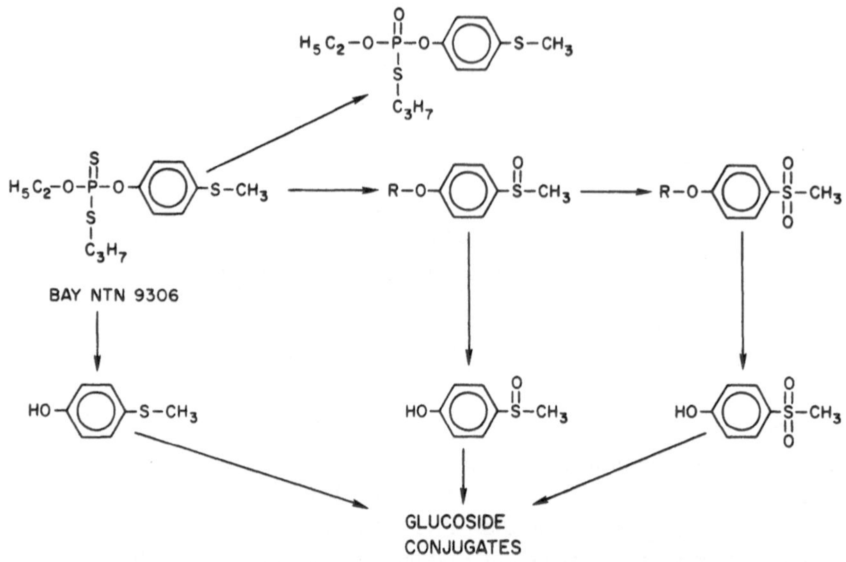

Figure 2.4. Oxidative metabolism of BAY NTN 9306® in cotton.

The oxidation of insecticides to their sulfoxides and sulfones occurs readily in plants (Casida and Lykken, 1969), but only limited examples are known of herbicides undergoing similar reactions. Prometryne was oxidized to its sulfoxide and sulfone before hydrolysis (Müller and Payot, 1966), but this reaction has not been confirmed (Fig. 2.5). Recent evidence indicates that the sulfoxide of a 2-methylmercapto-*s*-triazine is a good substrate for glutathione conjugation (Lamoureux and Frear, 1979). Therefore, oxidation to the sulfone may not occur with prometryne. EPTC was oxidized to its sulfoxide in corn (Lay and Casida, 1976) and mice (Casida *et al.*, 1975) before cleavage by glutathione *S*-transferase. This reaction is discussed further in the section on glutathione conjugation of pesticides. EPTC was oxidized to the sulfone and several hydroxylated metabolites by mice liver mfo (Chen and Casida, 1978).

The sulfoxidation of the insecticides phorate (Krueger, 1975) and aldicarb (Krueger, 1977) by root extracts of several crop plants has been demonstrated (Fig. 2.5). However, the properties of the enzymes catalyzing the above sulfoxidations were not consistent with known mfo systems. Aldicarb sulfoxidase was a soluble enzyme (105,000g supernatant), and phorate sulfoxidase was in the 25,000-g pellet. Piperonyl butoxide and SKF 525A inhibited phorate sulfoxidase but not aldicarb sulfoxidase (Krueger, 1975, 1977).

Oxidation of organophosphate insecticides to their sulfoxides and sulfones is required for insecticidal activity (Bull *et al.*, 1976; O'Brien, 1967). However,

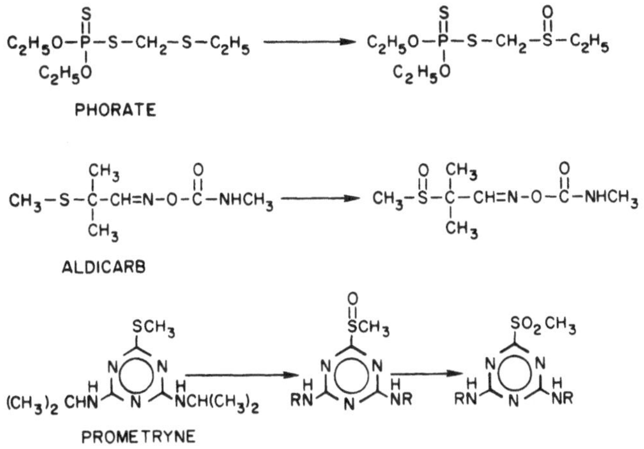

Figure 2.5. Sulfoxidation of phorate, aldicarb, and prometryne.

with herbicides such as prometryne, sulfoxidation is probably the initial step toward complete detoxication since the methylmercaptan is the herbicidally active molecule (Esser *et al.*, 1975).

Organophosphate insecticides are readily metabolized by apparent mfo-catalyzed hydrolysis and conjugation to water-soluble metabolites in plants (Bull, 1972; Bull *et al.*, 1976; McBain *et al.*, 1970; Narayan and Lichtenstein, 1973). In pea roots 81–91% of the recovered ^{14}C from [^{14}C]Dyfonate® was in the organosoluble fraction after 8 days of treatment. However, in the shoots 47–71% of the ^{14}C was in water-soluble metabolites and 19–47% was in a "bound" insoluble residue (Narayan and Lichtenstein, 1973). The water-soluble metabolites were associated primarily with proteins. Water-soluble metabolites of BAY NTN 9306® were primarily glycosides of the different phenols (Fig. 2.4), and they accounted for 34% of the ^{14}C in cotton leaf extracts after 16 days (Bull *et al.*, 1976).

The hydrolysis of the acid anhydride bond and *O*-dealkylation of ring substituents of phosphorothionates occur readily in plants (Casida and Lykken, 1969). These reactions were demonstrated with etrimfos in beans and corn (Fig. 2.6) (Akram *et al.*, 1978). Only small amounts of the *O*-analog of etrimfos were detected. Most of the EEHP (Fig. 2.6) may be derived after desulfuration of etrimfos (Casida and Lykken, 1969).

The removal of alkyl groups on substituted amide and amino nitrogens of pesticides is well-established in plants, insects, and mammals (Baldwin, 1977; Bull, 1972; Menzer, 1973). The *N*-hydroxymethyl intermediates of dicrotophos (Menzer and Casida, 1965) and carbaryl (Kuhr and Casida, 1967) have been isolated from plants. The *N*-demethylation of monuron in cotton is the one

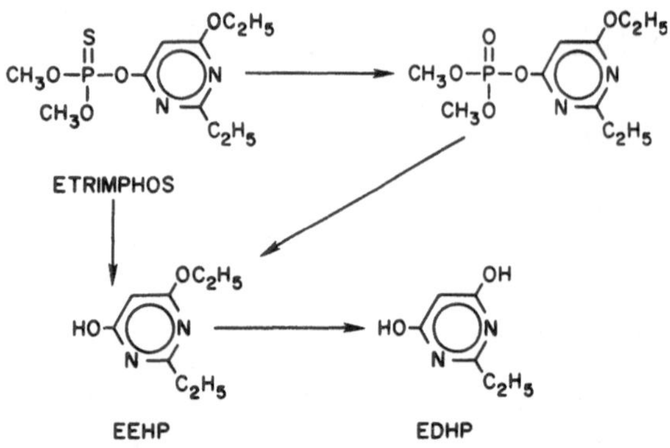

Figure 2.6. Apparent mixed function oxidase-catalyzed hydrolysis, O-dealkylation, and desulfuration of etrimfos in beans and corn.

example of pesticide metabolism in plants where an mfo system and its reaction mechanism have been demonstrated (Fig. 2.7) (Frear *et al.*, 1969, 1972*b*). Successive oxidative *N*-demethylation to monomethyl monuron and *p*-chlorophenylurea is the major monuron detoxication pathway in plants (Frear and Swanson, 1972; Frear *et al.*, 1972*b*). A minor pathway involved aryl hydroxylation followed by glucosylation of the phenolic intermediates (Frear and Swanson, 1974). The *N*-dealkylation reaction was catalyzed by an mfo system that required molecular oxygen and reduced pyridine nucleotides as cofactors (Fig. 2.8). When monuron was the substrate, the reaction products were monomethyl monuron and formaldehyde. An unstable *N*-hydroxymethyl intermediate was detected as a reaction product when monomethyl monuron was the substrate. This intermediate was not isolated, but it degraded stoichiometrically to *p*-chlorophenylurea and formaledhyde (Frear *et al.*, 1969, 1972*b*). The *N*-demethylase system had limited substrate specificity for dimethyl- and monomethylphenylurea herbicides and was strongly inhibited by carbamate insecticides (Frear *et al.*, 1969, 1972*b*).

N-Dealkylation may either detoxify or activate a pesticide. Generally, *N*-dealkylation of herbicides is a detoxication mechanism in contrast to some insecticides. Successive *N*-demethylation of monuron is a detoxication mechanism (C. R. Swanson and H. R. Swanson, 1968). Mono-*N*-dealkylation of atrazine is only a partial detoxication mechanism (Fig. 2.9) (Shimabukuro, 1967). Sandoz 6706®, a substituted phenyl pyridazinone herbicide, was successively demethylated by susceptible corn and soybeans to the more phytotoxic Sandoz 9789® (norflurazon) and to the nonphytotoxic demethylated metabolite (Fig. 2.9) (Strang and Rogers, 1974). Diphenamid was successively demethylated in plants, and the *N*-methyl-*N*-hydroxymethyl intermediate was detected in high concentrations

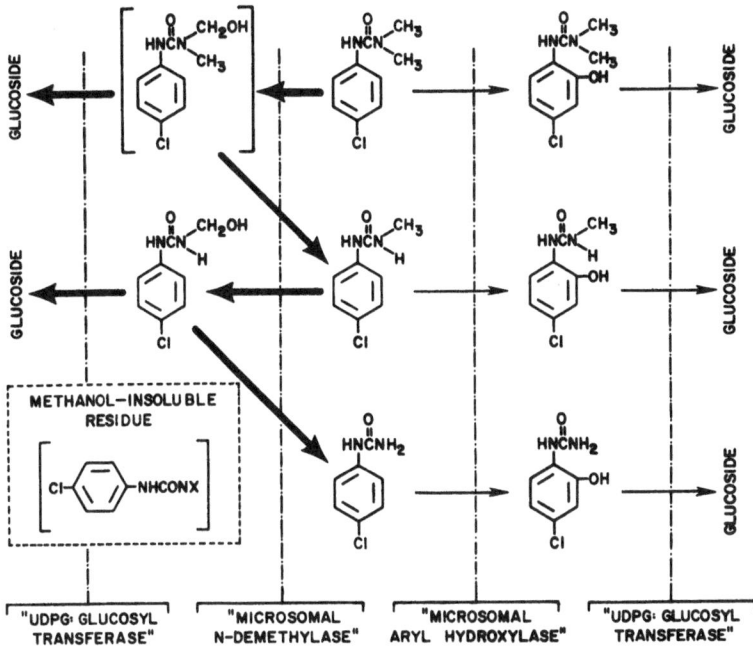

Figure 2.7. *N*-demethylation and aryl hydroxylation of monuron in cotton.

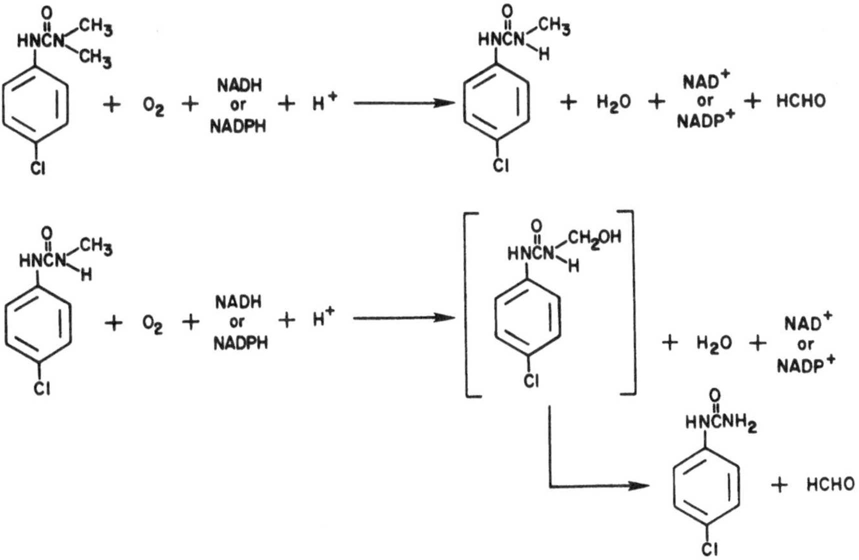

Figure 2.8. The mechanism of monuron *N*-demethylation by microsomal mfo from cotton.

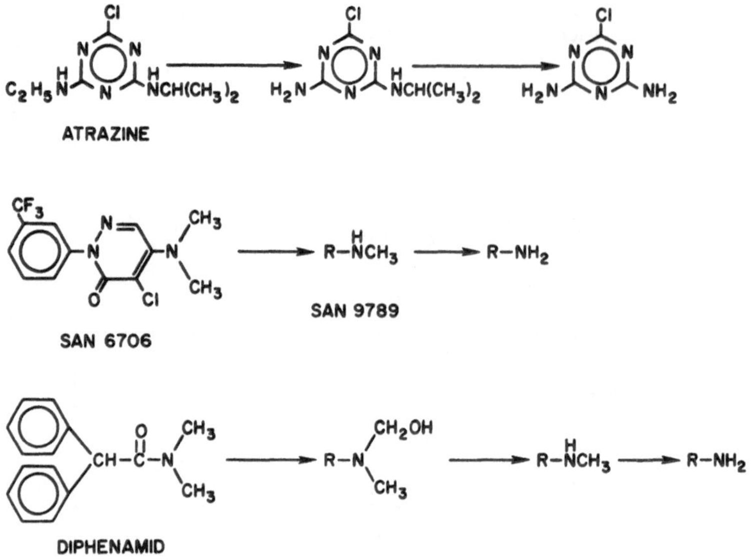

Figure 2.9.   *N*-dealkylation of atrazine, SAN 6706®, and diphenamid in plants.

in peppers (Hodgson and Hoffer, 1977) and soybean cell cultures (Fig. 2.9) (Davis *et al.*, 1978). Methazole was hydrolyzed to phytotoxic monomethyl diuron much faster in susceptible bean than in resistant cotton (Fig. 2.10) (Dorough *et al.*, 1973*b*). Subsequent detoxication by *N*-demethylation to 3,4-dichlorophenylurea was more rapid in cotton than in bean. The metabolism of monomethyl diuron appears to be similar to that of monomethyl monuron. The *N*-hydroxymethyl intermediates for SAN 6706® and methazole were not isolated in contrast to those of diphenamid (Hodgson and Hoffer, 1977; Davis *et al.*, 1978), dicrotophos (Biolrin®) (Menzer and Casida, 1965), and carbaryl (Kuhr and Casida, 1967). In contrast to the herbicides monuron and diuron, the insecticide dicrotophos was converted to successively more potent anticholinesterase agents by *N*-demethylation reactions (Menzer and Casida, 1965).

The *N*-dealkylated metabolites of pesticides are not the terminal residues in plants. Subsequent conjugation or further oxidation followed by conjugation generally yields significant amounts of water-soluble derivatives and insoluble residues (Frear *et al.*, 1972*a*).

Very little is known about the fate of DDT and Kelthane® (dicofol) in plants. Chlorinated hydrocarbon insecticides appear to be resistant to metabolism by all forms of plants. DDT was absorbed by barley plants, but no metabolism occurred (Upshall and Goodwin, 1964). DDT residues on the leaf surface of apples included traces of DDD and 4,4'-dichlorobenzophenone (DCBP) (Fig. 2.11) (Harrison *et al.*, 1967). DDD and the oxidatively dehalogenated DDE,

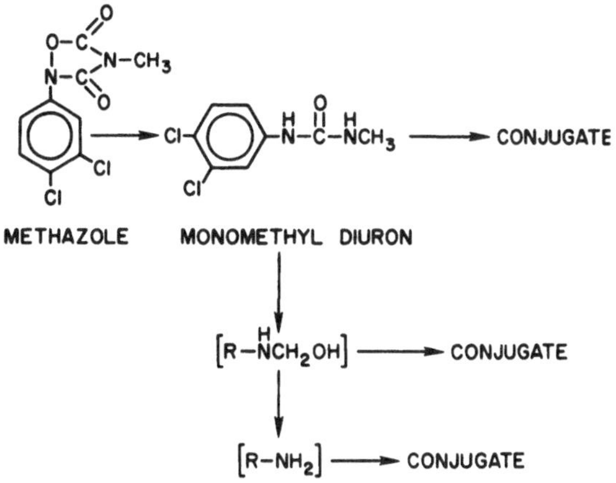

Figure 2.10. Hydrolysis and *N*-demethylation of methazole in cotton and beans.

but no DCBP, were detected in cottonseed (El Zorgani, 1975) and in extracts of cotton leaves that presumably included surface residues and tissue metabolites (Nash *et al.*, 1977). Kelthane was metabolized to at least three unknown polar products in a microsomal preparation from suspended parsley cells (Sandermann *et al.*, 1977).

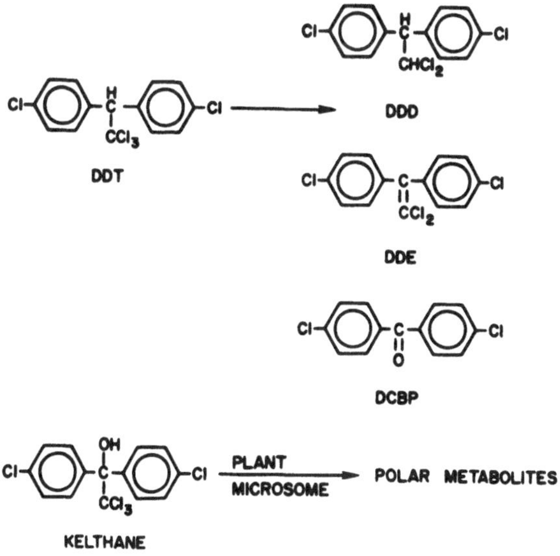

Figure 2.11. Metabolism of DDT and Kelthane® in plants.

DDT was highly resistant to metabolism by marine phytoplankton (Bowes, 1972). DDE was the only metabolite of DDT in seven marine phytoplankters with a conversion rate of 0–7.4% after 9 days of growth with DDT. Apparently, oxidation to DCBP did not occur. Metabolism by dehydrochlorination is not a detoxication mechanism as far as the effect on the noncyclic electron transport reaction in photosynthesis is concerned. Both DDT and DDE inhibited noncyclic electron transport in isolated chloroplasts with an I_{50} concentration of 20 μM (Bowes, 1972).

Examples of *in vitro* pesticide metabolism by plant mfo systems are limited (Lamoureux and Frear, 1979). The mixed function oxidases from plants may have narrow substrate specificities in contrast to animal mfo systems. Plants typically show levels of mfo activity with specific activities between 1.0 to 10 nmole product/mg protein per hour. Concentrations of P-450 in plants ranged from 0.007 to 0.02 nmole P-450/mg microsomal protein as compared to 0.8–1.1 nmole P-450/mg microsomal protein in rat liver (Markham *et al.*, 1972).

2.3.2. Reduction

Reduction is less prevalent than oxidation in the metabolism of pesticides by plants. Reduction of the sulfoxide of fensulfothion to the sulfide and the reductive dechlorination of tetrachlorvinphos in plants have been described (Fig. 2.12) (Eto, 1974). Aryl nitroreduction of fluorodifen was a minor metabolic pathway in the peanut (Eastin, 1971). However, aryl nitroreduction of the fungicide PCNB was a significant reaction in peanut root in the absence of root aeration (Fig. 2.12) (Lamoureux and Rusness, 1976). About 28% of the absorbed PCNB was converted to pentachloroaniline.

Aryl nitroreductase from roots and hypocotyls of peanut seedlings reduced PCNB under a nitrogen atmosphere with both FAD and NADPH as cofactors (Lamoureux and Rusness, 1976). The herbicide Dinoben® was also reduced to another herbicide, chloramben, by an aryl nitroreductase from soybean roots (Fig. 2.12) (Frear, 1975). This enzymatic reaction occurred under nitrogen with either NADPH or NADH as cofactors, but the more purified enzyme required FAD or FMN in addition to NADPH or NADH. The physiological significance of Dinoben® reduction is not clear, but it may be an activation mechanism influencing herbicidal selectivity of Dinoben®.

The reduction of the nitro groups in substituted dinitroaniline herbicides occurs in plants (Biswas and Hamilton, 1969; Probst *et al.*, 1976). The biotransformation of these herbicides in plant tissues has been questioned (Probst *et al.*, 1976), but published reports indicate that plants metabolize these compounds rapidly and extensively by reactions including nitroreduction, *N*-dealkylation, and cyclization (Biswas and Hamilton, 1969; Marquis *et al.*, 1979; Sumner *et al.*, 1976; Wright *et al.*, 1975).

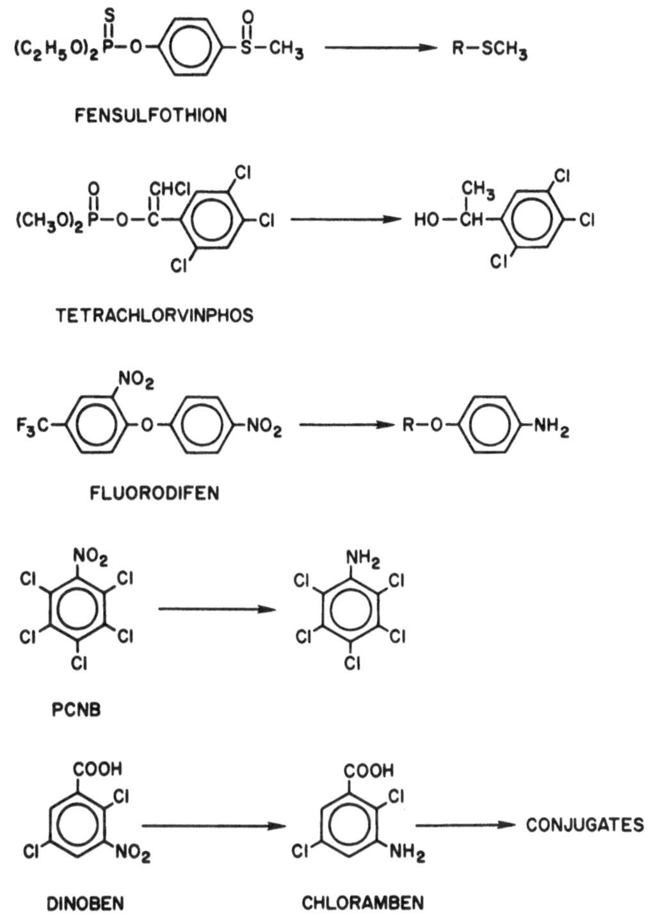

Figure 2.12. Reductive metabolism of fensulfothion, tetrachlorvinphos, fluorodifen, PCNB, and dinoben in plants.

2.3.3. Hydrolysis

Hydrolysis of esters, amides, and nitriles is a common reaction in plants. Hydrolysis appears to be a selective mechanism for some pesticides in plants.

The herbicide propanil was hydrolyzed by a particular enzyme, aryl acylamidase, from resistant rice (Fig. 2.13) (Frear and Still, 1968; Still and Kuzerian, 1967). This enzyme was associated with the chloroplast membrane from rice (Still and Kuzerian, 1967). The level of enzyme activity in resistant rice leaves was 60 times higher than in the leaves of susceptile barnyard grass. However,

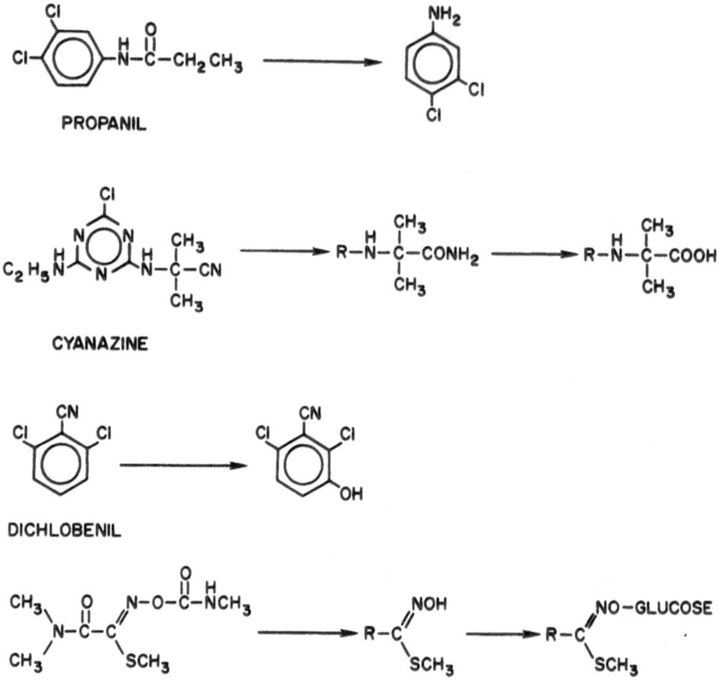

Figure 2.13. Hydrolytic reactions in the metabolism of propanil, dichlobenil, cyanazine, and oxamyl in plants.

the enzyme activity was equal in the roots of both species (Frear and Still, 1968). The enzyme was specific for the anilide linkage since the phenylurea, monuron (Fig. 2.7), and the phenylcarbamate, chlorpropham (Fig. 2.2), were not hydrolyzed to the chloroanilines.

The phosphorothionate insecticides parathion and fenitrothion acted as propanil synergists by causing increased injury to rice (Matsunaka, 1968). The oxon forms were 100–200 times more effective in inhibiting propanil hydrolysis than the thionate forms. Carbaryl was also a strong inhibitor of propanil hydrolysis (Frear and Still, 1968). The apparent K_m for propanil was 2.93×10^{-3} M as compared to an apparent K_i of 1.51×10^{-8} M for carbaryl (Frear and Still, 1968). Apparently, carbaryl and the phosphorothionate insecticides acted as strong synergists by inhibiting the hydrolytic detoxication of propanil in rice.

Compounds with cyano groups such as the s-triazine herbicide cyanazine are presumed to be hydrolyzed in plants to the amide and the acid (Fig. 2.13) (Beynon *et al.*, 1972a,b). However, the acids of the herbicide dichlobenil (Fig.

2.13) and 2,6-dichlorobenzamide have not been identified positively in plants. Instead, these compounds are aryl hydroxylated and conjugated (Frear, 1976). It is likely that steric hindrance by the adjacent chlorine atoms prevents hydrolysis of the cyano group.

Many carbamate insecticides and carbanilate herbicides that contain an aromatic moiety resist hydrolysis in plants (Kuhr and Casida, 1967; Still and Mansager, 1973). However, the insecticide oxamyl, which lacks an aromatic moiety, was readily metabolized in plants by hydrolysis of the methylcarbamoyl group, conjugated and incorporated into insoluble residue (Fig. 2.13) (Harvey *et al.*, 1978). In alfalfa, 98% of the extracted radioactivity from labeled oxamyl was in the form of polar metabolites. No sulfoxide or sulfone metabolites were detected in several plant species tested (Harvey *et al.*, 1978).

Many carboxylic acid esters are hydrolyzed readily to their free acids in plants. The free acid forms of herbicides are often presumed to be the active forms. Activation by hydrolysis of 2,4-D esters, amides, and nitriles to the free acid and by α- and β-oxidation of higher phenoxyalkanoic acids to active 2,4-D has been demonstrated (Loos, 1975; Wain and Smith, 1976). Hydrolysis of the wild oat herbicide benzoylprop-ethyl to the free acid form benzoylprop was shown to be an activation mechanism (Fig. 2.14) (Jeffcoat and Harries, 1973)

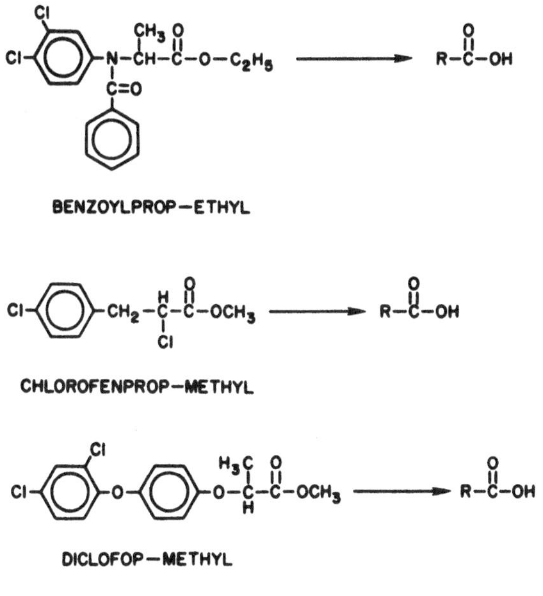

BENZOYLPROP—ETHYL

CHLOROFENPROP—METHYL

DICLOFOP—METHYL

Figure 2.14. Hydrolysis of the herbicidal esters, benzoylprop-ethyl, chlorfenprop-methyl, and diclofop-methyl.

analogous to the hydrolysis of 2,4-D esters. Hydrolysis of benzoylprop-ethyl to benzoylprop occurred very rapidly in susceptible oats but not in resistant wheat (Beynon *et al.*, 1974; Jeffcoat and Harries, 1973). Wheat coleoptiles were sensitive to benzoylprop but not to benzoylprop-ethyl. The carboxylesterase from wild oat that catalyzed the hydrolysis of benzoylprop-ethyl was a stable enzyme, required no cofactors, and had an apparent K_m for benzoylprop-ethyl of 3.8 × 10^{-6} M (Hill *et al.*, 1978). A similar carboxylesterase was not detected in wheat (Hill *et al.*, 1978). Other analogs of benzoylprop-ethyl are known to act similarly (Jeffcoat and Harries, 1975).

Not all pesticide esters appear to be activated by hydrolysis as with 2,4-D esters and benzoylprop-ethyl. Both resistant wheat and susceptible wild oat and cultivated oat hydrolyzed rapidly chlorfenprop-methyl and diclofop-methyl to their acids (Fig. 2.14) (Fedtke and Schmidt, 1977; Shimabukuro *et al.*, 1979). However, very little of both acids and parent esters remained in either plant species after 24–30 hr (Fedtke and Schmidt, 1977; Shimabukuro *et al.*, 1979). Chlorfenprop-methyl (Andreev and Amrhein, 1976; Collet and Pont, 1978) and diclofop-methyl (Shimabukuro *et al.*, 1978*b*) were stronger auxin antagonists (approximately two times stronger) than their free acids. In *in vitro* membrane experiments in which penetration into plant tissues by esters or acids was not a factor, bound auxin was displaced more effectively by the ester, chlorfenprop-methyl, than by the acid, chlorfenprop (Andreev and Amrhein, 1976). Intact susceptible plants were equally sensitive to the ester and acid forms when sprayed or injected with chlorfenprop-methyl (Fedtke and Schmidt, 1977) and diclofop-methyl (Donald and Shimabukuro, 1980), respectively. More of the esters of both herbicides were absorbed from leaf surfaces than the acids, but the absorption differences were minor (Fedtke and Schmidt, 1977; Shimabukuro and Walsh, unpublished data, 1978). It appears that the esters and acids of both herbicides are biologically active.

The organophosphorous insecticides, unlike the *N*-methyl and *N*,*N*-dimethylcarbamates, are readily cleaved in plants to form metabolites suggestive of hydrolytic reactions (Bull, 1972; Casida and Lykken, 1969). The alkyl phosphate and acid anhydride bonds of organophosphates are known to be cleaved in animals and insects by phosphotriesterases, NADPH-dependent mfo systems, and soluble glutathione *S*-transferases (Appleton and Nakatsugawa, 1977; Bull, 1972; Eto, 1974). It appears that cleavage by oxidative and glutathione conjugation mechanisms may be more significant than by a hydrolytic mechanism. In plants the mechanisms for cleavage have not been characterized.

Hydrolysis of BAY NTN 9306® (Fig. 2.4) yielded the free phenols that were conjugated subsequently with glucose. Hydrolysis of the conjugates yielded 23% phenol sulfide [*p*-(methylthio)phenol], 41% phenol sulfoxide [*p*-(methylsulfinyl)phenol], and 36% phenol sulfone [*p*-(methylsulfonyl)phenol] (Bull *et al.*, 1976). The pyrimidinyl bond of etrimfos was hydrolyzed to the pyrimidinol,

EEHP, in beans, cotton, and corn, but the formation of a glucoside conjugate was not established (Fig. 2.6) (Akram *et al.*, 1978). Dimethoate was rapidly hydrolyzed in corn, peas, potatoes, and cotton leaves (Dauterman *et al.*, 1960) and by wheat and soybean grains *in vitro* or *in vivo* (Fig. 2.15) (Rowlands, 1966). Desulfuration to dimethoxon was not a major reaction in both studies but was greater in leaf tissues than in the grains. The major products in leaves were mono-*O*-methyl-*S*-(*N*-methyl-carbamoylmethyl) phosphorothiolothionate, *O,O*-dimethyl phosphoric acid, and *O,O*-dimethyl phosphorothionate (Fig. 2.15) (Dauterman *et al.*, 1960; Rowlands, 1966). Almost no *O,O*-dimethyl phosphorothiolothionate was detected in plants, indicating that enzymatic or nonenzymatic cleavage of the P–S–C bond occurred at the P–S rather than at the S–C linkage (Dauterman *et al.*, 1960; Rowlands, 1966). Quantitative differences between species occurred in dimethoate metabolism. Hydrolysis of the methoxy group occurred in cotton, corn, and potato leaves after absorption of surface-applied dimethoate to give the mono-*O*-methyl derivative of dimethoate as the major metabolite. However, hydrolysis to phosphoric acid was a major reaction only on the leaf surfaces of peas. Subsequent absorption resulted in a high internal concentration of phosphoric acid in pea leaf tissue (Dauterman *et al.*, 1960). No evidence for enzymatic carbamoyl bond cleavage was observed in the leaves of several plant species (Dauterman *et al.*, 1960), but in wheat grains apparent cleavage by amidase reaction occurred to give traces of mono-*O*-methyl-*S*-carboxymethyl phosphorothiolothionate (Rowlands, 1966).

The apparent hydrolysis of malathion by phosphatase occurred in wheat

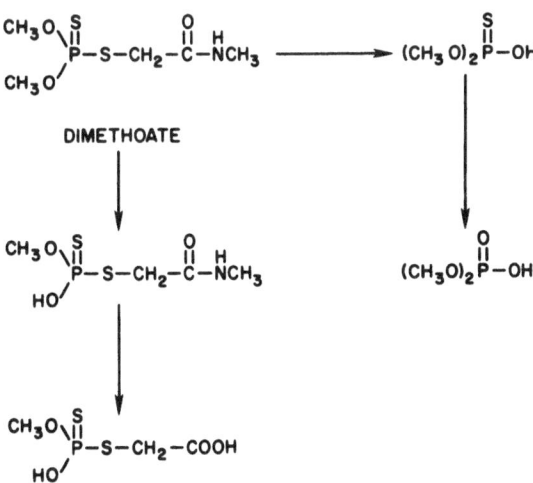

Figure 2.15. Apparent hydrolysis of the organophosphate insecticide dimethoate in plants.

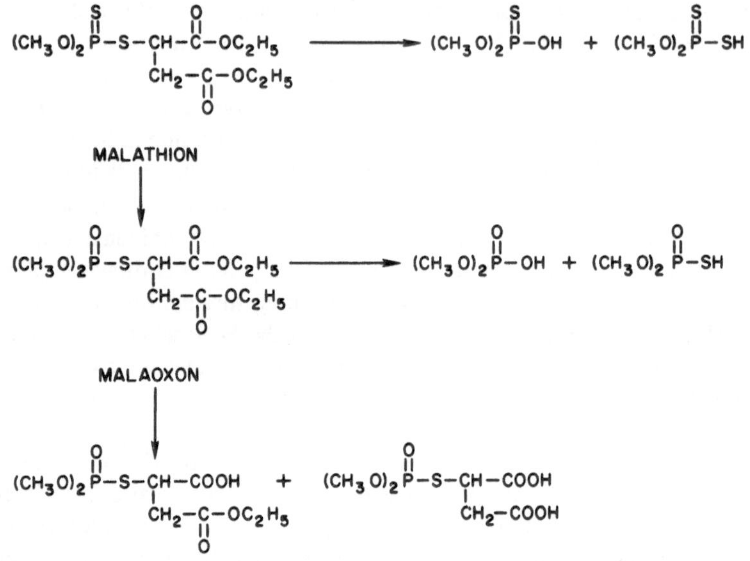

Figure 2.16.   Apparent hydrolysis of malathion in wheat grain.

grains with the formation of nontoxic dimethylphosphorothionate and dimethylphosphorothiolothionate (Fig. 2.16) (Rowlands, 1965). Activation of malathion by desulfuration to malaoxon was followed by hydrolysis and detoxication to dimethyl phosphoric acid, dimethylphosphorothiolate, and malaoxon mono-and diacids. Mechanisms for the metabolism of pesticides such as malathion and dimethoate have not been characterized in plants as they have been in animals and insects. The metabolism of organophosphorous insecticides by mixed function oxidases and glutathione S-transferases often results in some of the same products formed by esterases.

2.3.4. Conjugation

Conjugation, as applied to pesticide metabolism, is the *in vivo* reaction of a pesticide metabolite with an endogenous substrate to form a new compound of higher molecular weight (Dorough, 1976). Conjugation of pesticides is a mechanism for converting nonpolar compounds to more hydrophilic forms for elimination by biological organisms. In many cases conjugation may be considered a secondary reaction since conjugation often follows alteration of the parent molecule. In plants conjugation may determine the nature of the terminal residues since elimination is not a significant factor. Conjugation also plays a role in pesticide detoxication and selectivity in plants. The major pesticide conjugates in plants are simple and complex glucosides, glutathione conjugates and related products, and amino acid conjugates. In mammals the sulfate, glucuronic acid, and glutathione-related conjugates often predominate.

2.3.4.1. Glucose Conjugation

Conjugation of pesticides with glucose in plants usually involves oxidized, hydrolyzed, or reduced forms of the pesticide in which a free hydroxyl, carboxyl, or amino group has been exposed so that the conjugation reaction can occur. Many secondary metabolites of pesticides contain these functional groups that can be conjugated readily with glucose. Indeed, glucose conjugation is so prevalent with phenolic metabolites of pesticides that the free phenols are rarely observed in significant concentrations relative to the conjugate forms. The pesticides or their metabolites are normally conjugated as β-glucosides in plants and insects. The formation of O-, N-, and S-glucosides of pesticides has been demonstrated in plants (Baldwin, 1977; Frear, 1975). However, only a few of these conjugates have been identified unequivocally as glucosides (Frear, 1975). The primary mechanism for glucosylation appears to involve a UDPG-dependent glucosyl transferase reaction.

In bean plants, oxidation of the carbamate insecticides, carbaryl (Fig. 2.3), Baygon® (propoxur), and Banol® (carbanolate) was followed by glucosylation of the phenol and alcohol metabolites (Kuhr and Casida, 1967). Oxidation and hydrolysis of the organophosphate BAY NTN 9306® in cotton resulted in the formation of several phenolic derivatives (Fig. 2.4) that were rapidly conjugated to apparent glucosides (Bull *et al.*, 1976). Examples of O-glucosylated herbicides include chlorprophamm (Still and Mansager, 1972), cisanilide (Frear and Swanson, 1975), and perfluidone (Lamoureux and Stafford, 1977) (Fig. 2.17).

O-glucosylation of oxidized phenolic metabolites of pesticides appears to be an effective detoxication mechanism. Hydroxylated metabolites of carbamate insecticides with anticholinesterase activity were inactivated by glucosylation (Kuhr and Cadisa, 1967). The aryl hydroxylated metabolites of chlorpropham were reported to be equally active to, or more active than, the parent herbicide in the inhibition of respiration and phosphorylation activities in isolated plant mitochondria and the inhibition of firefly luciferase activity (Still *et al.*, 1974). The O-glucosides of the hydroxylated metabolites had no inhibitory activity. Generally, very little of the free phenol forms of pesticides are found in both susceptible and resistant plants (Frear and Swanson, 1975; Lamoureux and Stafford, 1977; Shimabukuro *et al.*, 1979; Still *et al.*, 1974).

Examples of pesticide N- and S-glucosylation in plants are limited (Frear, 1975). The substituted aniline herbicide, chloramben (Amiben®), and other arylamines were glucosylated by a UDP-glucosyl transferase from soybeans that were specific for the glycosyl donors UDPG and TDPG (Fig. 2.18) (Frear, 1968).

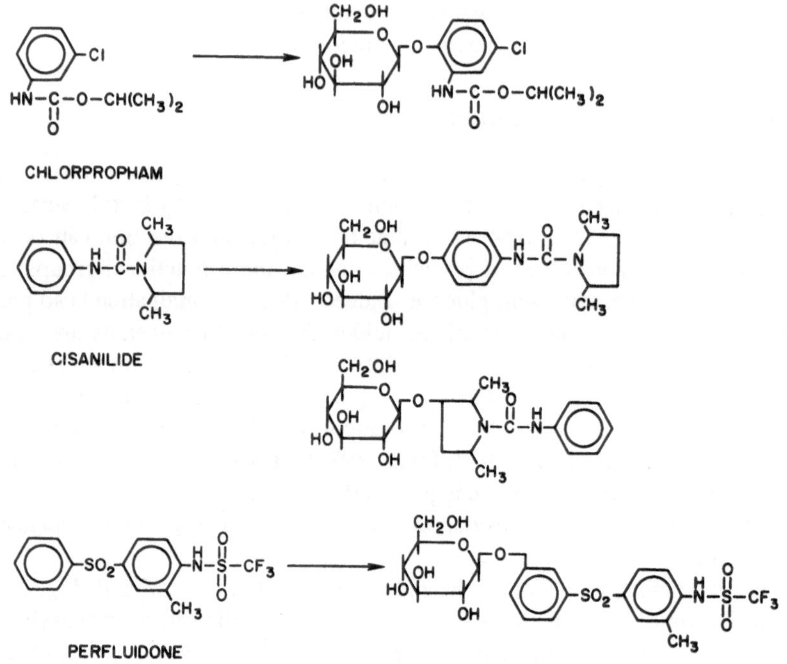

Figure 2.17. *O*-glucoside metabolites of chlorpropham, cisanilide, and perfluidone.

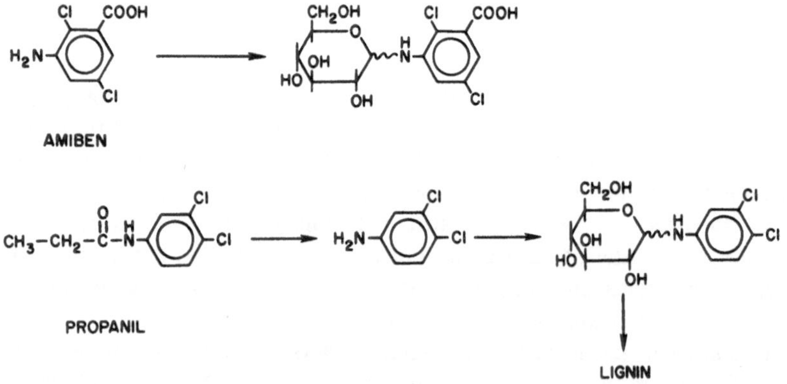

Figure 2.18. *N*-glucoside metabolites of chloramben (Amiben®) and propanil.

The formation of the *N*-glucoside and glycosyl ester of chloramben appears to be a significant mechanism for chloramben selectivity (Frear, 1975; Frear *et al.*, 1978). Enzymatic hydrolysis of propanil (Frear and Still, 1968; Still and Kuzerian, 1967) in rice yielded 3,4-dichloroaniline (Fig. 2.18). This metabolite was subsequently glucosylated to the *N*-(3,4-dichlorophenyl) glucosylamine (Still, 1968). The 3,4-dichloroaniline appears to be further metabolized to insoluble lignin or ligninlike products (Balba and Still, 1977; Yih *et al.*, 1968).

The formation of glucose esters of pesticides and plant growth regulators appears to be an increasingly important mechanism for the bioregulation of plant hormone levels and the selective toxicity of some herbicides. The glucosyl esters of 2,4-D (Thomas *et al.*, 1964) and indole acetic acid (IAA) (Zenk, 1961) have been identified (Fig. 2.19). Many phytotoxic forms of pesticides are acids or readily hydrolyzable esters. The glucose ester of chloramben (Fig. 2.19) (Frear *et al.*, 1978), the complex glucosyl ester of flamprop-methyl (Dutton *et al.*, 1976), and the apparent glucose ester of diclofop-methyl (Fig. 2.19) (Shimabukuro *et al.*, 1979) have been identified. The identification of the glycosyl moiety of the diclofop-methyl metabolite is only tentative. It may be similar to the complex glucosyl ester of flamprop-methyl (Fig. 2.20).

A large proportion of the IAA is bound as inactive glucose ester conjugates (Bandurski and Schulze, 1977). Changes in free IAA and IAA-ester levels with concomitant changes in the growth rate of corn seedlings have been demonstrated (Bandurski *et al.*, 1977). The *N*-glucosyl chloramben was not hydrolyzed in plant tissues, but the glucose ester of chloramben was hydrolyzed readily to regenerate chloramben (Frear *et al.*, 1978). Very little of either the methyl ester or the acid of diclofop-methyl and chlorfenprop-methyl remained in resistant and susceptible plants (Fedtke and Schmidt, 1977; Shimabukuro *et al.*, 1979). However, a large concentration of an apparent glucose ester conjugate of diclofop accumulated in susceptible wild oats, whereas resistant wheat formed predominantly phenolic conjugates of the aryl hydroxylated metabolite (Fig. 2.2) (Shimabukuro *et al.*, 1979). The regeneration of the acid, diclofop, from the glucose ester has not been demonstrated, but a bioregulation mechanism similar to that of IAA and chloramben may also be an important selective mechanism for diclofop-methyl. The glucose ester of chloramben was identified as the α-anomer and not the β-anomer as with most glucosides from plants (Frear *et al.*, 1978). The physiological significance of the α-configuration and the mechanism of its formation have not been determined.

The gentiobioside of diphenamid (Hodgson *et al.*, 1973) and several malonate hemiesters of β-glucosides have been reported (Dutton *et al.*, 1976; Hoffer and Hodgson, 1978; Shimabukuro *et al.*, 1975). The proposed biosynthetic pathways for these complex glycosides include reactions catalyzed by UDP-glucosyl transferase and malonyl CoA transferase (Frear, 1976). Diphenamid was oxidized to its *N*-hydroxymethyl-*N*-methyl derivative (Fig. 2.9) and con-

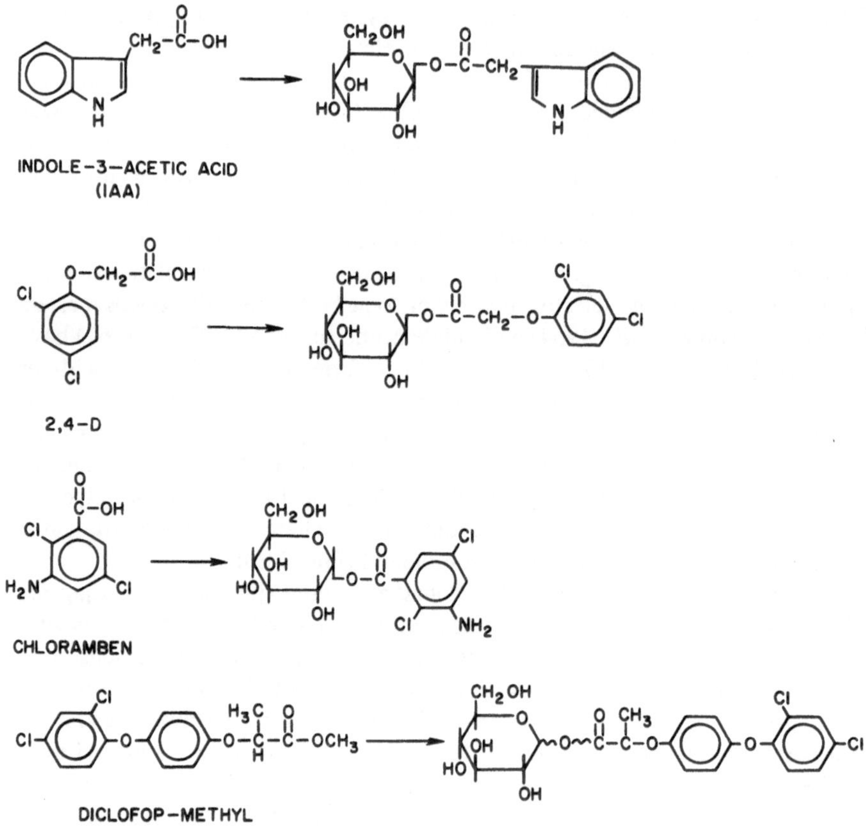

Figure 2.19.   Glucosyl esters of IAA, 2,4-D, chloramben, and diclofop-methyl.

jugated both as a β-glucoside and a β-gentiobioside (Fig. 2.20) (Hodgson *et al.*, 1973). A recent report indicated the acylation of the β-glucoside to a malonyl glucoside in resistant soybeans (Hoffer and Hodgson, 1978). The cleavage of fluorodifen by glutathione *S*-transferase gave free *p*-nitrophenol (Shimabukuro *et al.*, 1973a) that was conjugated as the β-glucoside and a malonyl glucoside (Shimabukuro *et al.*, 1975). Flamprop-methyl was hydrolyzed in wheat and conjugated as a glucose ester followed by acylation to a malonyl glucose ester (Fig. 2.20) (Dutton *et al.*, 1976). Complex acidic glucosides of insecticides have not been detected in plants, but an acidic metabolite of tetrachlorvinphos that readily hydrolyzed to the β-glucoside has been reported (Beynon *et al.*, 1973). However, the acidic conjugate has not been characterized.

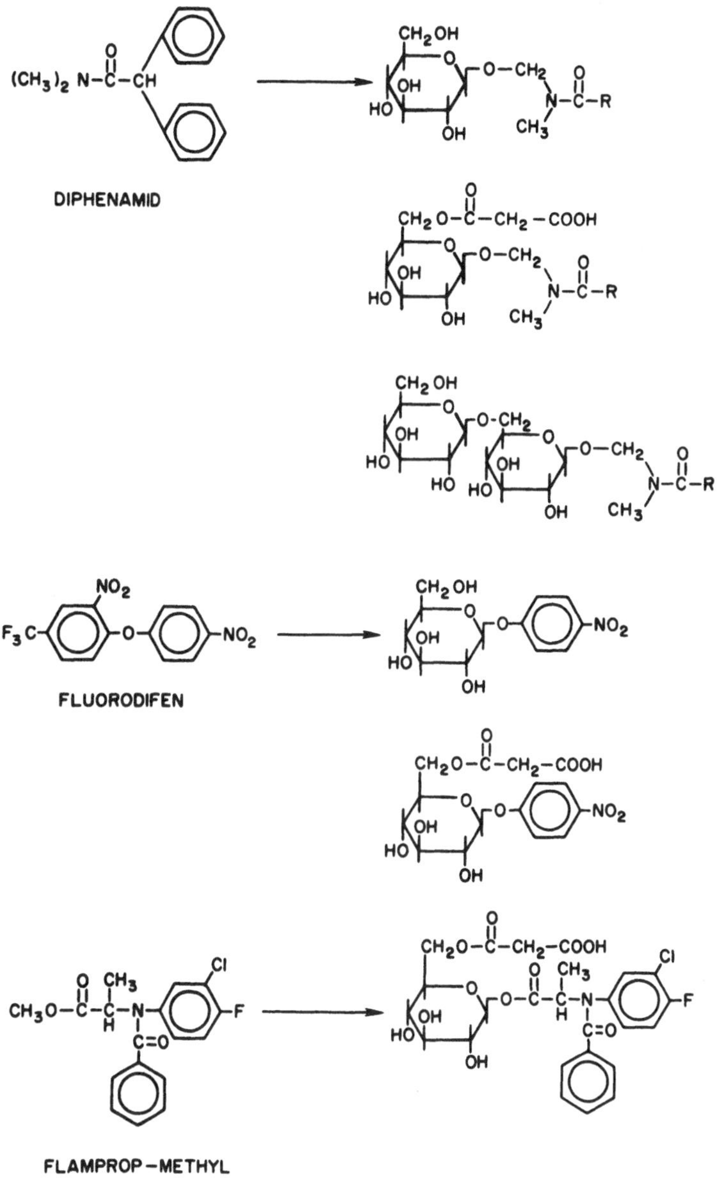

Figure 2.20. Complex glycoside metabolites of diphenamid, fluorodifen, and flamprop-methyl.

   The formation of simple and complex glucosides and other glycosides is
a major mechanism for pesticide metabolism and detoxication in plants. Glucose
metabolites are involved in the bioregulation of pesticide availability in plants
and may act also as intermediates in the formation of terminal pesticide residues.

2.3.4.2. Amino Acid Conjugation

   Pesticides that are known to form amino acid conjugates through an α-
amide bond in plants have been predominantly acidic herbicides (Mumma and
Hamilton, 1976). The most extensive work on amino acid conjugation has been
reported for 2,4-D, IAA, and auxinlike plant growth regulators (Mumma and
Hamilton, 1976).

   The amino acid conjugates of 2,4-D, IAA, and 2,4,5-T have been characterized primarily from callus cultures (Arjmand *et al.*, 1978; Feung *et al.*,
1971, 1975, 1976), but similar metabolites of 2,4-D and IAA have been detected
in plant tissues (Fig. 2.21) (Andreae and Good, 1955; Loos, 1975). The major
metabolite of 2,4-D in bean plants was the β-glucoside of 4-OH-2,5-D (Fig. 2.2)
(Hamilton *et al.*, 1971). The amino acid conjugates were not characterized in
bean plants, but only trace amounts of these ether-soluble conjugates may have
been formed (Hamilton *et al.*, 1971). In plant callus culture, large amounts of
amino acid conjugates were formed. These conjugates ranged from 84% of the
^{14}C from [^{14}C]-2,4-D in susceptible carrot callus tissue to 26% in resistant corn
callus tissue (Feung *et al.*, 1975). Callus tissues of carrots, jackbeans, sunflow-
ers, tobacco, and corn all formed 2,4-D conjugates of glutamic (2,4-D-Glu) and
aspartic (2,4-D-Asp) acids with 2,4-D-Glu predominating (Fig. 2.21) (Feung *et
al.*, 1975).

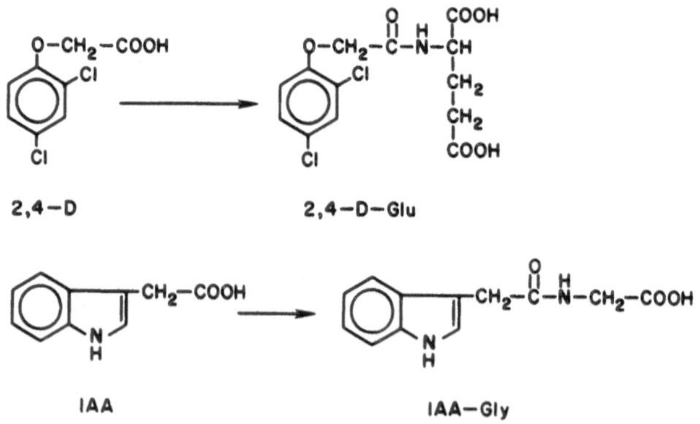

Figure 2.21.   Amino acid conjugates of 2,4-D and IAA in plant callus tissue.

Minor 2,4-D conjugates of alanine, valine, leucine, phenylalanine, and tryptophan have been identified in soybean callus tissue (Feung *et al.*, 1973). The glutamic and aspartic acid conjugates of IAA were minor metabolites in crown gall callus (Feung *et al.*, 1976). Major metabolites were conjugates of glycine, alanine, and valine. The significance of the differences between species and pesticides in the formation of amino acid conjugates has not been determined.

Amino acid conjugates of 2,4-D display typical auxin activity by stimulating cell elongation in *Avena* coleoptile sections and growth of soybean callus tissue (Feung *et al.*, 1974). It appears that the conjugate 2,4-D-Glu and other amino acid conjugates are biologically active as the conjugated molecule and not necessarily as the free acid 2,4-D. Both 2,4-D-Glu and 2,4-D-methionine stimulated callus growth by more than 50% over that of 2,4-D at the optimum 2,4-D concentration of 0.1 μM (Feung *et al.*, 1974). Soybean callus tissue incubated with [^{14}C]-2,4-D-Glu hydrolyzed only 4% of the absorbed [^{14}C]-2,4-D-Glu, but 55% was oxidized to biologically inactive 4-OH-2,5-D and 4-OH-2,3-D (Feung *et al.*, 1973). Amino acid conjugation may be an activation mechanism for the expression of biological activity by 2,4-D.

2.3.4.3. Glutathione Conjugation

Glutathione conjugation is becoming recognized as a major metabolic reaction for pesticide degradation in plants. The significance of glutathione conjugation and biosynthesis of mercapturic acids in mammals has been recognized for a long time. The importance of this reaction in all biological systems is reflected in the numerous reviews on this subject (Arias and Jacoby, 1976; Boyland and Chasseaud, 1969; Hutson, 1976; Jacoby, 1978; Lamoureux and Frear, 1979; Shimabukuro *et al.*, 1978*a*). Glutathione conjugation in plants is extremely important because of (1) the wide range of potential substrates, (2) its role as a detoxication mechanism and a major factor in herbicide selectivity, and (3) its influence on the nature of terminal pesticide residues that remain in plants.

Glutathione conjugation is the initial reaction that leads to the synthesis of mercapturic acids in mammals (Boyland and Chasseaud, 1969). This is illustrated in the formation of the mercapturic acid of 3,4-dichloronitrobenzene (Fig. 2.22). Conjugation with reduced glutathione (GSH) is catalyzed by glutathione *S*-transferases with different substrate specificities (Boyland and Chausseaud, 1969; Hutson, 1976; Jacoby, 1978). The initial reaction involves an enzyme-catalyzed nucleophilic displacement with the formation of the GSH conjugate. Sequential removal of the glutamic acid and glycine residues gives the *S*-cysteine conjugate that is then *N*-acetylated to yield the mercapturic acid, the terminal excretion product in mammals.

Few examples of pesticides metabolized by GSH conjugation are known in

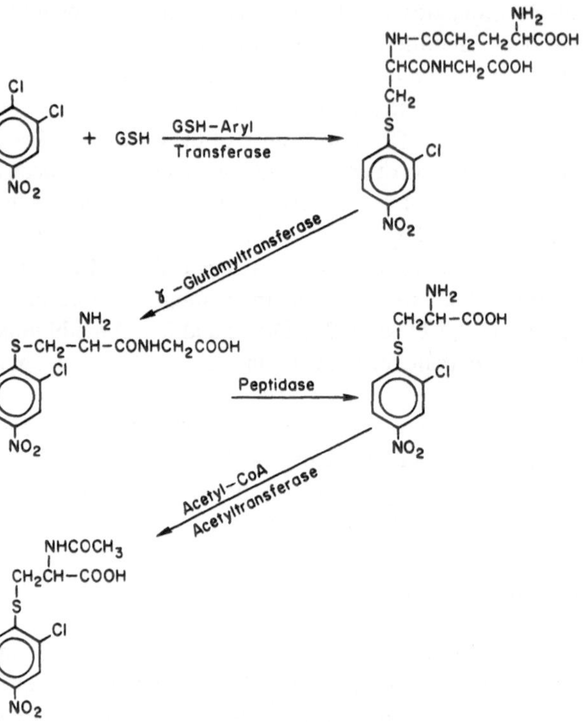

Figure 2.22.   Mercapturic acid pathway in mammals.

plants (Lamoureux and Frear, 1979; Shimabukuro *et al.*, 1978*a*). Insecticides such as parathion and its *O*-analog, tetrachlorvinphos, diazinon, and other phosphoric acid triesters are known to be metabolized by glutatione *S*-transferases in mammals and insects (Eto, 1974). None of these insecticides has been shown to be metabolized by GSH conjugation in plants. However, further research may prove otherwise.

The initial conjugation reaction with GSH occurs in both plants and mammals. However, limited studies with herbicides indicate that, unlike in mammals, the terminal products in plants may not be mercapturic acids. Atrazine, the first herbicide reported to be metabolized by GSH conjugation in plants (Lamoureux *et al.*, 1970), is catabolized to the lanthionine conjugate and other unknown soluble and insoluble products in sorghum (Fig. 2.23) (Lamoureux *et al.*, 1973; Shimabukuro *et al.*, 1973*b*). The GSH conjugate of atrazine was catabolized to the *S*-cysteine conjugate by the sequential loss of glycine and glutamic acid. The order of amino acid cleavage was the reverse of that in mammals (Fig. 2.22). The *S*-cysteine conjugate was not acetylated to yield the mercapturic acid as

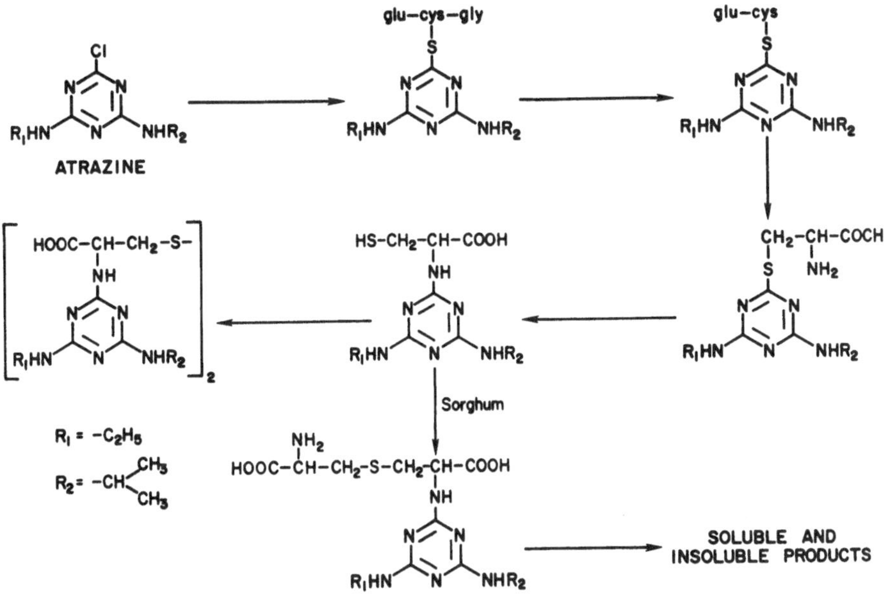

Figure 2.23.   Metabolism of atrazine by glutathione conjugation.

expected in mammals, but a rearrangement to the N-cysteine derivative and subsequent metabolism to the lanthionine conjugate occurred (Lamoureux *et al.*, 1973). Atrazine (Bakke *et al.*, 1972*a*), simazine (Hutson, 1976), and cyprazine (Larsen and Bakke, 1975) were not metabolized to their GSH conjugates when fed to rats. However, all three compounds formed GSH conjugates in several plant species (Lamoureux *et al.*, 1972).

Glutathione conjugation of atrazine is a major mechanism for detoxication and selectivity in resistant plants such as corn and sorghum (Shimabukuro *et al.*, 1978*a*). Photosynthesis was inhibited by atrazine in both resistant and susceptible species. However, recovery of photosynthetic activity to nearly normal rates occurred within 6–7 hr in resistant species concomitant with a rapid detoxication of atrazine by glutathione conjugation (Shimabukuro *et al.*, 1978*a*). Metabolism of atrazine was negligible, and no photosynthetic recovery occurred in susceptible species.

Cyanazine, another 2-chloro-*s*-triazine herbicide, was metabolized by GSH conjugation to its mercapturic acid in the rat (Crayford and Hutson, 1972). No GSH conjugate was detected in corn grown in cyanazine-containing soil (Beynon *et al.*, 1972*a*). However, the GSH conjugate of cyanazine was detected in several plant species including corn when the herbicide was absorbed from nutrient solution (Thompson, 1974) (Fig. 2.24).

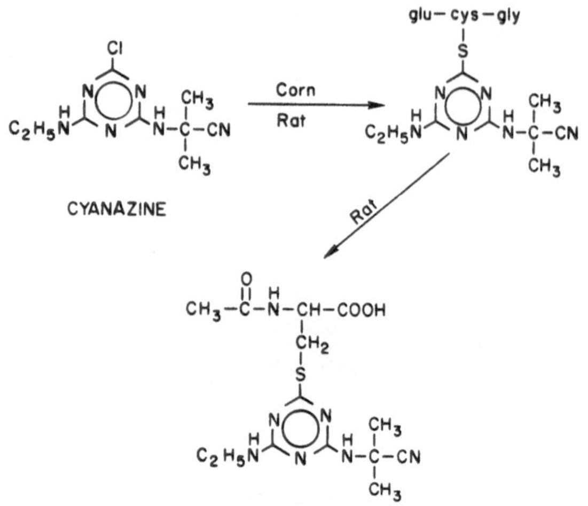

Figure 2.24.   Metabolism of cyanazine by glutathione conjugation in corn and rats.

GSH conjugation and catabolism of flurodifen occurred in both mammals (Lamoureux and Davison, 1975) and plants (Fig. 2.25) (Shimabukuro *et al.*, 1973*a*). The initial GSH-dependent cleavage of the diphenylether as catalyzed by a glutathione *S*-aryl transferase from rat liver (Lamoureux and Davison, 1975), and from several plant species (Frear and Swanson, 1973). In rats the resultant mercapturic acid was excreted in the urine (Lamoureux and Davison, 1975). However, unlike atrazine in sorghum (Fig. 2.23) flurodifen was not metabolized to its lanthionine conjugate. Instead, the *S*-cysteine conjugate of flurodifen was acylated in peanuts to yield *S*-(2-nitro-4-trifluoromethylphenyl)-*N*-malonylcysteine, an analog of the *N*-acetylated mercapturic acid (Shimabukuro *et al.*, 1976*b*).

Other herbicides known to be metabolized by GSH conjugation are propachlor (Lamoureux *et al.*, 1971), CDAA (Lamoureux *et al.*, 1971), and barban (Fig. 2.26) (Lamoureux *et al.*, 1971; Shimabukuro *et al.*, 1976*a*). The γ-glutamylcysteine conjugate of propachlor was characterized in corn (Lamoureux *et al.*, 1971), but the mercapturic acids of propachlor and CDAA were identified only in the rat (Lamoureux and Davison, 1975). *In vitro* and *in vivo* conjugation with glutathione occurred with the fungicide PCNB in peas (Fig. 2.26) (Lamoureux and Rusness, 1976) and the aryl hydroxylated metabolites of chlorpropham (Fig. 2.27) and cisanilide in oats (Rusness and Still, 1977).

Direct conjugation of 4-hydroxychlorpropham with cysteine was also demonstrated (Fig. 2.27) (Still and Rusness, 1977). Conjugation occurred enzymatically without the loss of either the halogen or the hydroxyl group. The

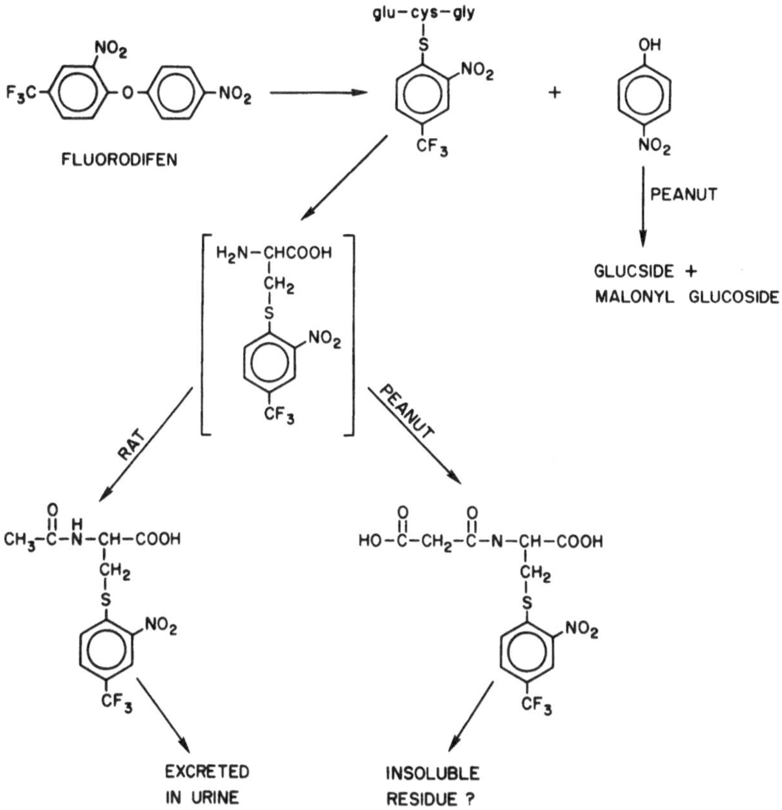

Figure 2.25. Metabolism of fluorodifen by glutathione conjugation in peanuts and rats.

detoxication of chlorfenprop-methyl in resistant wheat coleoptiles was postulated to be a direct displacement of the alkyl chlorine by cysteine (Collet and Pont, 1978) following partial detoxication by deesterification. The cysteine conjugation showed very little physiological activity as compared to the parent methyl ester and free acid (Collet and Pont, 1978). No mercapturic acids were identified as metabolites of the two cysteine conjugates.

The limited number of examples indicates that because an appropriate substrate is metabolized by an initial reaction with glutathione in one system, e.g., an animal system, it is no assurance that it will be metabolized in a corresponding manner in another system, e.g., a plant system. The chloro-*s*-triazines are metabolized to a large extent in plants by glutathione conjugation, and animals appear to have the necessary enzymes to metabolize these compounds similarly. However, glutathione conjugation is not a general method of metabolism of 2-

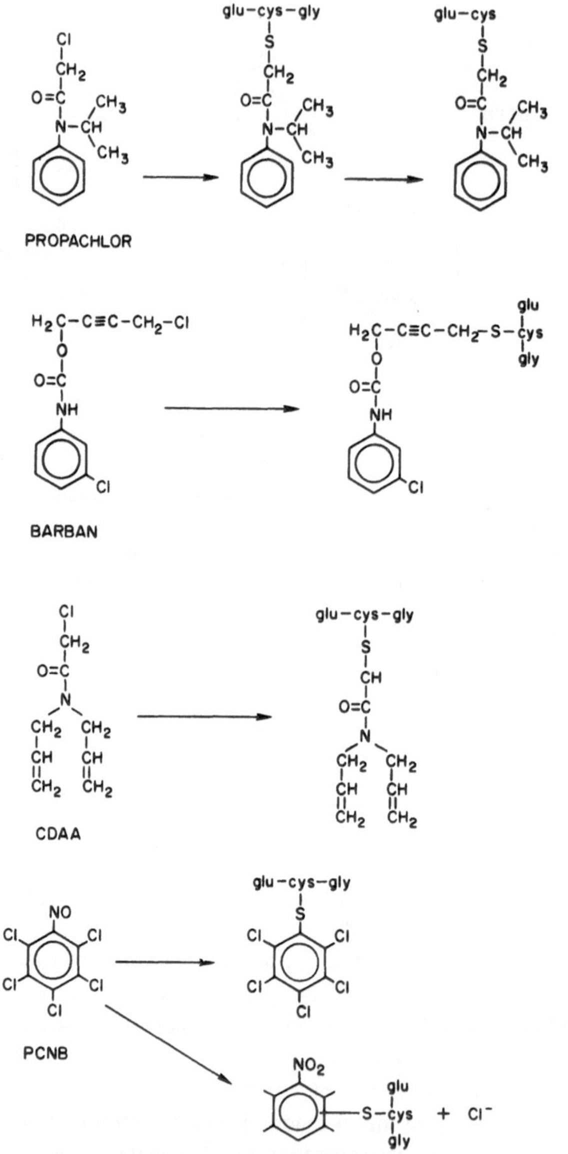

Figure 2.26.   Glutathione conjugation of propachlor, barban, CDAA, and PCNB in plants.

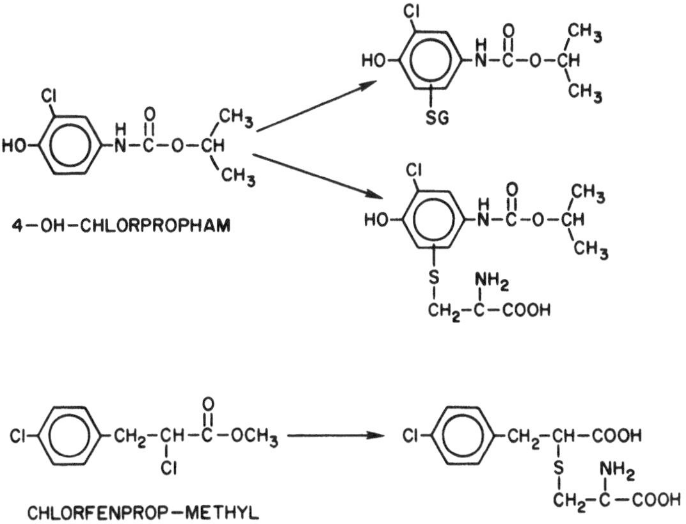

Figure 2.27.   Direct cysteine conjugation of 4-hydroxychlorpropham and chlorfenprop-methyl.

chloro-*s*-triazines in animals. In this case, alternate methods of metabolism may exist in animals. These alternate methods may be relatively more active or more accessible and hence compete favorably with glutathione conjugation. This is further demonstrated with propachlor, which was metabolized primarily by GSH conjugation in certain excised plant tissues (Lamoureux *et al.*, 1971), but only 25% of the propachlor was metabolized directly by GSH conjugation in the rat (Lamoureux and Davison, 1975). Other pesticides such as insecticides may be metabolized via GSH conjugation in animals, but the necessary GSH transferases may be absent in plants.

The role of glutathione conjugation in herbicide detoxication and selectivity has been clearly demonstrated (Shimabukuro *et al.*, 1978a). Generally, resistant plants have the necessary glutathione *S*-transferase to detoxify the herbicide when glutathione conjugation is the selective mechanism. Recent reports indicate that glutathione conjugation also plays a role in the mechanism of action of the herbicide antidote R-25788 (Lay and Casida, 1976, 1978). Corn is normally susceptible to injury by the herbicide EPTC. However, injury was greatly reduced when corn seeds were treated with the antidote (Lay and Casida, 1978). GSH conjugation of EPTC sulfoxide, the apparent active form of EPTC, was enhanced by treatment with the antidote due to increased concentrations of both glutathione *S*-transferase and total GSH content (Fig. 2.28) (Lay and Casida, 1976, 1978). The *S*-carbamyl-GSH derivative was metabolized to the mercapturic acid in the

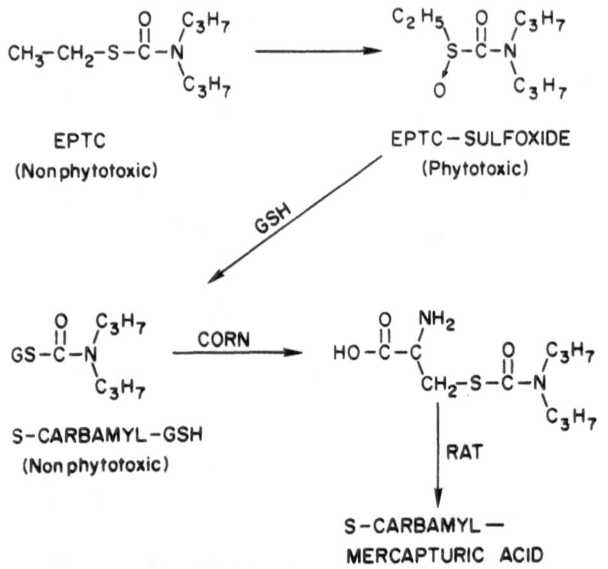

Figure 2.28. Antidote-enhanced detoxication of EPTC by glutathione conjugation.

rat, but only the S-cysteine conjugate and other unidentified products were detected in corn (Hubbell and Casida, 1977).

Glutathione S-transferases have been detected in 21 plant species, and they appear to be widespread in the plant kingdom (Lamoureux and Frear, 1979). Some of the properties and substrate specificities of these soluble plant enzymes are discussed in a recent review (Lamoureux and Frear, 1979).

2.3.5. Bound or Insoluble Residues

It is increasingly evident that most pesticides are not eliminated totally from plants by either complete oxidation to CO_2 or by secretion. Studies with radioactively labeled compounds indicate that the aromatic or heterocyclic moieties of most pesticides are not readily cleaved but remain in plants as conjugated soluble metabolites or insoluble bound residues (Baldwin, 1977; Frear and Shimabukuro, 1970; Frear *et al.*, 1972a; Kaufman *et al.*, 1976; Kearney and Kaufman, 1975). Little is known about the chemistry and biosynthesis of bound pesticide residues in plants (Kaufman *et al.*, 1976).

The diverse nature of the pesticides that eventually become associated with bound residues makes it unlikely that all bound residues would be in the same chemical fraction or have the same chemical composition. In fact, it is probable that several different bound forms of the same pesticide may exist in plants.

Recent studies with chloroanilines derived from herbicides indicate that these metabolites are associated mostly with the lignin fraction (Balba and Still, 1977). It is reasonable to expect many of the phenolic residues from herbicides and insecticides to be found also in the same lignin fraction. However, it is difficult to speculate how products metabolized via glutathione conjugation might be incorporated into lignin. Perhaps products from glutathione conjugation are incorporated into various protein fractions. The study of insoluble pesticide residues is an area of pesticide metabolism that is in need of additional research, but it is one of the most difficult to study.

Several examples of high insoluble residue formation in plants from different pesticides have been cited (Baldwin, 1977). However, only a few of the reported residues have been tested for their bioavailability. Generally, the insoluble residues of pesticides in plants appear to be highly stable and are not readily degraded for absorption in the gastrointestinal tract of animals.

About 21% of the absorbed radioactivity from ring-labeled [^{14}C]atrazine was in the insoluble residue fraction of sorghum. This residue was highly stable and resisted digestion by the rat and ruminant sheep, which excreted 88% and 100%, respectively, of the bound residue in the feces (Bakke *et al.*, 1972*b*). In alfalfa, 26% and 77% of the ^{14}C found in the shoots and roots, respectively, from root-absorbed [^{14}C]propham was incorporated into insoluble residue after 7 days. When the insoluble residue was fed to rats, 86% of the ^{14}C was excreted in the feces and less than 3% remained in the carcass 96 hr after treatment (Paulson *et al.*, 1975). Bean plants incorporated 51% and 7% of ring ^{14}C-labeled carbaryl and carbofuran, respectively, into insoluble residues 20 days after treatment (Marshall and Dorough, 1977). Water-soluble conjugates from carbaryl and carbofuran accounted for 30% and 67% of the ^{14}C, respectively (Marshall and Dorough, 1977). When the insoluble residues of carbaryl and carbofuran were fed to rats, 98% and 85%, respectively, of the doses were excreted in the feces. In contrast, rats fed ^{14}C water-soluble metabolites of carbaryl and carbofuran excreted 80% to 90%, respectively, of the radiocarbon in the urine (Marshall and Dorough, 1977).

2.4. CONCLUSION

This review is not a complete compilation of pesticide metabolism in plants. Important pesticide compounds such as the synthetic pyrethroids (Gaughan and Casida, 1978; Ruzo and Casida, 1977) and other naturally occurring plant insecticides such as nicotine and rotenone have not been discussed. However, these compounds, especially the pyrethroids, should not be overlooked because of their potential use as important insecticides.

This short discussion on pesticide metabolism in plants indicates that most

Table 2.2. Generalized Summary of Pesticide Behavior and Fate in Plants

Characteristics	Phase I	Phase II		Phase III
Reactions	Pesticide ⟶	Oxidation; reduction; hydrolysis ⟶	Conjugation ⟶	Secondary conjugation or incorporation into biopolymers (insoluble residues)
Solubility	Lipophilic	Amphophilic	Hydrophilic	Hydrophilic and insoluble
Transport	Selective mobility	Modified or reduced mobility	Limited or immobile	Immobile
Phytotoxicity	Toxic	Modified or less toxic	Greatly reduced or nontoxic	Nontoxic
Bioavailability[a]	+ + +	+ + +	+ +	+ or Unavailable

[a] + + +, Readily absorbed in GI tract of animals; + +, less absorption in GI tract of animals; +, limited absorption.

biological organisms, including plants, animals, and microorganisms, appear to metabolize foreign compounds or xenobiotics in the same general way. The common objective in all biological organisms appears to be the conversion of xenobiotics into some innocuous forms that may be excreted or stored as inactive materials in the organism. Pesticides and other xenobiotics appear to be metabolized in two phases in animals (Table 2.2) (Williams, 1959). Phase I metabolism involves oxidation, reduction or hydrolysis reactions followed by phase II, in which products from phase I are conjugated and detoxified before excretion. In plants, excretion of the conjugated pesticide metabolites is not significant. Therefore, these metabolites must either be compartmentalized within plant cells or removed from further metabolic activity by other mechanisms. This may be accomplished by a phase III-type metabolism that appears to be peculiar to plants (Table 2.2).

Phase I metabolism is probably the most important phase of pesticide metabolism in plants. Phase I reactions often decrease or modify the biological activity of pesticides and predispose the compounds to phase II conjugation reactions which yield nontoxic, water-soluble metabolites that are relatively immobile in the plant. Secondary conjugations or incorporation into insoluble pesticide residues with limited bioavailability are common in phase III reactions.

REFERENCES

Akram, M., Ahmad, S., and Forgash, A. J., 1978, Metabolism of phosphorothioic acid, *O,O*-dimethyl-*O*-(6-ethoxy-2-ethyl-4-pyrimidinyl) ester (etrimfos), in bean and corn plants, *J. Agric. Food Chem.* **26:**925.

Andreae, W. A., and Good, N. E., 1955, The formation of indole-acetylaspartic acid in pea seedlings, *Plant Physiol.* **30**:380.

Andreev, G. K., and Amrhein, N., 1976, Mechanism of action of the herbicide 2-chloro-3(4-chlorophenyl)propionate and its methyl ester: Interaction with cell responses mediated by auxin, *Physiol. Plant* **37**:175.

Appleton, H. T., and Nakatsugawa, T., 1977, The toxicological significance of paraoxon deethylation, *Pestic. Biochem. Physiol.* **7**:451.

Arias, J. M., and Jacoby, W. B., 1976, *Glutathione Metabolism and Function*, Kroc Foundation Series, Vol. 6, Raven Press, New York.

Arjmand, M., Hamilton, R. H., and Mumma, R. O., 1978, Metabolism of 2,4,5-trichlorophenoxyacetic acid. Evidence for amino acid conjugates in soybean callus tissue, *J. Agric. Food Chem.* **26**:1125.

Bakke, J. E., Larsen, J. D., and Price, C. E., 1972*a*, Metabolism of atrazine and 2-hydroxyatrazine by the rat, *J. Agric. Food Chem.* **20**:602.

Bakke, J. E., Shimabukuro, R. H., Davison, K. L., and Lamoureux, G. L., 1972*b*, Sheep and rat metabolism of the insoluble ^{14}C-residues present in ^{14}C-atrazine treated sorghum, *Chemosphere* **1**:21.

Balba, H. M., and Still, G. G., 1977, Studies of bound residues of chloroanilines in plants, Abstract, 174th National Meeting, American Chemical Society, Chicago.

Baldwin, B. C., 1977, Xenobiotic metabolism in plants, in: *Drug Metabolism: From Microbe to Man* (D. V. Parke and R. L. Smith, eds.), pp. 191–217, Taylor and Francis, London.

Bandurski, R. S., and Schulze, A., 1977, Concentration of indole-3-acetic acid and its derivatives in plants, *Plant Physiol* **60**:211.

Bandurski, R. S., Schulze, A., and Cohen, J. D., 1977, Photoregulation of the ratio of ester to free indole-3-acetic acid, *Biochem. Biophys. Res. Commun.* **79**:1219.

Beynon, K. I., Stoydin, G., and Wright, A. N., 1972*a*, A comparison of the breakdown of the triazine herbicides cyanazine, atrazine and simazine in soils and maize, *Pestic. Biochem. Physiol.* **2**:153.

Beynon, K. I., Stoydin, G., and Wright, A. N., 1972*b*, The breakdown of the triazine herbicide cyanazine in wheat and potatoes grown under indoor conditions in treated soils, *Pestic. Sci.* **3**:379.

Beynon, K. I., Hutson, D. H., and Wright, A. N., 1973, The metabolism and degradation of vinyl phosphate insecticides, *Res. Rev.* **47**:55.

Beynon, K. I., Roberts, T. R., and Wright, A. N., 1974, The degradation of the herbicide benzoylprop ethyl following its application to wheat, *Pestic. Sci.* **5**:429.

Biswas, P. K., and Hamilton, W., Jr., 1969, Metabolism of trifluralin in peanuts and sweet potatoes, *Weed Sci.* **17**:206.

Bowes, G. W., 1972, Uptake and metabolism of 2,2-bis(*p*-chlorophenyl)-1,1,1-trichloroethane (DDT) by marine phytoplankton and its effect on growth and chloroplast electron transport, *Plant Physiol.* **49**:172.

Boyland, E., and Chasseaud, L. F., 1969, The role of glutathione and glutathione *S*-transferases in mercapturic acid biosynthesis, *Adv. Enzymol.* **32**:173.

Brain, K. R., and Lines, D. S., 1977, Uptake and metabolism of aldrin in plant tissue culture, in: *Plant Tissue Culture and Its Bio-Technical Application* (W. Barz, E. Reinhard, and M. W. Zenk, eds.), pp. 197–203, Springer-Verlag, New York.

Brooks, G. T., 1974, *Chlorinated Insecticides*, Vol. II, CRC Press, Cleveland.

Bukovac, M. T., 1976, Herbicide entry into plants, in: Herbicides: *Physiology, Biochemistry, Ecology*, Vol. 1 (L. J. Audus, ed.), pp. 335–364, Academic Press, New York.

Bull, D. L., 1972, Metabolism of organophosphorus insecticides in animals and plants, *Res. Rev.* **43**:1.

Bull, D. L., Whitten, C. J., and Ivie, G. W., 1976, Fate of O-ethyl-[4-(methylthio)phenyl]-S-propyl phosporodithioate (BAY NTN 9306) in cotton plants and soil, *J. Agric. Food Chem.* **24**:601.

Casida, J. E., and Lykken, L., 1969, Metabolism of organic pesticide chemicals in higher plants, *Annu. Rev. Plant Physiol.* **20**:607.

Casida, J. E., Kimmel, E. C., Ohkawa, H., and Ohkawa, R., 1975, Sulfoxidation of thiocarbamate herbicides and the metabolism of thiocarbamate sulfoxides in living mice and liver enzyme systems, *Pestic. Biochem. Physiol.* **5**:1.

Chen, Y. S., and Casida, J. E., 1978, Thiocarbamate herbicide metabolism: Microsomal oxygenase metabolism of EPTC involving mono- and dioxygenation at the sulfur and hydroxylation at each alkyl carbon, *J. Agric. Food Chem.* **26**:263.

Collett, G. F., and Pont, V., 1978, Le rôle de la cystéine dans la dé toxification d'un herbicide, *C.R. Acad. Sci. Ser. D* **286**:681.

Crafts, A. S., and Crisp, C. E., 1971, *Phloem Transport in Plants*, W. H. Freeman, San Francisco.

Crayford, J. V., and Hutson, D. H., 1972, The metabolism of the herbicide, 2-chloro-4-(ethylamino)-6-(1-cyano-1-methylethylamino)-s-triazine, in the rat, *Pestic. Biochem. Physiol.* **2**:295.

Crosby, D. G., 1973, The fate of pesticides in the environment, *Annu. Rev. Plant Physiol.* **24**:467.

Dauterman, W. C., Viado, G. B., Casida, J. E., and O'Brien, R. D., 1960, Persistence of dimethoate and metabolites following foliar application to plants, *J. Agric. Food Chem.* **8**:115.

Davis, D. G., Hodgson, R. H., Dusbabek, K. E., and Hoffer, B. L., 1978, The metabolism of the herbicide diphenamid (*N,N*-dimethyl-2,2-diphenylacetamide) in cell suspensions of soybean (*Glycine max*), *Physiol. Plant* **44**:87.

Donald, W. W., and Shimabukuro, R. H., 1980, Selectivity of diclofop-methyl between wheat and wild oat: Growth and herbicide metabolism, *Physiol. Plant* **49**:459.

Dorough, H. W., Whitacre, D. M., and Cardona, R. A., 1973*a*, Metabolism of the herbicide methazole in cotton and beans, and fate of certain of its polar metabolites in rats, *J. Agric. Food Chem.* **21**:7.

Dorough, H. W., 1976, Biological activity of pesticide conjugates, in: *Bound and Conjugated Pesticide Residues* (D. D. Kaufman, G. G. Still, G. D. Paulson, and S. K. Bandal, eds.), pp. 11–34, ACS Symposium Series 29, American Chemical Society, Washington, D.C.

Dutton, A. J., Roberts, T. R., and Wright, A. N., 1976, Characterization of acidic conjugates of flamprop in wheat, *Chemosphere* **3**:195.

Dutton, A. J., Roberts, T. R., and Wright, A. N., 1976, Characterization of acidic conjugates of flamprop in wheat, *Chemosphere* **3**:195.

Earl, J. W., and Kennedy, I. R., 1975, Aldrin epoxidase from pea roots, *Phytochemistry* **14**:1507.

Eastin, E. F., 1971, Fate of fluorodifen in resistant peanut seedlings, *Weed Sci.* **19**:261.

El Zorgani, G. A., 1975, Residues of DDT in cottonseed after spraying with DDT and torbidan, *Pestic. Sci.* **6**:457.

Esser, H. O., Dupuis, G., Ebert, E., Marco, G., and Vogel, C., 1975, S-triazines, in: *Herbicides: Chemistry, Degradation, and Mode of Action*, Vol. 1 (P. C. Kearney and D. D. Kaufman, eds.), pp. 129–208, Marcel Dekker, New York.

Eto, M., 1974, *Organophosphorous Pesticides: Organic and Biological Chemistry*, CRC Press, Cleveland.

Fedtke C., and Schmidt, R. R., 1977, Chlorfenprop-methyl: Its hydrolysis *in vivo* and *in vitro* and a new principle for selective herbicidal action, *Weed Res.* **17**:233.

Feung, C. S., Hamilton, R. H., and Witham, F. H., 1971, Metabolism of 2,4-dichlorophenoxyacetic acid by soybean cotyledon callus tissue cultures, *J. Agric. Food Chem.* **19**:475.

Feung, C. S., Hamilton, R. H., and Mumma, R. O., 1973, Metabolism of 2,4-dichlorophenoxyacetic acid. V. Identification of metabolites in soybean callus tissue cultures, *J. Agric. Food Chem.* **21**:637.

Feung, C. S., Mumma, R. O., and Hamilton, R. H., 1974, Metabolism of 2,4-dichlorophenoxyacetic acid. VI. Biological properties of amino acid conjugates, *J. Agric. Food Chem.* **22**:307.

Feung, C. S., Hamilton, R. H., and Mumma, R. O., 1975, Metabolism of 2,4-dichlorophenoxyacetic acid. VII. Comparison of metabolites from five species of plant callus tissue cultures, *J. Agric. Food Chem.* **23**:373.

Feung, C. S., Hamilton, R. H., and Mumma, R. O., 1976, Metabolism of indole-3-acetic acid, III. Identification of metabolites isolated from crown gall callus tissue, *Plant Physiol.* **58**:666.

Frear, D. S., 1968, Herbicide metabolism in plants. I. Purification and properties of UDP-glucose: Arylamine N-glucosyl-transferase from soybean, *Phytochemistry* **7**:381.

Frear, D. S., 1975, The benzoic acid herbicides, in: *Herbicides: Chemistry, Degradation, and Mode of Action*, Vol. 2 (P. C. Kearny and D. D. Kaufman, eds.), pp. 541–607, Marcel Dekker, New York.

Frear, D. S., 1976, Pesticide conjugates—glycosides, in: *Bound and Conjugated Pesticide Residues* (D. D. Kaufman, G. G. Still, G. D. Paulson, and S. K. Bandal, eds.), pp. 35–54, ACS Symposium Series 29, American Chemical Society, Washington, D.C.

Frear, D. S., and Shimabukuro, R. H., 1970, Metabolism and effects of herbicides in plants, Technical Papers of FAO Int. Conf. Weed Control, pp. 560, Weed Science Society America, Champaign, Illinois.

Frear, D. S., and Still, G. G., 1968, The metabolism of 3,4-dichloropropionanilide in plants: Partial purification and properties of an aryl acylamidase from rice, *Phytochemistry* **7**:913.

Frear, D. S., and Swanson, H. R., 1972, New metabolites of monuron in excised cotton leaves, *Phytochemistry* **11**:1919.

Frear, D. S., and Swanson, H. R., 1973, Metabolism of substituted diphenylether herbicides in plants. I. Enzymatic cleavage of fluorodifen in peas (*Pisum sativum* L.), *Pestic. Biochem. Physiol.* **3**:473.

Frear, D. S., and Swanson, H. R., 1974, Monuron metabolism in excised *Gossypium hirsutum* leaves: Aryl hydroxylation and conjugation of 4-chlorophenylurea, *Phytochemistry* **13**:357.

Frear, D. S., and Swanson, H. R., 1975, Metabolism of cisanilide (*cis*-2,5-dimethyl-1-pyrrolidinecarboxanilide) by excised leaves and cell suspension cultures of carrot and cotton, *Pestic. Biochem. Physiol.* **5**:73.

Frear, D. S., Swanson, H. R., and Tanaka, F. S., 1969, N-demethylation of substituted 3-(phenyl)-1-methylureas: Isolation and characterization of a microsomal mixed function oxidase from cotton, *Phytochemistry* **8**:2157.

Frear, D. S., Hodgson, R. H., Shimabukuro, R. H., and Still, G. G., 1972*a*, Behavior of herbicides in plants, *Adv. Agron.* **24**:328.

Frear, D. S., Swanson, H. R., and Tanaka, F. S., 1972*b*, Herbicide metabolism in plants, in: *Recent Advances in Phytochemistry*, Vol. 5 (V. C. Runeckles and T. S. Tso, eds.), pp. 225–246, Academic Press, New York.

Frear, D. S., Swanson, H. R., Mansager, E. R., and Wien, R. G., 1978, Chloramben metabolism in plants: Isolation and identification of glucose ester, *J. Agric. Food Chem.* **26**:1347.

Gaughan, L. C., and Casida, J. E., 1978, Degradation of *trans*- and *cis*-permethrin on cotton and bean plants, *J. Agric. Food Chem.* **26**:525.

Gorbach, S. G., Kuenzler, K., and Asshauer, J., 1977, On the metabolism of HOE-23408 OH in wheat, *J. Agric. Food Chem.* **25**:507.

Guroff, G., Daly, J. W., Jerina, D. M., Renson, J., Witkop, B., and Undenfriend, S., 1967, Hydroxylation-induced migration: The NIH shift, *Science* **157**:1524.

Hamilton, R. H., Hurter, J., Hall, J. K., and Ercegovich, C. D., 1971, Metabolism of 2,4-dichlorophenoxyacetic acid and 2,4,5-trichlorophenoxyacetic acid by bean plants, *J. Agric. Food Chem.* **19**:480.

Harrison, R. B., Holmes, D. C., Roburn, J., and Tatton, J. O'G., 1967, The fate of some orga-nochlorine pesticides on leaves, *J. Sci. Food Agric.* **18**:10.

Harvey, John, Jr., C.-Y. Han, J., and Reiser, R. W., 1978, Metabolism of oxamyl in plants, *J. Agric. Food Chem.* **26**:529.

Hay, J. R., 1976, Herbicide transport in plants, in: *Herbicides: Physiology, Biochemistry, Ecology*, Vol. 1 (L. J. Audus, ed.), pp. 365–396, Academic Press, New York.

Hill, B. D., Stobbe, E. H., and Jones, B. L., 1978, Hydrolysis of the herbicide benzoylprop ethyl by wild oat esterases, *Weed Res.* **18**:149.

Hodgson, R. H., and Hoffer, B. L., 1977, Diphenamid metabolism in pepper and an ozone effect. II. Herbicide metabolite characterization, *Weed Sci.* **25**:331.

Hodgson, R. H., Frear, D. S., Swanson, H. R., and Regan, L. A., 1973, Alteration of diphenamid metabolism in tomato by ozone, *Weed Sci.* **21**:542.

Hoffer, B. L., and Hodgson, R. H., 1978, Evidence for formation of a glucosyl-malonyl ester of diphenamid in soybeans, Weed Science Society of America, Abstr. 154, Dallas.

Hubbell, J. P., and Casida, J. E., 1977, Metabolic fate of the *N,N*-dialkylcarbamoyl moiety of thiocarbamate herbicides in rats and corn, *J. Agric. Food Chem.* **25**:404.

Hussain, M., Fukuto, T. R., and Reynolds, H. T., 1974, Physical and chemical basis for systemic movement of organophosphorus esters in the cotton plant, *J. Agric. Food Chem.* **22**:225.

Hutson, D. H., 1976, Glutathione conjugates, *in: Bound and Conjugated Pesticide Residues* (D. D. Kaufman, G. G. Still, G. D. Paulson, and S. K. Bandal, eds.), pp. 103–131, ACS Symposium Series 29, American Chemical Society, Washington, D.C.

Jacoby, W. B., 1978, The glutathione *S*-transferases: A group of multifunctional detoxification proteins, *Adv. Enzymol.* **46**:383.

Jeffcoat, B., and Harries, W. N., 1973, Selectivity and mode of action of ethyl (±)-2-(*N*-3-benzoyl-3,4-dichloroanilino)propionate in the control of *Avena fatua* in cereals, *Pestic. Sci.* **4**:891.

Jeffcoat, B., and Harries, W. N., 1975, Selectivity and mode of action of flamprop-isopropyl, isopropyl (±)-2-[*N*-(3-chloro-4-flurophenyl)benzamido] propionate, in the control of *Avena fatua* in barley, *Pestic. Sci.* **6**:282.

Jerina, D. M., and Daly, J. W., 1974, Arene oxides: A new aspect of drug metabolism, *Science* **185**:573.

Kaufman, D. D., Still, G. G., Paulson, G. D., and Bandal, S. K. (eds.), 1976, *Bound and Conjugated Pesticide Residues*, ACS Symposium Series 29, American Chemical Society, Washington, D.C.

Kearney, P. C., and Kaufman, D. D. (eds.), 1975, *Herbicides: Chemistry, Degradation, and Mode of Action*, Vols. 1 and 2, Marcel Dekker, New York.

Krueger, H. R., 1975, Phorate sulfoxidation by plant root extracts, *Pestic. Biochem. Physiol.* **5**:396.

Krueger, H. R., 1977, Aldicarb sulfoxidation by plant root extracts, *Pestic. Biochem. Physiol.* **7**:154.

Kuhr, R. J., and Casida, J. E., 1967, Persistent glycosides of metabolites of methylcarbamate insecticide chemicals formed by hydroxylation in bean plants, *J. Agric. Food Chem.* **15**:814.

Lamoureux, G. L., and Davison, K. L., 1975, Mercapturic acid formation in the metabolism of propachlor, CDAA, and fluorodifen in the rat, *Pestic. Biochem. Physiol.* **5**:497.

Lamoureux, G. L., and Frear, D. S., 1979, Pesticide metabolism in higher plants: *In vitro* enzyme studies, in: *Xenobiotic metabolism, in vitro methods* (G. D. Paulson, D. S. Frear, And E. P. Marks, eds.), pp. 77–128, ACS Symposium Series 97, American Chemical Society, Washington, D.C.

Lamoureux, G. L., and Rusness, D. G., 1976, Pentachloronitrobenzene (PCNB) metabolism in peanuts, 172nd National Meeting, American Chemical Society, San Francisco.

Lamoureux, G. L., and Stafford, L. E., 1977, Translocation and metabolism of perfluidone (1,1,1-trifluoro-*N*-[2-methyl-4-(phenylsulfonyl)phenyl]methanesulfonamide) in peanuts, *J. Agric. Food Chem.* **25**:512.

Lamoureux, G. L., Shimabukuro, R. H., Swanson, H. R., and Frear, D. S., 1970, Metabolism of 2-chloro-4-ethylamino-6-isopropylamino-*s*-triazine (atrazine) in excised sorghum leaf sections, *J. Agric. Food Chem.* **18**:81.

Lamoureux, G. L., Stafford, L. E., and Tanaka, F. S., 1971, Metabolism of 2-chloro-*N*-isopropylacetanilide (propachlor) in the leaves of corn, sorghum, sugarcane and barley, *J. Agric. Food Chem.* **19**:346.

Lamoureux, G. L., Stafford, L. E., and Shimabukuro, R. H., 1972, Conjugation of 2-chloro-4,6-bis(alkylamino)-*s*-triazines in higher plants, *J. Agric. Food Chem.* **20**:1004.

Lamoureux, G. L., Stafford, L. E., Shimabukuro, R. H., and Zaylskie, R. G., 1973, Atrazine metabolism in sorghum: Catabolism of the glutathione conjugate of atrazine, *J. Agric. Food Chem.* **21**:1020.

Larsen, G. L., and Bakke, J. E., 1975, Metabolism of 2-chloro-4-cyclopropylamino-6-isopropylamino-*s*-triazine (cyprazine) in the rat, *J. Agric. Food Chem.* **23**:388.

Lay, M. M., and Casida, J. E., 1976, Dichloroacetamide antidotes enhance thiocarbamate sulfoxide detoxication by elevating corn root glutathione content and glutathione *S*-transferase activity, *Pestic. Biochem. Physiol.* **6**:442.

Lay, M. M., and Casida, J. E., 1978, Involvement of glutathione and glutathione *S*-transferases in the action of dichloroacetamide antidotes for thiocarbamate herbicides, in: *Chemistry and Action of Herbicide Antidotes* (F. M. Pallos and J. E. Casida, eds.), pp. 151–160, Academic Press, New York.

Loos, M. S., 1975, Phenoxyalkanoic acids, in: *Herbicides: Chemistry, Degradation, and Mode of Action*, Vol. 1 (P. C. Kearney and D. D. Kaufman, eds.), pp. 1–128, Marcel Dekker, New York.

Makeev, A. M., Makoviechuk, A. I. U., and Chkanikov, D. C., 1977, Microsomal hydroxylation of 2,4-dichlorophenoxyacetic acid herbicide in plants, cucumbers and peas, *Dokl. Akad. Nauk. SSSR* **233**:1222.

Markham, A., Hartman, G. C., and Parke, D. V., 1972, Spectral evidence for the presence of cytochrome P-450 in microsomal fractions obtained from some higher plants, *Biochem. J.* **130**:90.

Marquis, L. Y., Shimabukuro, R. H., Stolzenberg, G. E., Feil, V. J., and Zaylskie, R. G., 1979, Metabolism and selectivity of fluchloralin in soybean roots, *J. Agric. Food Chem.* **27**:1148.

Marshall, T. C., and Dorough, H. W., 1977, Bioavailability in rats of bound and conjugated plant carbamate insecticide residues, *J. Agric. Food Chem.* **25**:1003.

Matsumura, F., and Boush, G. M., 1967, Dieldrin: Degradation by soil microorganisms, *Science* **156**:959.

Matsumura, F., Boush, G. M., and Tai, A., 1968, Breakdown of dieldrin in the soil by a microorganism, *Nature (London)* **219**:965.

Matsunaka, S., 1968, Propanil hydrolysis: Inhibition in rice plants by insecticides, *Science* **160**:1360.

McBain, J. B., Hoffman, L. J., and Menn, J. J., 1970, Metabolic degradation of O-ethyl S-phenyl ethylphosphonodithionate (dyfonate) in potato plants, *J. Agric. Food Chem.* **18**:1139.

McKinney, J. D., and Mehendale, H. M., 1973, Formation of polar metabolites from aldrin by pea and bean root preparations, *J. Agric. Food Chem.* **21**:1079.

Menzer, R. E., 1973, Biological oxidation and conjugation of pesticide chemicals, *Res. Rev.* **48**:79.

Menzer, R. E., and Casida, J. E., 1965, Nature of toxic metabolites formed in mammals, insects, and plants from S-(dimethoxyphosphinyloxy)-*N*,*N*-dimethyl-*cis*-crotonamide and its *N*-methyl analog, *J. Agric. Food Chem.* **13**:102.

Montgomery, M. L., Chang, Y. L., and Freed, V. H., 1971, Metabolism of 2,4-D by bean and corn plants, *J. Agric. Food Chem.* **19**:1219.

Müller, P. W., and Payot, P. H., 1966, Studies on the fate of C^{14}-labeled triazine herbicides in plants, in: *Isotopes in Weed Research*, pp. 61–70, International Atomic Energy Agency, Vienna.

Mumma, R. O., and Hamilton, R. H., 1976, Amino acid conjugates, in: *Bound and Conjugated Pesticide Residues* (D. D. Kaufman, G. G. Still, G. D. Paulson, and S. K. Bandal, eds.), pp. 68–85, ACS Symposium Series 29, American Chemical Society, Washington, D.C.

Mumma, R. O., Khalifa, S., and Hamilton, R. H., 1971, Spectroscopic identification of metabolites of carbaryl in plants, *J. Agric. Food Chem.* 19:445.

Narayan, S. T., and Lichtenstein, E. P., 1973, Influence of mineral nutrients on the penetration, translocation, and metabolism of [^{14}C]dyfonate in pea plants, *J. Agric. Food Chem.* 21:851.

Nash, R. G., Beall, M. L. Jr., and Harris, W. G., 1977, Toxaphene and 1,1,1-trichloro-2,2-bis(*p*-chlorophenyl)ethane (DDT) losses from cotton in agroecosystem chamber, *J. Agric. Food Chem.* 25:336.

O'Brien, R. D., 1967, *Insecticides: Action and Metabolism,* Academic Press, New York.

Oloff, P. C., and Lichtenstein, E. P., 1969 Epoxidation of aldrin by excised pieces of plant tissue, *J. Agric. Food Chem.* 17:143.

Paulson, G. D., Jacobsen, A. M., and Still, G. G., 1975, Animal metabolism of propham (isopropyl carbanilate): The fate of residues in alfalfa when consumed by the rat and sheep, *Pestic. Biochem. Physiol.* 5:523.

Pree, D. J., and Saunders, J. L., 1974, Metabolism of carbofuran in mugho pine, *J. Agric. Food Chem.* 22:620.

Probst, G. W., Golab, T., Wright, W. L., 1975, Dinitroanilines, in: *Herbicides: Chemistry, Degradation, and Mode of Action,* Vol. 1 (P. C. Kearney and D. D. Kaufman, eds.), pp. 453–500, Marcel Dekker, New York.

Rowlands, D. G., 1965, The *in vitro* and *in vivo* oxidation and hydrolysis of malathion by wheat grain esterases, *J. Sci. Food Agric.* 16:325.

Rowlands, D. G., 1966, The *in vitro* and *in vivo* metabolism of dimethoate by stored wheat and sorghum grains, *J. Sci. Food Agric.* 17:90.

Rusness, D. G., and Still, G. G., 1977, Partial purification and properties of *S*-cysteinyl-hydroxychlorpropham transferase from oat (*Avena sativa*, L.), *Pestic. Biochem. Physiol.* 7:220.

Russell, D. W., 1971, The metabolism of aromatic compounds in higher plants. X. Properties of the cinnamic acid 4-hydroxylase of pea seedlings and some aspects of its metabolic and developmental control, *J. Biol. Chem.* 246:3870.

Russell, D. W., and Conn, E. E., 1967, The cinnamic acid 4-hydroxylase of pea seedlings, *Arch. Biochem. Biophys.* 122:256.

Ruzo, L. O., and Casida, J. E., 1977, Metabolism and toxicology of pyrethroids with dihalovinyl substituents, *Environ. Health Perspec.* 21:285.

Sanderman, H., Jr., Diesperger, H., and Scheel, D., 1977, Metabolism of xenobiotics by plant cell cultures, in: *Plant Tissue Culture and Its Biotechnological Application* (W. Barz, E. Reinhard, and M. H. Zenk, eds.), pp. 178–196, Springer-Verlag, New York.

Shimabukuro, R. H., 1967, Atrazine metabolism and herbicidal selectivity, *Plant Physiol.* 42:1269.

Shimabukuro, R. H., and Walsh, W. C., 1979, Xenobiotic metabolism in plants: *In vitro* tissue, organ and isolated cell techniques, in: *Xenobiotic metabolism: In vitro methods* (G. D. Paulson, D. S. Frear, and E. P. Marks, eds.), pp. 3–34, ACS Symposium Series 97, American Chemical Society, Washington, D.C.

Shimabukuro, R. H., Lamoureux, G. L., Swanson, H. R., Walsh, W. C., Stafford, L. E., and Frear, D. S., 1973a, Metabolism of substituted diphenylether herbicides in plants. II. Identification of a new fluorodifen metabolite, *S*-(2-nitro-4-trifluoromethylphenyl)-glutathione in peanuts, *Pestic. Biochem. Physiol.* 3:483.

Shimabukuro, R. H., Walsh, W. C., Lamoureux, G. L., and Stafford, L. E., 1973b, Atrazine metabolism in sorghum: Chloroform-soluble intermediates in the *N*-dealkylation and glutathione conjugation pathways, *J. Agric. Food Chem.* 21:1031.

Shimabukuro, R. H., Walsh, W. C., Stolzenberg, G. E., and Olson, P. A., 1975, Metabolism of fluorodifen in peanuts, Weed Science Society of America, Abst. 171, Washington, D.C.

Shimabukuro, R. H., Walsh, W. C., and Hoerauf, R. A., 1976a, The role of coleoptile on barban selectivity between wild oat and wheat, *Pestic. Biochem. Physiol.* 6:115.

Shimabukuro, R. H., Walsh, W. C., Stolzenberg, G. E., and Olson, P. A., 1976b, Metabolism of fluorodifen to S-(2-nitro-4-trifluoromethylphenyl-N-malonylcysteine in peanuts, Weed Science Society of America, Abstr. 196, Denver.

Shimabukuro, R. H., Lamoureux, G. L., and Frear, D. S., 1978a, Glutathione conjugation: A mechanism for herbicide detoxication and selectivity in plants, in: *Chemistry and Action of Herbicide Antidotes* (F. M. Pallos and J. E. Casida, eds.), pp. 133–149, Academic Press, New York.

Shimabukuro, M. A., Shimabukuro, R. H., Nord, W. S., and Hoerauf, R. A., 1978b, Physiological effects of methyl 2-(4-[2,4-dichlorophenoxy]phenoxy)propanoate on oat, wild oat and wheat, *Pestic. Biochem. Physiol.* 8:199.

Shimabukuro, R. H., Walsh, W. C., and Hoerauf, R. A., 1979, Metabolism and selectivity of diclofop-methyl in wild oat and wheat, *J. Agric. Food Chem.* 27:615.

Still, G. G., 1968, Metabolism of 3,4-dichloropropionanilide in plants: The metabolic fate of the 3,4-dichloroaniline moiety, *Science* 159:992.

Still, G. G., and Kuzerian, O., 1967, Enzyme detoxication of 3',4'-dichloropropionanilide in rice and barnyard grass, a factor in herbicide selectivity, *Nature* (London) 216:799.

Still, G. G., and Mansager, E. R., 1972, Aryl hydroxylation of isopropyl-3-chlorocarbanilate by soybean plants, *Phytochemistry* 11:515.

Still, G. G., and Mansager, E. R., 1973, Soybean shoot metabolism of isopropyl-3-chlorocarbanilate: Ortho and para aryl hydroxylation, *Pestic. Biochem. Physiol.* 3:87.

Still, G. G., and Rusness, D. G., 1977, S-cysteinyl-hydroxychlorpropham: Formation of the S-cysteinyl conjugate of isopropyl-3'-chloro-4'-hydroxycarbanilate in oat (*Avena sativa* L.), *Pestic. Biochem. Physiol.* 7:210.

Still, G. G., Rusness, D. G., and Mansager, E. R., 1974, Carbanilate herbicides and their metabolic products: Their effect on plant metabolism, in: *Mechanism of Pesticide Action* (G. K. Kohn, ed.), pp. 117–129, ACS Symposium Series 2, American Chemical Society, Washington, D.C.

Strang, R. H., and Rogers, R. L., 1974, Behavior and fate of two phenylpyridazinone herbicides in cotton, corn and soybean, *J. Agric. Food Chem.* 22:1119.

Sumner, D. D., Cassidy, J. E., and Marco, G. J., 1976, Metabolism of profluralin in soybeans, Weed Science Society of America, Abst. 33, Denver.

Swanson, C. R., and Swanson, H. R., 1968, Inhibition of degradation of monuron in cotton leaf tissue by carbamate insecticides, *Weed Sci.* 16:481.

Thiman, K. V., 1977, *Hormone Action in the Whole Life of Plants*, University of Massachusetts Press, Amherst, Mass.

Thomas E. W., Loughman, B. C., and Powell, R. G., 1964, Metabolic fate of some chlorinated phenoxyacetic acids in the stem tissue of *Avena sativa*, *Nature* (London) 204:286.

Thompson, R. P., 1974, A comparative study on the fate of cyanazine and atrazine in plants, Ph.D. Thesis, University of Illinois, Xerox University Microfilms, Ann Arbor, Michigan.

United States Department of Agriculture, 1977, Agricultural Stabilization and Conservation Service, *Pestic. Rev.*, July 1976.

Upshall, D. G., and Goodwin, T. W., 1964, Biochemical investigations into the susceptibility of barley varieties of DDT, *J. Sci. Food Agric.* 15:846.

Wain, R. L., and Smith, M. S., 1976, Selectivity in relation to metabolism, in: *Herbicides: Physiology, Biochemistry, Ecology* (L. J. Audus, ed.), pp. 279–302, Academic Press, New York.

Williams, R. T., 1959, *Detoxication Mechanisms: The Metabolism and Detoxication of Drugs, Toxic Substances and Other Organic Compounds*, Chapman and Hall, London.

Woolhouse, H. W., 1974, Longevity and senescence in plants, *Sci. Progr.* **61**:123.

Wright, T. H., Rieck, C. E., and Harger, T. R., 1975, Metabolism of profluralin in peanuts and soybeans, *Weed Sci. Soc. Am. Abstr.* No. 169.

Yih, R. Y., McRae, D. H., and Wilson, H. F., 1968, Metabolism of 3',4'-dichloropropionanilide: 3,4-dichloroaniline-lignin complex in rice plants, *Science* **161**:376.

Yu, S. J., Kiigemagi, U., and Terriere, L. C., 1971, Oxidative metabolism of aldrin and isodrin by bean root fractions, *J. Agric. Food Chem.* **19**:5.

Zenk, M. H., 1961, 1-*O*-(Indole-3-acetyl)-beta-*D*-glucose, a new compound in the metabolism of indole-3-acetic acid in plants, *Nature (London)* **191**:493.

Zimmerman, M. H., and Milburn, J. A. (eds.), 1975, Transport in plants. I. Phloem transport, in: *Encyclopedia of Plant Physiology* (N.S.), Vol. 1, Springer-Verlag, Heidelberg.

3

Degradation of Pesticides in the Environment by Microorganisms and Sunlight

Fumio Matsumura

3.1. INTRODUCTION

It may be generalized that pesticide contamination problems in the environment are directly related to their persistent nature, the most important factor determining the degree of persistence being the chemical characteristics of the pesticidal compound itself.

It is generally agreed that the two most important degradation forces operating on chemicals in the environment are microorganisms and sunlight. A few reasons are offered to justify the above conclusion: first, most pesticides are known to end up in soil whether they are aimed at crops or not; second, they are spread in the environment at relatively low concentrations; third, soil and aquatic sediments are generally loaded with microorganisms; and fourth, many of the pesticides have some degree of volatility to escape into the atmosphere depending on whether they are exposed to, for example, sunlight.

Many excellent books and reviews are available to cover various aspects of the subject. Examples are those by Hill and Wright (1978), Khan (1977), Matsumura *et al.* (1972), and Zabik *et al.* (1976). The purpose of this chapter,

Fumio Matsumura • Pesticide Research Center, Michigan State University, East Lansing, Michigan 48824.

therefore, is not to give an encyclopedic coverage of the subject areas, but rather to give the basic concept of the general mechanisms of pesticidal degradation in the environment. Examples are usually cited to clarify the point of interest. Also, the contributions of plants and animals in the overall metabolic changes of pesticide residues in the environment are not considered, since they are covered by other contributors. However, some nonenzymatic reactions which often contribute to the overall degradation of pesticides in the environment are described.

3.2.   CHARACTERISTICS OF MICROBIAL METABOLISM

It was originally assumed by many pesticide scientists that the patterns of microbial metabolism were in general very similar to the ones already found in animals, particularly the mammalian species, since studies on microbial metabolism of pesticides were lagging far behind the comparable studies in mammalian species. However, as knowledge on microbial degradation has advanced, it has become apparent that in many cases the patterns of degradation in these two different groups of organisms are often very different.

First of all, the purpose of all metabolic reactions on xenobiotics in higher animals is to eventually convert them into polar and therefore excretable forms. Second, in higher animals the processes of primary metabolism of xenobiotics are centralized in a few specialized organs. In the case of the liver, its metabolic pattern is largely determined by the activity of an oxidative detoxification system, generally termed *mixed-function oxidase*.

On the contrary, the predominant metabolic activities in the microbial world are meant for production of energy. In this respect, it is not even possible to define xenobiotics here, since most organic materials can serve as the source of energy to at least some microorganisms. Here only a few groups of chemicals may be regarded as foreign to microorganisms. Among insecticidal compounds, the halogen-containing chemicals, particularly halogenated aromatics, must be regarded as foreign (or unusable) material to microorganisms.

Another characteristic or microbial metabolism is the adaptability of microorganisms to changing environments through mutation and induction, particularly toward chemicals that are initially toxic to them. The case of penicillin resistance in bacteria through induction of penicillinase is well known.

The metabolic activities of microorganisms encompass many different types of biological processes not found in any other organisms. They include fermentation, some types of anaerobic metabolism, chemolithotrophic metabolism, and metabolism through exoenzymes.

In general, microbial contributions to metabolic alteration of insecticides may be classified in several categories as shown in Table 3.1.

Table 3.1. General Classification of Microbial Metabolism of Pesticides[a]

I. *Enzymatic*
  A. Incidental metabolism: Pesticides themselves cannot serve as energy sources
    1. Metabolism by generally available enzymes
      a. Metabolism due to generally-present broad-spectrum enzymes (hydrolases, oxidases, etc.)
      b. Metabolism due to specific enzymes present in many microbe species
    2. Analog-induced metabolism (cometabolism)
      c. Metabolism by enzymes utilizing substrates structurally similar to pesticides
  B. Catabolism: Pesticides serve as energy sources
      d. Pesticides or a part of the molecule are the readily available source of energy for microbes
      e. Pesticides are not readily utilized. Some specific enzymes must be induced.
  C. Detoxification metabolism
      f. Metabolism by resistant microbes
II. *Nonenzymatic*
  A. Participation in photochemical reactions
  B. Contribution through pH changes
  C. Through production of organic and inorganic reactants
  D. Through production of cofactors

[a] Modified from Benezet and Matsumura (1973).

3.2.1. Enzymatic Degradation

It must be stressed that the main purpose of the following classification effort is to present clearly the types of microbial degradation according to their final manifestations. They are not classified according to the intrinsic mechanisms by which they degrade pesticides. Various reactions which involve different enzymatic mechanisms and yet are known to behave in similar patterns have been grouped together.

3.2.1.1. Incidental Metabolism

The key characteristic of *incidental metabolism* is that the pesticides themselves, including any part of the pesticide molecules, do not serve as the energy and carbon source for the microorganisms. Therefore, addition of pesticides does not affect their growth, which is always controlled by other nutrients. Two completely different subgroups of metabolic activities are present in this type. In the first subgroup, pesticides are degraded by enzymes which are not specifically related to pesticidal molecules (reactions a and b). In these cases pesticides are degraded by either broad-spectrum enzymes such as hydrolases, reductases, and oxidases or by specific enzymes commonly present in high percentages of microorganisms. In either case the pesticidal substrates are metabolized as a result of general microbial activities. In the environment, therefore, those types of reactions are observed in which microbial activities are stimulated by the availability of nutrients and moisture, and by the right temperature and pH.

3.2.1.2. Analog-Induced Metabolism

The term *cometabolism* has been used in the past to include all a, b, and c types of metabolism. However, in this chapter I have decided to apply the term in a more restricted manner to include only the cases where the microorganisms are induced by chemicals which structurally resemble the pesticide molecules. Thus, to avoid confusion, I shall use the term *analog-induced metabolism* here. In such a case the microorganisms can grow on the given chemical (analog) but not on the pesticide, despite their capability to at least partially metabolize the latter. Good examples are those produced by Focht and Alexander (1970*a–c*), who obtained DDT-degrading *Hydrogenomonas* sp. (*Pseudomonas* sp.) by using diphenylmethane as a carbon source, and those produced by Ahmed and Focht (1972) and Furukawa and Matsumura (1975), who selected PCB-metabolizing microorganisms by using biphenyl as a carbon source. The important feature distinguishing this type from other incidental metabolisms is that these microorganisms are purposely selected by nonpesticidal analogs. The enzyme systems induced do not initially recognize the difference in the substrate molecules and therefore partially degrade the pesticide molecules. However, in such cases the microorganisms are incapable of completing the metabolism necessary to receive energy for growth.

3.2.1.3. Catabolism

In *catabolism* microorganisms are capable of deriving energy from the pesticide molecules and therefore can grow on them. I include here cases in which only a part of the pesticide molecule is utilized for growth from a practical standpoint. Thus a complete mineralization of the pesticide is not the absolute requirement so long as growth is observed by using the pesticide as a sole carbon source.

3.2.2. Criteria for Distinguishing One Type of Metabolism from Another

It is also important to realize that in the case of types a and b metabolism microorganisms depend for their survival upon other more accessible carbon sources such as glucose, which should increase their general metabolic activities. Thus one could control the rate of microbial metabolism by changing the amounts of either pesticide or other carbon sources added, depending upon the types of microbial degradation activities (Table 3.2).

It may be also generalized that incidental metabolism is the more prevalent form of microbial metabolism, when the amount of pesticides is low in comparison with other carbon sources. Catabolic metabolism could occur when the amount of pesticide is high, coupled with the favorable chemical structure of the insecticide that allows it to be microbially degradable and utilizable as a carbon source.

Another way to distinguish these classes of metabolic activities is to induce insecticide-metabolizing microbes by the use of insecticides themselves (in the presence and absence of other carbon sources). Strictly speaking, in the absence of other carbon sources only the microbes performing types d and e metabolism should be inducible and able to flourish by using the insecticide as a sole carbon source. In the presence of other carbon sources, administration of high doses of pesticides can cause two different types of responses. If the pesticide is toxic to the organisms, it may stimulate the growth of resistant strains which can either metabolically or otherwise detoxify it or withstand the toxic-action type f metabolism, (Table 3.1). If the pesticide is not toxic to the microbes, types a and b metabolism will continue, depending upon the availability of other carbon sources.

This classification is not made on the basis of microbial species or individual pesticides. On the contrary, the nature of metabolism can be influenced largely by environmental factors, which in turn affect the physiological conditions of the microbes. It is therefore possible that the same microorganisms might metabolize a pesticide differently according to environmental conditions.

Certain degradation activities on pesticides may be stimulated by the ad-

Table 3.2. Various Characteristics and Responses to Specific Treatments of the Metabolic Types

Metabolic types	Did pesticides induce growth?	Does metabolic activity increase or decrease by the addition of glucose?	Is induction time needed?	Is mixed culture metabolic activity proportional to number of cells?	Pesticide concentration for optimum metabolism
a	No	Increase	No	Yes	Low
b	No	Variable[a]	No	Yes	Low
c	No	Decrease	Yes	No	Low
d	Yes	Decrease	No	No	High
e	Yes	Decrease	Yes	No	High
f	No	Variable	Yes	No	Independent

[a] Usually require specific carbon source which will produce the substrate for the specific enzyme.

dition of extra nutrient to increase microbial growth, and yet other circumstances exist where the addition of the same nutrient can shut off the degradation activities. Generally speaking, the more specific the metabolic route and the more difficult in developing the metabolizing microbes, the less likely it is that the addition of nutrients would help degradation activities.

The cases of resistance development would be more prevalent with fungicides: the phenomena could well lead to the failure of crop protection or any other intended result.

Nonenzymatic Processes. The processes by which microbial activities contribute to the overall alteration of insecticidal molecules by nonenzymatic mechanisms are less well studied than those involving enzymatic reactions. It is known that some pesticidal chemicals can be photochemically altered in the environment, and microbial products can promote photochemical reactions in two ways. First, microbial products can act as photosensitizers by absorbing the energy from light and transmitting it to the insecticidal molecule. We have been able to show, for instance, that an aqueous extract from heat-sterilized blue-green algal cultures promoted photochemical degradation of DDT (Esaac and Matsumura, 1979). Another way that microbial products can facilitate such photochemical reactions is to serve as donors or acceptors of electrons and/or reacting groups of chemicals, for example, hydrogen and OH^-, which are often needed for photochemical reactions.

Recently Esaac and Matsumura (1980) demonstrated that ferridoxin and flavoproteins isolated from algae are powerful photosensitizers. These are known to play important roles in electron transfer systems in algae. Since they are quite stable molecules, it would not be suprising if they persist long enough in the environment after the death and lysing of algae cells to become a factor in pesticide degradation.

The effect of pH is often neglected in the field of pesticide metabolism despite numerous reports on the pH-dependent reactions of relatively labile molecules, both in soil and *in vitro.* Large pH changes are often associated with microbial activities together with changes in nutritional sources, particularly in aqueous media. Initially degradation of proteins causes alkaline pHs, and with carbohydrate metabolism the pH becomes acid. While the actual occurrence of microbial pH effects in nature might be difficult to document, it is certainly easy to demonstrate the phenomenon *in vitro,* where during the decay period the pH of spent culture media often becomes very low. Incubation of labile insecticides such as tetraethyl pyrophosphate (TEPP) with such spent medium under sterile conditions would certainly cause breakdown of the insecticides.

Little attention has been paid so far to the importance of the microbial formation of organic products capable of reacting with pesticides. Such reactants of microbial origin can be postulated to include amino acids, peptides, alkylating agents such as acetylCoA, methylcobalamine, S-adenosylmethionine, and organic acids. Conceivably, organic amines and nucleic acids could also react with some pesticidal chemicals, but no such incidence has been reported. Some pesticidal chemicals are known to react with amino acids, particularly with an -SH moiety.

Much less is known about the contribution of inorganic reactants to the alteration of insecticides or derivatives. Certainly various metallic and some nonmetallic ions and gasses, such as H_2S, O_2, and H_2, are known to react with organic chemicals, though some of the reactions require rather extreme conditions of, for example, light, heat, and pressure. Walker and Stojanovic (1973) reported that most of the microbial metabolic products of malathion in an *Arthrobacter* sp. were in the form of potassium salts. Hydrogen sulfide is known to react with mercuric and other metallic ions which are also used as insecticides.

Finally, microbial production of cofactors used in both enzymatic and nonenzymatic reactions should not be overlooked. *Cofactors* are here defined as the organic molecules which promote the overall reactions involving an organic chemical without becoming a part of the reaction product derived from that chemical. For example, Miskus *et al.* (1965) found that dechlorination of DDT to form TDE (DDD) proceeded nonenzymatically in the presence of reduced porphyrins added to lake water. The presence of such porphyrin residues in natural lake water could certainly be traced to microbial activities, particularly to those of photosynthetic microorganisms. Other possible candidates are glutathione, NAD^+, $NADP^+$, NADH, NADPH, and cytochromes.

It must be pointed out that many reductive reactions proceed nonezymatically under anaerobic conditions (Esaac and Matsumura, 1980). The details of such reactions will be covered in the section dealing with reductive reactions in this chapter.

3.3. COMMONLY OCCURRING METABOLIC PROCESSES IN MICROORGANISMS

3.3.1. Hydrolytic Processes

As mentioned earlier, one of the moieties most commonly present in pesticides is the ester linkage. This includes all of the organophosphate and carbamate insecticides as well as pyrethroids. Hydrolysis of ester, halide, ether, and amide bonds usually gives rise to nontoxic products.

There is a considerable body of evidence that hydrolytic activities are much more prevalent in the microbial world than in any other biological group. For instance, the normal environmental and microbial metabolic product of carbaryl

(1-naphthyl methylcarbamate) is 1-naphthol (Matsumura, 1974) in contrast to the mammalian metabolism of this insecticide.

In the case of organophosphates, which are largely degraded via hydrolytic processes, this general trend is clearly observable. The major microbial degradation product of diazinon [*O,O*-diethyl *O*-(2-isopropyl-6-methyl-4-pyrimidinyl)phosphorothioate] is 2-isopropyl-6-methyl-4-hydroxypyrimidine, a product of hydrolysis at the P–O bond, and not the hydroxylation products or the glutathione *S*-aryltransferase products that are prevalent in animal species. Indeed, there have been almost no records of microbial activities to form P=O analogues from P=S compounds, reactions extremely common throughout the animal and plant kingdoms. Thus, in animals diazinon is expected to become diazoxon, which is actually the toxic principle of the insecticide, owing to its high cholinesterase inhibitory property. The lack of reports of this effect in the microbial world is indeed striking in view of the existence of a wide variety of biological systems that carry out such a reaction.

Perhaps the reason for such hydrolytic reactions being common in the microbial world is that many of the organisms excrete hydrolytic enzymes outside the cells *(exoenzymes)*, particularly the fungi. Nearly all the exoenzymes liberated by microorganisms seem to be related to the metabolism of large molecules, so that such compounds may be reduced to smaller fragments to permit their passage through the cell membrane. Various soils also contain exoenzymes that are hydrolytic in nature. Thus by definition most of the hydrolytic reactions belong to type a metabolism (Figure 3.1), where incidental metabolism takes place by the action of broad-spectrum enzymes.

Other types of pesticides having hydrolyzable bonds are subject to metabolic attack via esterases. These include phenoxyalkanoates and chlorinated pesticides, particularly aliphatics, phenylamides, phenylureas, triazines, and thiophenates.

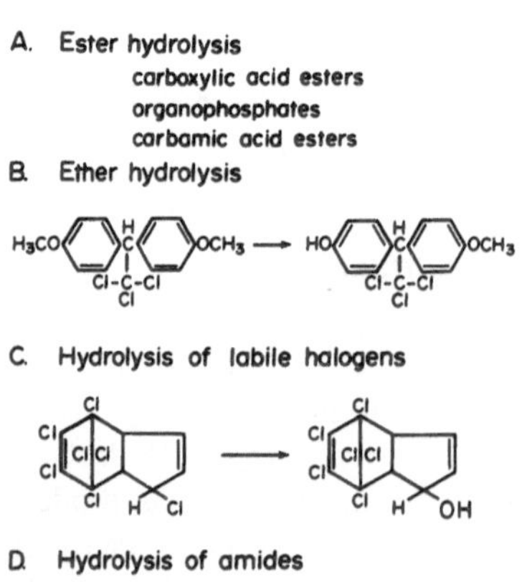

Figure 3.1.   Examples of the most commonly observed hydrolytic processes of insecticides.

$$(EtO)_2 \ P(S)OphNO_2 \xrightarrow{\text{microorganisms}} (EtO)_2 \ P(S)OphNH_2$$

$$(EtO)_2 \ P(S)OphNO_2 \xrightarrow{\text{animals}} (EtO)_2 \ P(O)OphNO_2$$

$$\xrightarrow{\text{animals}} (EtO)_2 \ P(S)OH$$

Figure 3.2. Comparison of metabolic patterns between higher animals and microorganisms.

3.3.2. Reductive Systems

Another class of important microbial reactions on pesticidal chemicals is the reductive processes. The work that first showed the importance of reductive systems in microorganisms was done by Cook (1957), who demonstrated that the major conversion product of parathion in microorganisms is aminoparathion, and not the products of oxidative reactions such as para-oxon diethylthiophosphoric acid. Similarly both fenitrothion and EPN are converted to their corresponding aminoanalogs by *Bacillus subtilis* (Miyamoto *et al.*, 1966) (Fig. 3.2).

One of the most common types of reductive reactions is dehalogenation. The importance of this type of reaction is that many environmentally problematic chemicals are halogenated chemicals and, moreover, in many instances dehalogenation is a rate-limiting reaction.

The reaction proceeds by replacing a halogen atom such as chlorine on a nonaromatic carbon with a hydrogen; the most well known case is the conversion of DDT to TDE (= DDD) (Fig. 3.3).

French and Hoopingarner (1970) found that in *Escherichia coli* this reaction is stimulated by the presence of reduced FAD (+FADH). This enzyme system is located in the cell membrane, but the presence of the cytoplasmic supernatant also increased the rate of dechlorination. The addition of TCA cycle intermediates, which shift the overall state of metabolism to more oxidative ones, results in the loss of dechlorination activities.

Other insecticides known to go through such dechlorination reactions are γ-BHC (Ruzo *et al.*, 1974; Benezet and Matsumura, 1973; Jagnow *et al.*, 1977; Mathur and Saha, 1977) and endrin (Matsumura *et al.*, 1971). Other reductive

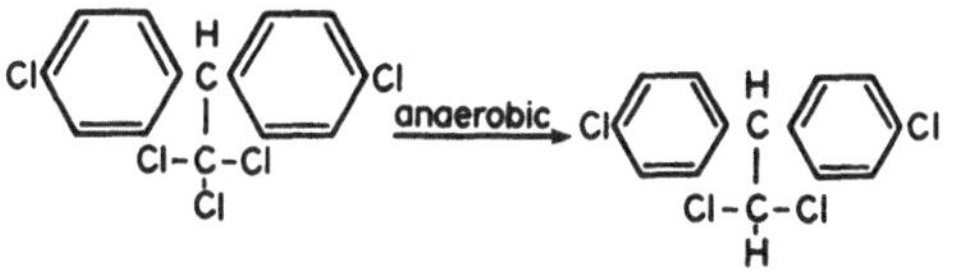

Figure 3.3. Metabolic conversion of DDT to TDE by microorganisms.

reactions recently found to be active are *N*-desmethylation and sulfones to give sulfides. The example of the former case is mexacarbate, which has been shown to undergo 4-*N*-desmethylation by preparations from *Anacystis nudilans* and *Pseudomonas putida* under anaerobic conditions (Esaac and Matsumura, 1979). The occurrence of the latter type of reaction has not been documented in the microbial world, but it has been shown to occur in an animal system (DeBaun and Menn, 1976).

Although the mechanisms of all the reductive systems active in degrading pesticides have not been elucidated, at least three major classes of reactions seem to be dominant. The first one is the system coupled with the mixed-function oxidase. In this system the substrates for reduction bind directly in the reduced cytochrome P-450 (Esaac and Matsumura, 1979). The presence of oxygen is detrimental to the reaction, as the entire reductive cycle is carried out by the reduced cytochrome (Fig. 3.4). Though the comparable system has not been studied in microorganisms, the chances are good that such a system does operate there in view of the presence of cytochrome P-450 in some of the microorganisms. The second system is the one found in our laboratory (Esaac and Matsumura, 1978) involving flavoprotein–flavin cofactors. The system is nonenzymatically operated, and the scheme by which it reduces the substrates is illustrated in Fig. 3.5. The system is characteristically resistant to heat and protease treatments

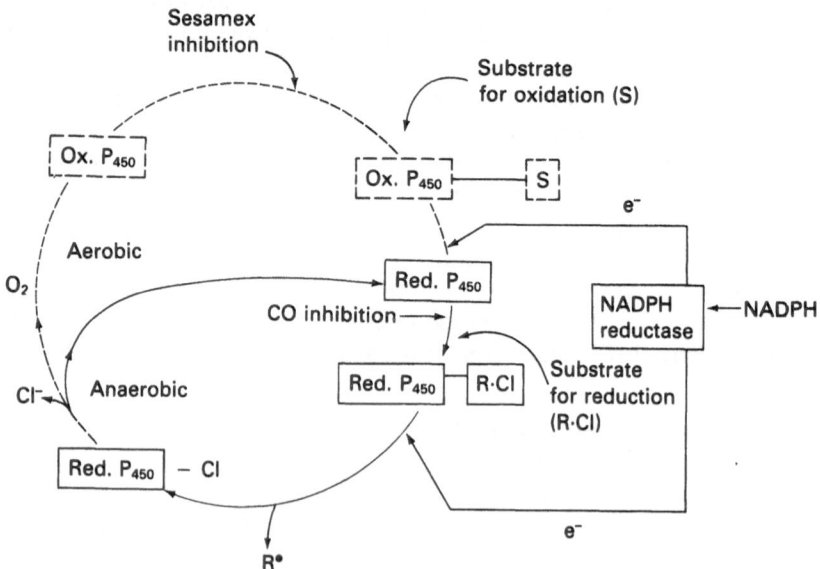

Figure 3.4. Proposed reductive metabolic pathway for pesticidal substrates via the mixed-function oxidase system under anaerobic conditions.

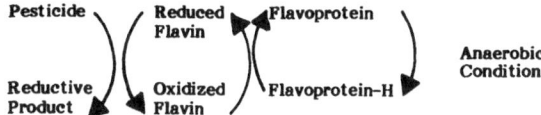

Figure 3.5. Reductive degradation of pesticides by flavoprotein–flavin cofactor systems.

and is stimulated by a flavin cofactor such as FAD, FMN, or riboflavin. A third class of reductive systems involves porphyrin-containing materials. According to Castro (1964), the system (here an example of reductive dechlorination has been adopted) works according to the scheme shown in Fig. 3.6.

3.3.3. Oxidative Reactions

While the extent of reports on oxidative metabolism in the microbial world is somewhat less than may be found in other biological systems, many oxidative reactions occur widely among microorganisms. They are (1) *epoxidation of cyclodienes* such as aldrin and heptachlor to corresponding epoxides (e.g., dieldrin and heptachlor epoxide), (2) *oxidation of thioethers* to sulfoxides and sulfones (e.g., phorate), (3) *oxidative dealkylation of alkylamines* (e.g., mexacarbate), (4) *ring opening* (e.g., 2,4-D), and (5) *decarboxylation*.

One very important reaction that takes place only in the microbial world is the aromatic ring-opening process. The system is operated by a series of oxidative ring hydroxylation (including epoxidation) reactions. The ring hydroxylation can occur even at the chlorine-attached aromatic carbon, in contrast to reductive dechlorination reactions on chlorinated hydrocarbons. The rate of such hydroxylation reactions decreases drastically as the number of chlorine substitutions on any given aromatic ring. Thus, 2,4,5-T is almost always more persistent than 2,4-D, and PCB members with fewer chlorines degrade faster than the highly chlorinated ones.

Focht and Alexander (1970*a*–*c*) selected a species of *Pseudomonas (Hydrogenomonas)* by using diphenyl methane (true metabolism) and found that more chlorinated analogs such as bis-(*p*-chlorophenyl) methane (DDM) are less vigorously metabolized. The final product of DDM degradation was *p*-chloro-

$$RCl = Fe^{II} \rightleftharpoons (RCl) \, Fe^{II} \rightleftharpoons R + ClFe^{II}$$

$$R + Fe^{II} + HOH \rightleftharpoons RH + Fe^{III} + OH$$

Figure 3.6. Nonenzymatic reduction of pesticides by iron–porphyrin systems.

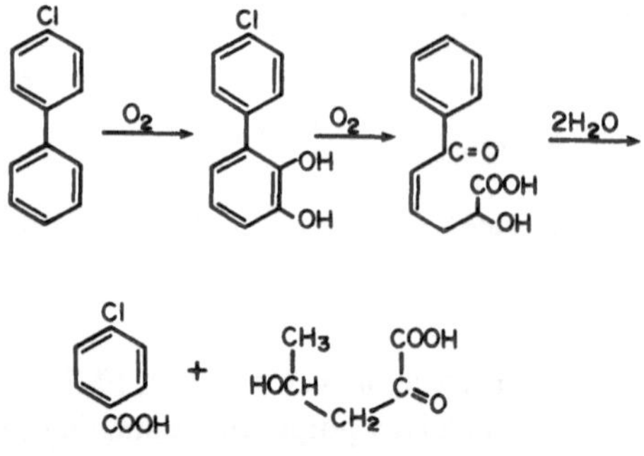

Figure 3.7. Oxidative degradation of PCB by microbial systems.

phenylacetic acid, indicating the opening of one of the chlorinated aromatic rings. Similarly, Ahmed and Focht (1972) could demonstrate a ring-opening process in two species of *Achromobacter,* originally selected by nonchlorinated biphenyl or *p*-chlorobiphenyl. The process of the ring opening on *p*-chlorobiphenyl has been proposed by these workers as shown in Fig. 3.7. Furukawa and Matsumura (1975) and Furukawa *et al.* (1978) found *Alcaligenes* and *Acinetobacter* strains that actively degrade PCB isomers via similar ring-opening mechanisms. The degree of degradation was found to be inversely correlated to the degree of chlorination on the biphenyl ring. *p*-Nitrophenol, a degradation product of parathion, can also be degraded through a ring operation (Munnecke and Hsieh, 1974).

Decarboxylation reactions are common oxidative reactions. Miyazaki *et al.* (1969), for instance, found that 4,4′-dichlorobenzilic acid (DBA), a hydrolysis product of both chlorobenzilate and chloropropylate, gives rise to 4,4-dichlorobenzophone (DBP) in a yeast strain of *Rhodotorula gracilis* (Fig. 3.8). The process was stimulated when citric acid was added to the culture medium and inhibited when 2-ketoglutaric acid was given, indicating the necessity of promoting an oxidative activity in decarboxylating this intermediate.

Other common oxidative reactions are β-oxidation, conversion of alcohols and aldehydes to acids, and dehydrogenation, but they are much less frequently observed among metabolic activities on pesticides.

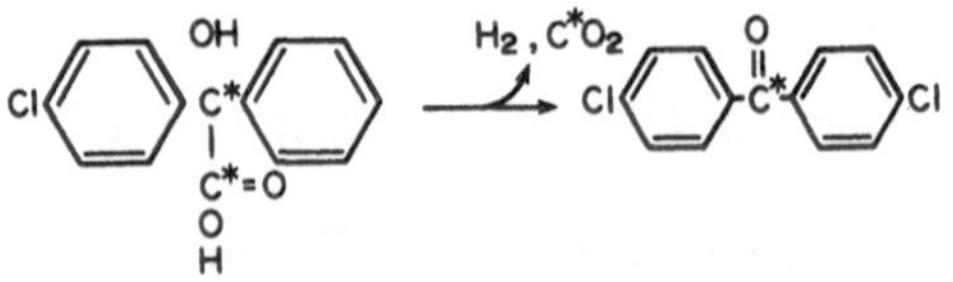

Figure 3.8. Formation of DBP from DBA by *R. gracilis.*

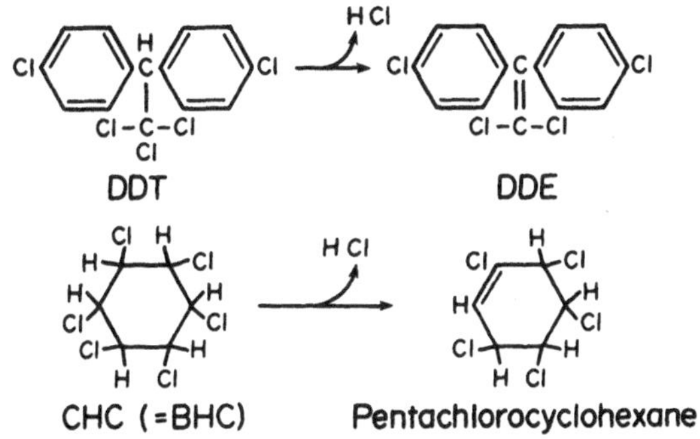

Figure 3.9. Examples of dehydrochlorination reactions.

3.4. OTHER METABOLIC REACTIONS RELATED TO PESTICIDE DEGRADATION

3.4.1. Dehydrochlorination

It is well known that DDT is dehydrochlorinated to give DDE. The reaction involves an elimination of HCl, and hence is called dehydrochlorination. In higher animals the reaction is mediated by GSH, but evidence is lacking in the microbial world as to whether GSH plays any significant role. Typically, the reaction takes place between the saturated chlorinated carbon and the adjacent hydrogen on the neighboring carbon, the net result being an appearance of olefinic compounds. Examples of dehydrochlorination reactions are shown in Fig. 3.9.

3.4.2. Isomerization

It has been observed accidentally that various cyclodiene compounds go through isomerization reactions to yield more stable products. For example, Matsumura *et al.* (1970) observed that dieldrin is converted to photodieldrin by the formation of an intramolecular bridge in several microbial species. Similarly, ketoendrin is formed from endrin (Matsumura *et al.*, 1971) (Fig. 3.10). It is not at all clear why microorganisms go through such an isomerization reaction, which does not yield any energy. However, from the viewpoint of environmental toxicology, such reactions are very important, since they give rise to other unsuspected environmental contaminants, the toxicity and hazards of which are often unknown (Matsumura, 1974).

Another important isomerization reaction is the formation of α-HCH (α-

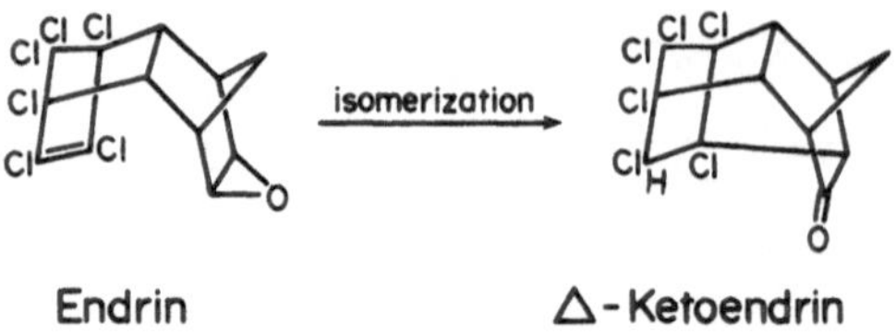

Endrin   △-Ketoendrin

Figure 3.10.   Isomerization of endrin.

BHC) from γ-HCH as shown to occur in *P. putida* (Benezet and Matsumura, 1973) and by other microbes under anaerobic conditions (Jagnow *et al.*, 1977; Mathur and Saha, 1977).

3.4.3. Synthetic Metabolism

In some cases microbial systems add certain ligands to pesticides or their metabolic intermediates. The results of such synthetic reactions are formations of metabolic products that are larger in molecular size than the starting material.

The most commonly occurring reactions are acetylation and methylation. Cserjesi and Johnson (1972), for instance, found that *Trichoderma virgatum* methylates pentachlorophenol to form a stable methyl ether, and Tweedy *et al.* (1970) demonstrated that *p*-bromoaniline undergoes acetylation in *Talaromyces wartmanii* and *Fusarium oxysporum* to form an *N*-acetyl product. Though no enzymatic explanations of these events have been offered, chances are that reactive systems such as *S*-adenosylmethionine, methylcobalamine, and acetylCoA are the possible sources of ligands in the microbial world. Also, CoA is known to react with dichlone in *Neurospora stiophila* (Owens and Novotny, 1958) and trichloroacetic acid in a *Pseudomonas* species (Kearney *et al.*, 1969*a*)

3.4.4. Polymerization

Polymerization reactions are best known to occur among chlorinated anilines. In these cases two molecules of substituted anilines form an azobenzene as has been shown to occur in soil (Kearney *et al.*, 1969*b*) (Fig. 3.11).

In the case of *F. oxysporum* more complex reactions may take place, de-

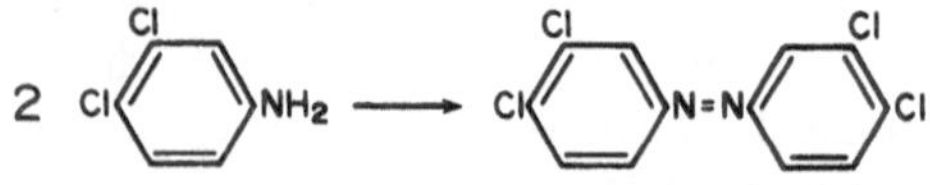

Figure 3.11.   Dimerization of dichloroaniline.

pending upon the physiological state of the organisms (Kaufman *et al.*, 1972), involving azoxybenzene and triazene, as shown in Fig. 3.12.

3.5. DEGRADATION BY SUNLIGHT AND OTHER PHYSICAL FACTORS

Among the physical factors known to influence the residual fate of pesticides in nature (e.g., light, air surfaces, moisture, and pH), sunlight, particularly the ultraviolet portion of sunlight, appears to make the most significant contribution. The sunlight reaching the surface of the earth does not have any ultraviolet component below 280 nm because the atmosphere effectively eliminates such short-wave ultraviolet rays. It is possible, therefore, that artificial ultraviolet radiation, produced for instance by an intense mercury lamp (253.7 nm), can create degradation products not produced by the action of natural sunlight. Theoretically, compounds which do not show absorption in any given range of wavelength are not supposed to go through photochemical reactions, and yet we know that even such a compound as dieldrin can be affected by sunlight. Several factors may contribute to this phenomenon.

One of the most important factors affecting the rate of sunlight degradation of pesticides and other organic chemicals is the presence of *photosensitizers*, compounds that facilitate the transfer of the energy of light into the receptor chemicals. In the past, photolytic research has been carried out in the presence and absence of photosensitizers, although no significant qualitative differences have been found in the metabolic (photolytic) routes. It is known that various photosensitizers facilitate photolysis of pesticidal compounds. Rosen and Carey (1968) and Rosen *et al.* (1970) used both benzophenone and riboflavin-5'-phosphate as sensitizers for their studies on photodecomposition of pesticides. Ivie and Casida (1971*a,b*) found rotenone and other pesticides and nonpesticides to be sensitizers for degradation of various insecticides. In addition to rotenone, good photosensitizers included some aromatic amines, anthraquinone (which showed the broadest spectrum), and benzophenone. Insecticidal combinations

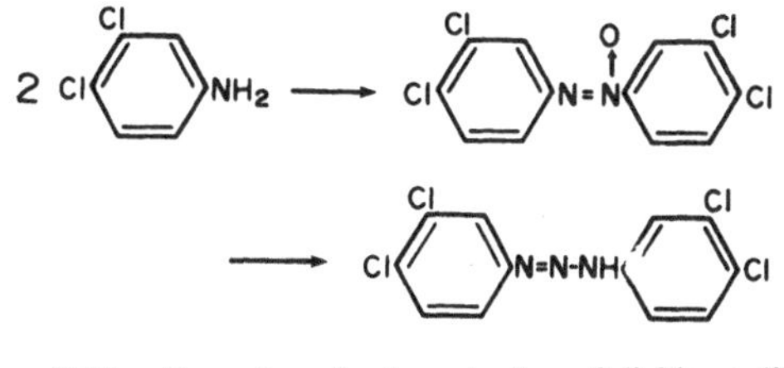

Figure 3.12.   Examples of polymerization of dichloroanilines.

which synergistically acted as sensitizers were Abate®–dieldrin, carbyne(12E)–Sumithion®, phenothiazine–DDT, and rotenone–dieldrin. The same authors (Ivie and Casida, 1971b) also reported that substituted 4-chroman-ones and rotenone-sensitized dieldrin converted to photodieldrin on bean leaves. Chlorophyll from spinach chloroplasts plus rotenone acted as a sensitizer for organophosphates, carbamates, pyrethroids, and dinitrophenol insecticides.

Another important factor affecting the nature of photochemical reactions is the medium in which the reacting substance is dissolved or suspended. In laboratory tests, the effect of solvents becomes an important factor in deciding either the speed of the reaction or the nature of the reaction products. The medium and the solvent can influence the outcome of photochemical reactions in two different ways: (1) they can be photosensitizers or (2) they can act as the reaction partner to the pesticide molecule energized by light. The difference may be best expressed in the following equations:

$$A + B \xrightarrow{\text{Light}} A + B^* \to (AB) \to A' + B' \tag{1}$$

$$A + B \xrightarrow{\text{Light}} A^* + B \to A' + B' \tag{2}$$

where A is a pesticide molecule and B is the substance which promotes pho-tochemical reactions. In equation (1), B is the photosensitizer and therefore is energized by light first. It in turn reacts with the pesticide to form the photo-chemical reaction product A'. In equation (2), B is the reacting agent (e.g., solvent or medium) for the pesticide that has been energized by light to produce the product A'.

3.5.1. Hydrolysis: Nucleophilic Reaction

An example of a photonucleophilic reaction is the displacement of a chlorine atom on a benzene ring with -OH in aqueous solution containing nucleophilic agents (Cserjesi and Johnson, 1972) (Fig. 3.13). In the range of sunlight irra-diation (above 280 nm), the H–OH bond is not expected to break up to provide

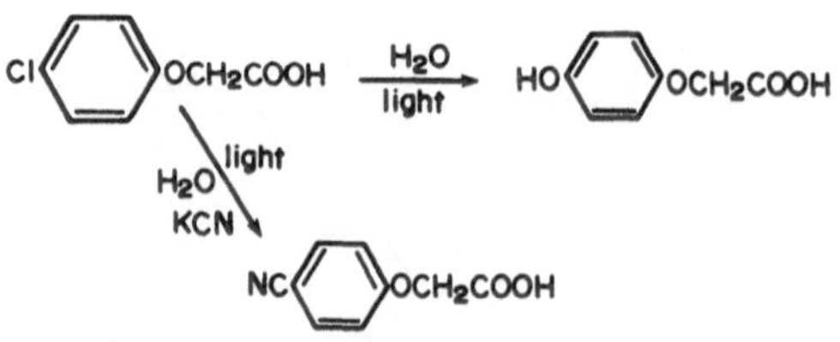

Figure 3.13. Nucleophilic photochemical reactions.

the nucleophil needed for reaction (Castro, 1964). The most likely source of the nucleophilic agent in this case is the hydroxide ion (OH⁻), which can be replaced by the cyanide ion (CN⁻) to yield the corresponding *p*-cyanophenol product.

In aqueous solution the most predominant photochemical reaction on organophosphates and carbamates is hydrolysis. Thus many of the substrates for hydrolysis cited in Section 3.3.1 would also be expected to be photochemically attacked.

3.5.2. Dehalogenation

Dehalogenation is a rather commonly occurring photochemical reaction. Because of the high energy involved, UV irradiation can directly dehalogenate even stable halogens attached to aromatic rings—a capability that has not been found in microorganisms. For example, it has been shown that photolysis of PCB gives monochlorobiphenyl (Ruzo *et al.*, 1974). Other examples of aromatic dechlorination are monuron (Crosby and Leitis, 1969) and PCP (pentachlorophenol). Dechlorination from alkyl carbons takes place with relative ease. The 1-exo-chlorine of heptachlor, for instance, is released by UV irradiation at 300 nm (McGuire *et al.*, 1970) (Fig. 3.14). Other examples are BHC isomers, mirex, and chlordane isomers. It must be pointed out here that when there is an abundance of proton donors such as saturated alkanes and flavoproteins, the end result of dehalogenation resembles reductive reactions. Whether or not these should be called reductive reactions is a matter of choice.

3.5.3. Oxidation

Photochemical oxidation usually takes place as a result of reactions between photoactivated pesticidal molecules and oxygen. Thus the reactions are usually carried out in atmospheric conditions rather than in aqueous solutions, although dissolved oxygen in some cases can react with pesticides to give oxidation products. Perhaps the most frequently encountered photooxidative reaction in the pesticide field is the conversion of P=S to P=O in the case of organo-

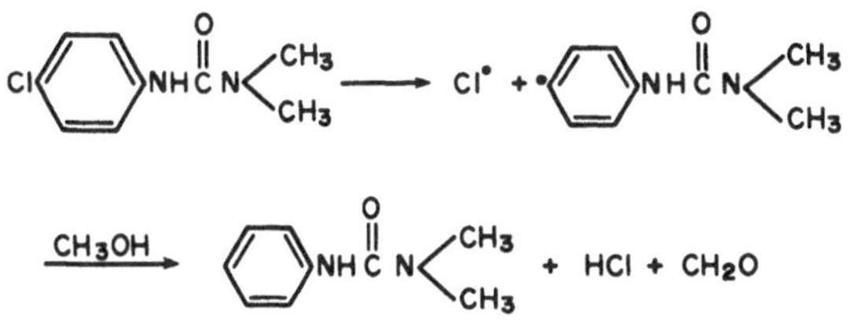

Figure 3.14. Dechlorination reaction catalyzed by photochemical reactions.

phosphates. This is analogous to the activation process by higher organisms to give more toxic (= antichlorergic potency) products (Grumwell and Erickson, 1973).

Pyrethroids are known to undergo photooxidative reactions (e.g., Tweedy *et al.*, 1970), although in this case the reactions are complex and one can only guess the nature of the reactions involved by the products formed, e.g., benzaldehyde, benzoic acid, and 5-hydroxy-3-oxo-4-phenyl-1-cyclopentenyl methanol, from resmethrin.

Pyridines are also known to go through oxidative transformation. For instance, diquat and paraquat give a carbonyl and carboxylic acid, respectively, as a result of photoxidation. It must be pointed out here that many of the reaction products of biological oxidation, such as epoxides for cycladienes, *N*-oxides for amines, sulfoxides, and sulfones from sulfides, have not been observed among photolytic products.

3.5.4. Isomerization and Polymerization

Intramolecular rearrangements occur quite frequently by photochemical reactions, which often yield isomerized products. The first observation of such a case was made by two groups of scientists (Robinson *et al.*, 1966; Rosen *et al.*, 1966) on dieldrin (Fig. 3.15). Soon many other cyclodiene insecticides were found to go through similar isomerization processes (see Ueda *et al.*, 1974). Examples are heptachlor, heptachlor epoxide, *trans*- and *cis*-chlordane, aldrin, and endrin.

Complex polymerization reactions are known to take place with substituted anilines and pentachlorophenol. From anilines, corresponding azo and anilinoazobenzenes are formed (Rosen *et al.*, 1970).

3.6. CONCLUSION

In the above description of photochemical and microbial conversion of pesticidal chemicals I have deliberately omitted the description of complicated

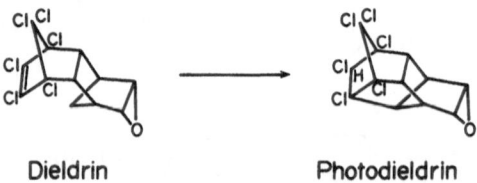

Dieldrin   Photodieldrin

Figure 3.15.   Isomerization of dieldrin by a photochemical reaction.

degradation pathways of individual compounds. Rather, the classes of reactions and similar interactions were grouped together for the sake of clarity. Naturally many of the reactions may occur on one compound, and as a result could yield complicated interacting reaction patterns. Furthermore, in the environment other factors—such as redox potential, nutritional state of soil, availability of catalytic material, pH, physical adsorption and absorption, and physiochemical changes (e.g., emulsification and liposolubilization)—would greatly affect the eventual outcome of the expression of the degradative activities. What one has to re-member, however, is the simple fact that certain chemical properties make the compounds susceptible to these degradative forces. For instance, the *N*-chlorine atoms of triazine herbicides are labile, and so are the carboxyl esters of malathion. Thus, the advantage of studying basic reaction mechanisms is that the patterns of degradation of chemicals in the environment become explainable and even predictable as such knowledge accumulates. Well-informed scientists in this field should be capable of examining the molecular structure of a new compound, identifying its labile moieties, and coming up with a reasonable prediction of the pattern and mechanisms of its degradation.

REFERENCES

Ahmed, M. K., and Focht, D. D., 1972, Degradation of polychlorinated biphenyls by two species of *Achromobacter, Can. J. Microbiol.* **19**:47.

Benezet, H., and Matsumura, F., 1973, Isomerization of γ-BHC to α-BHC in the environment, *Nature (London)* **243**:480.

Castro, C. E., 1964, The rapid oxidation of iron (II) porphyrines by alkyl halides. A possible mode of intoxication of organisms by alkyl halides, *J. Am. Chem. Soc.* **86**:2310.

Cook, J. W., 1957, *In vitro* destruction of some organophosphate pesticides by bovine rumen fluid, *J. Agric. Food Chem.* **5**:859.

Crosby, D. G., and Leitis, E., 1969, Photolysis of chlorophenylacetic acids, *J. Agric. Food Chem.* **17**:1036.

Cserjesi, A. J., and Johnson, E. L., 1972, Methylation of pentachlorophenol by *Trichoderma virgatum, Can. J. Microbiol.* **18**:45.

DeBaun, J. R., and Menn, J. J., 1976, Sulfoxide reduction in relation to organosphosphorus insecticide detoxication, *Science* **191**:187.

Esaac, E. G., and Matsumura, F., 1978, A novel reduction system involving flavoprotein in the rat intestine, *Bull. Environ. Contam. Toxicol.* **19**:15.

Esaac, E. G., and Matsumura, F., 1979, Mechanisms of reductive dechlorination of DDT by rat liver microsomes, *Pestic. Biochem. Physiol.* **13**:81.

Esaac, E. G., and Matsumura, F., 1980, Metabolism of insecticides by reductive systems, *Pharmacol. Ther.* **9**:1.

Focht, D. D., and Alexander, M., 1970a, DDT metabolites and analogs: Ring fission by *Hydrogenomonas, Science* **170**:91.

Focht, D. D., and Alexander, M., 1970b, Aerobic cometabolism of DDT analogues by Hydrogenomonas sp., *J. Agric. Food Chem.* **19**:20.

Focht, D. D., and Alexander, M., 1970c, Bacterial degradation of diphenylmenthane, a DDT model substrate, *Appl. Microbiol.* **20:**608.

French, A. L., and Hoopingarner, R. A., 1970, Dechlorination of DDT by membranes isolated from *Escherichia coli, J. Econ. Entomol.* **63:**756.

Furukawa, K., and Matsumura, F., 1975, Microbial metabolism of PCBs: Studies of the relative degradability of PCB components by *Alcaligenes* sp., *J. Agric. Food Chem.* **24:**251.

Furukawa, K., Matsumura, F., and Tonomura, K., 1978, *Alcaligenes* and *Acinetobacter* strains capable of degrading polychlorinated biphenyls, *Agric. Biol. Chem.* **42:**543.

Grumwell, J. R., and Erickson, R. H., 1973, Photolysis of parathion, *O,O*-diethyl-*O*-(4-nitrophenyl) thiophosphate. New products, *J. Agric. Food Chem.* **21:**929.

Hill, I. R., and Wright, S. J. L., 1978, *Pesticide Microbiology*, Academic Press, New York.

Ivie, G. W., and Casida, J. E., 1971a, Sensitized photodecomposition and photosensitizer activity of pesticide chemicals exposed to sunlight of silica gel chromatographic plates, *J. Agric. Food Chem.* **19:**40.

Ivie, G. W., and Casida, J. E., 1971b, Photosensitizers for the accelerated degradation of chlorinated cyclodienes and other insecticide chemicals exposed to sunlight on bean leaves, *J. Agric. Food Chem.* **19:**410.

Jagnow, G., Haider, K., and Ellwardt, P. C., 1977, Anaerobic dechlorination and degradation of hexachlorocyclohexane isomers by anaerobic and facultative anaerobic bacteria, *Arch. Microbiol.* **115:**285.

Kaufman, D. D., Plimmer, J. R., Iwan, J., and Klingebiel, U. I., 1972, 3,3′,4,4′-tetrachloroazoxybenzene from 3,4-dichloroaniline in microbial culture, *J. Agric. Food Chem.* **20:**916.

Kearney, P. C., Kaufman, D. D., von Endt, D. W., and Guardia, F. S., 1969a, TCA metabolism by soil microorganisms, *J. Agric. Food Chem.* **17:**1418.

Kearney, P. C., Kaufman, D. D., von Ednt, D. W., and Guardia, F. S., 1969b, Mixed chloroaxobenzene formation in soil, *J. Agric. Food Chem.* **17:**581.

Khan, M. A. Q., 1977, *Pesticides in Aquatic Environments*, Plenum Press, New York.

Mathur, S. P., and Saha, J. G., 1977, Degradation of lindane ^{14}C on a mineral soil and an organic soil, *Bull. Environ. Contam. Toxicol.* **17:**424.

Matsumura, F., 1974, Microbial degradation of pesticides, in: *Survival in Toxic Environments* (M. A. Q. Khan and J. P. Berderka, eds.), pp. 129–54, Academic Press, New York.

Matsumura, F., Patil, K. C., and Boush, G. M., 1970, Formation of "photodieldrin" by microorganisms, *Science* **170:**1206.

Matsumura, F., Khanvilkar, V. G., Patil, K. C., and Boush, G. M., 1971, Metabolism of endrin by certain soil microorganisms, *J. Agric. Food Chem.* **19:**27.

Matsumura, F., Boush, G. M., and Misato, T., 1972, *Environmental Toxicology of Pesticides*, Academic Press, New York.

McGuire, R. R., Zabik, M. J., Schuetz, R. D., and Flotard, R. D., 1970, Photochemistry of bioactive compounds. Photolyses of 1,4,5,6,7,8,8-heptachlor-3a-4,7,7a-tetrahydro-4,7-methanoindene, *J. Agric. Food Chem.* **18:**319.

Miskus, R. P., Blair, D. P., and Casida, J. E., 1965, Conversion of DDT to DDD by bovine rumen fluid, lake water, and reduced porphyrins, *J. Agric. Food Chem.* **13:**481.

Miyamoto, J., Kitagawa, K., and Sato, Y., 1966, Metabolism of organophosphorus insecticides by *Bacillus subtilis* with special emphasis on sumithion, *Jpn. J. Exp. Med.* **36:**211.

Miyazaki, S., Boush, G. M., and Matsumura, F., 1969, Metabolism of ^{14}C-Chloropropylate by *Rodotorula gracilis, Appl. Microbiol.* **28:**212.

Munnecke, D. M., and Hsieh, D. P. H., 1974, Microbial decontaminations of parathion and *p*-nitrophenol in aqueous media, *Appl. Microbiol.* **28:**212.

Owens, R. G., and Novotny, H. M., 1958, Mechanism of action of the fungicide dichlone (2,3-dichloro-1,4-naphthoquinone), *Contrib. Boyce Thompson Inst.* **19:**463.

Robinson, J., Richardson, A., Busch, B., and Elgar, K. E., 1966, Photoisomerization products of dieldrin, *Bull. Environ. Contam. Toxicol.* 1:127.

Rosen, J. D., and Carey, W. F., 1968, Preparation of the photoisomers of aldrin and dieldrin, *J. Agric. Food Chem.* 116:536.

Rosen, J. E., Sutherland, D. J., and Lipton, G. R., 1966, The photochemical isomerization of dieldrin and endrin and effects on toxicity, *Bull. Environ. Contam. Toxicol.* 4:133.

Rosen, J. D., Siewierski, M., and Winnett, G., 1970, FMN-sensitized photolysis of chloroanilines, *J. Agric. Food Chem.* 18:494.

Ruzo, L. O., Zabik, M. J., and Schuetz, R. D., 1974, Photochemistry of bioactive compounds, Photochemical processes of polychlorinated biphenyls, *J. Am. Chem. Soc.* 96:3809.

Tweedy, B. G., Loeppky, C., and Ross, J. A., 1970, Metobromuron: Acetylation of the aniline moiety as a detoxification mechanism, *Science* 168:482.

Ueda, K., Gaughan, L. C., and Casdia, J. E., 1974, Photodecomposition of resmethrin and related pyrethroids, *J. Agric. Food Chem.* 22:213.

Walker, W. W., and Stojanovic, B. J., 1973, Microbial versus chemical degradation of malathion in soil, *J. Environ. Qual.* 2:229.

Zabik, M. J., Leavitt, R. A., and Su, G. C. C., 1976, Photochemistry of bioactive compounds: A review of pesticide photochemistry, *Annu. Rev. Entomol.* 21:61.

Application of the Principles of Biodegradation of Pesticides

PART II

Application of the Principles of
Biodegradation of Pesticides

4

Microbial Degradation of Pesticides in Tropical Soils

N. Sethunathan, T. K. Adhya, and K. Raghu

4.1. INTRODUCTION

Hot and humid conditions of the tropical and subtropical environments, as exist in most developing countries, favor the buildup of a myriad of insect pests and disease pathogens harmful to man and his agriculturally important crops. Furthermore, in recent years, intensive and extensive cultivation of new high-yielding crop varieties with high nitrogen input in several tropical countries has led to serious outbreaks of certain insect pests that were previously considered minor pests, such as brown planthoppers *(Nilaparvata lugens)* in rice (Kulshreshtha *et al.*, 1974). Consequently, there has been a steady increase in the use of pesticides in most tropical countries in recent years. Pesticide use in most developing countries is still very low, with an input of 330 g/ha in India as compared to 1490 g/ha in a developed country such as Japan (Anonymous, 1979*a*). However, there are localized areas of heavy pesticide use, such as in cotton, tea, and cocoa and in irrigated rice culture, raising problems of environmental contamination.

In developed countries, herbicides constitute a major portion of all pesticides used. But, for most tropical countries, insecticides are the most important, accounting for, as in India (Anonymous, 1979*a*), more than 65% of all pesticides used.

In recent years, the use of certain chlorinated hydrocarbon pesticides has been banned in almost all developed countries because of concern over their

N. Sethunathan and T. K. Adhya ● Laboratory of Soil Microbiology, Central Rice Research Institute, Cuttack 753006, India.   *K. Raghu* ● Biology and Agriculture Division, Bhabha Atomic Research Centre, Bombay 400085, India.

recalcitrance to degradation processes and subsequent biomagnification through the food chain. But chlorinated hydrocarbon insecticides are of great importance to the public health and agriculture of most tropical countries in view of their indigenous availability, low cost, and broad-spectrum activity of long duration. In 1978, about 5000 tons of various pesticides were produced in India with imports of less than 2000 tons; hexachlorocyclohexane (HCH), a chlorinated hydrocarbon, alone accounted for more than 67% of all pesticides produced (Anonymous, 1979b). Price considerations and nonavailability of less-persistent substitutes would certainly delay the replacement of chlorinated hydrocarbon pesticides in the tropics. However, there are instances of banning or restricting the use of certain persistent insecticides, for example endrin, in tropical agriculture. This is consistent with the strategy followed in developed countries. But the loss of organic pesticides, through processes involving volatilization, photodecomposition, and more importantly microbial degradation, is expected to be more rapid under tropical and subtropical conditions than in temperate environments. Moreover, the persistence of pesticides is largely influenced by the conditions and cultural practices used for specific crops. Thus, γ-HCH (lindane), known for its long-term persistence under aerobic and temperate conditions, undergoes fairly rapid decomposition in tropical soils upon flooding, the most widely used cultural practice in rice cultivation (Raghu and MacRae, 1966).

These results emphasize the importance of realistically assessing the persistence of pesticides and their impact on the ecosystem under actual tropical conditions before restricting the use of economically important pesticides based on literature of no relevance to tropical conditions. Studies on the dynamics of pesticides in tropical ecosystems are relatively few, recent, and restricted almost entirely to microbial degradation in rice soils, as reflected in this review of available literature.

4.2. RESIDUES IN SOIL

Although persistent chlorinated hydrocarbon insecticides are used regularly and on a large scale in most tropical countries, information on their residues in the tropical environment is fragmentary and far from conclusive. Moreover, meaningful interpretation of the available data on pesticide residues in tropical ecosystems (Bindra and Kalra, 1973; Agnihothrudu and Mithyantha, 1978) has been difficult because of the unreliable and less-sophisticated techniques employed in most studies. In a few instances, however, residues have been determined with the help of sophisticated techniques after known applications of pesticides under field conditions.

In a long-term field experiment, γ-HCH reached nonsignificant levels of less than 0.02 ppm in soil and water within 20–30 days of its application, even at high doses, to submerged rice fields in the Philippines (Anonymous, 1966) in contrast to its reported residual life of 2–10 years in more aerobic upland soils (Kearney *et al.*, 1969). Moreover, even repeated additions of this insecticide to the same submerged field plot did not lead to any significant residue buildup in the soil. γ-HCH levels in the field soils that received a total of 48 and 12 kg/ ha in four crop seasons were comparable with values of 0.018 and 0.014 ppm, respectively, when analyzed 30 days after the last application. Irrespective of the dose of HCH applied, within 20–30 days after its application the residues declined to less than 0.02 ppm in both soil and water. Likewise, accumulation of diazinon was negligible upon its repeated applications to submerged rice fields in the Philippines (Sethunathan *et al.*, 1971).

In a long-term field experiment, residues of DDT and dieldrin decreased to 20 and 30% of the original levels in the fall and winter months in an upland soil under subtropical conditions in Taiwan; no accumulation of these residues occurred with further additions in spring and summer (Talekar *et al.*, 1977). Also, fonofos, phorate, and carbofuran, which decreased to 8, 0.4, and 32% of the original levels in the fall and winter months, disappeared even faster during the hot and rainy conditions of spring and summer. Application of carbofuran and chlordimeform to the root zone in the reduced soil layer of flooded rice paddies, in lieu of the conventional practice of broadcasting to the standing water or spraying to the foliage, reduced the concentration of the insecticides in the flood water and thereby the surface losses (Aquino and Pathak, 1976). Besides, root-zone application of the insecticides increased their uptake by the rice plants and stretched their efficiency in controlling brown planthoppers over a prolonged duration. A meaningful conclusion from most field studies essentially involving the monitoring of only the parent compounds, and not their degradation products, is difficult since transport losses through volatilization are considerable under tropical and subtropical conditions. Under flooded conditions, as in paddy fields, substantial volatilization of pesticides such as HCH may occur even more readily (Siddaramappa and Sethunathan, 1976). Also, in the tropics, increased loss of soil-applied pesticides can occur through translocation from the roots to the foliage and subsequent transpiration from the leaf surface, especially under conditions of excess water, as in paddy ecosystems. More recently, Siddaramappa and Watanabe (1979) showed, by radioautography, fairly rapid translocation of carbofuran in significant amounts to the foliage of rice seedlings after its application to flooded soils. However, actual measurements are not available to indicate the quantities involved in such losses under tropical field conditions.

4.3. MICROBIAL DEGRADATION

Pesticides applied to the environment are acted upon by several forces— physical, chemical and biological—independently or in combination. Since the classical demonstration of microbial breakdown of the hormonal herbicide 2,4-

D (Audus, 1951), it has become well established that the major, or frequently the only, means of degradation for several pesticides in the environment is microbial. In biological reactions essentially involving constitutive and adaptive enzyme systems, stepwise degradation of pesticide molecules is accomplished, often with the formation of inorganic end products; but, in nonbiological reactions, the degradation is less extensive and far from complete.

Microbial involvement in pesticide degradation is generally established by (1) more rapid degradation in nonsterile than in sterile soil samples; (2) an initial lag in the degradation followed by a more rapid loss attributed to the adaptation of microorganisms; (3) the initial lag becoming shorter with successive additions of pesticides due to the enrichment of pesticide-degrading microorganisms; (4) evolution of $^{14}CO_2$ from ring-^{14}C-labeled pesticides applied to biological systems; and (5) final and conclusive demonstration of the degradation of pesticides in isolated cultures of microorganisms. Using one or more of these methods, microbial participation has been demonstrated, with some degree of confidence, in the degradation of some pesticides, insecticides in particular, in tropical soils.

4.3.1. Chlorinated Hydrocarbon Insecticides

Although chlorinated hydrocarbon insecticides are used regularly in most tropical countries, in-depth information on their metabolic fate in soils is not available, with the exception of HCH.

4.3.1.1. Hexachlorocyclohexane

Commercial formulations of HCH generally contain α-, β-, δ-, and γ-isomers, of which the γ-isomer is the most insecticidal and the β-isomer is the most persistent. Although the β-isomer is a minor constituent in the commercial formulations of HCH, its entry, through persistence, into the food chain following its intensive use has caused concern in Japan (Tomizawa, 1977). Considerable work is available on the fate of HCH in tropical rice soils because of its continued extensive use for controlling common rice insect pests. Extensive studies at the International Rice Research Institute in the Philippines and elsewhere consistently showed fairly rapid degradation of α-, β-, δ-, and γ-isomers of HCH in tropical soils upon flooding (Raghu and MacRae, 1966; MacRae et al., 1967).

The advantage of flooding the soil as an effective means of accelerating the degradation of HCH isomers was demonstrated more convincingly by Yoshida and Castro (1970). During 30-day incubation, γ-HCH decreased to very low levels in all four soils under flooding while virtually no degradation occurred under upland conditions. The degradation of all four isomers of HCH was much faster in nonsterile than in sterile soils (MacRae et al., 1967; Castro and Yoshida, 1974). Also, the evolution of $^{14}CO_2$ from [^{14}C]-γ-HCH from nonsterile samples, although in small quantities of less than 1% of added ^{14}C, did implicate microbial participation (MacRae *et al.*, 1967). Moreover, several bacteria isolated from flooded soil treated with HCH attacked γ-HCH with ease, but only under anaerobic conditions (Anonymous, 1966). The most active bacterium (MacRae *et al.*, 1969), identified as *Clostridium sphenoides* (Heritage and MacRae, 1977), metabolized α- and γ-HCH, but not β- and δ-HCH, under anaerobic conditions (MacRae *et al.*, 1969; Sethunathan *et al.*, 1969; Heritage and MacRae, 1977, 1979). During bacterial degradation, γ-HCH was converted to γ-3,4,5,6,-tetrachloro-1-cyclohexene (TCCH) and α-HCH to δ-TCCH (Heritage and MacRae, 1977, 1979); γ- and δ-TCCH were further metabolized, leading to a nearly complete dechlorination of γ-HCH with the formation of chloride ions in stoichiometric amounts (MacRae *et al.*, 1969; Jagnow *et al.*, 1977). Temperature and pH optima for the metabolism of γ-HCH by washed cell suspensions of *C. sphenoides* were 40°C and 8.0, respectively, (Heritage and MacRae, 1979). The γ-HCH-adapted cells also metabolized the β-, δ-, and γ-isomers of TCCH, 2,3,4,5,6-pentachloro-2-cyclohexen-1-ol and γ-1,2,3,4,5-pentachlorocyclohex-1-ene, and 1,2,3,4,5-pentachlorocyclohexane, but not a selection of chlorinated benzenes, dichlorocyclohexane and chlorocyclohexane. Carbon dioxide and methane, the common end products of carbon metabolism, were not detected. Anaerobic degradation of γ-HCH in flooded Japanese soils, activated sludge, and rumen fluid has also led to the formation of γ-TCCH (Tsukano and Kobayashi, 1972; Beland *et al.*, 1976; Haider *et al.*, 1976), but γ-TCCH formation in tropical rice soils is yet to be reported.

Other microorganisms actively implicated in the anaerobic degradation of γ-HCH included *Clostridium butyricum, Clostridium pasteurianum, Citrobacter freundii* (Jagnow *et al.*, 1977), and *Clostridium rectum* (Ohisa and Yamaguchi, 1978a). Interestingly, γ-HCH was decomposed by both growing and resting cells of *C. sphenoides* (Heritage and MacRae, 1977) and only by growing cells of *C. rectum* (Ohisa and Yamaguchi, 1978a). Addition of peptone, but not γ-HCH, to the flooded soil significantly increased the population of γ-HCH-decomposing microorganisms, *Clostridium* sp. in particular (Ohisa and Yamaguchi, 1978b). Besides, no proliferation of *C. rectum* occurred during γ-HCH degradation, suggesting cometabolism (Ohisa and Yamaguchi, 1978a). Although all four isomers of HCH are almost equally biodegradable in predominantly anaerobic flooded soils, degradation of β- and δ-isomers in isolated cultures of microorganisms is yet to be demonstrated. More in-depth studies on the stepwise degradation of the β-isomer in pure and/or mixed cultures of microorganisms are warranted in view of the concern over its entry into the food chain.

4.3.1.2. Other Chlorinated Hydrocarbons

As with HCH isomers, several related chlorinated hydrocarbon insecticides, known to persist for several years in aerobic environments, showed a relatively short residual life of less than 3 to 6 months in flooded soils. Thus, more rapid degradation of DDT, methoxychlor, and heptachlor in four Philippine rice soils occurred under flooded than under nonflooded conditions (Castro and Yoshida, 1971). In some soils, these insecticides almost completely disappeared within 30 days of flooding; during this period the loss from nonflooded soils was negligible. Only nonsterile soil samples exhibited the striking capacity to degrade these insecticides (Castro and Yoshida, 1974). Furthermore, washed cell suspensions of *C. sphenoides*, isolated from γ-HCH-amended flooded soil, also metabolized DDT, methoxychlor, and heptachlor under anaerobic conditions (Sethunathan and Yoshida, 1973a). However, DDD, the major product formed by reductive dechlorination of DDT both in flooded soils (Castro and Yoshida, 1974) and in bacterial culture (Sethunathan and Yoshida, 1973a), resisted further degradation. Despite the extreme instability of DDT in anaerobic ecosystems, its use even in such systems still poses serious problems of environmental contamination from its more persistent metabolite, DDD, which is also used as an insecticide.

Endrin, a widely used insecticide until recently and now banned in many tropical countries, decomposed rapidly in one of four Philippine soils under flooded conditions (Castro and Yoshida, 1974). But endrin showed relatively low persistence and reached low levels within 55 days of flooding except in a sandy soil of eight selected Indian soils (Gowda and Sethunathan, 1976). Most rapid degradation occurred in an acid sulfate *Pokkali* soil. Six stable products were formed from endrin in most soils except in acid sulfate *Kari* soil, where five products were formed, and in sandy soil where three products were formed. More rapid degradation of endrin in three soils under fooded than under nonflooded conditions led to the formation of six compounds in flooded soils and four compounds in nonflooded soils (Gowda and Sethunathan, 1977). The degradation of endrin in flooded soils is both chemical and biological, but biological degradation is much faster and more extensive, with distinct formation of six products in nonsterile soils and three products in sterile soils (Gowda and Sethunathan, 1977). Microorganisms capable of degrading endrin have been isolated from several terrestrial and aquatic ecosystems, including marine environments in tropical Hawaii (Matsumura et al., 1971; Patil et al., 1970), but not yet from flooded soils. Although endrin is relatively short-lived in microbially active flooded soils, its degradation products could persist in the environment. It would be incorrect to conclude that all pesticides are unstable in flooded soils and other anoxic systems since aldrin, dieldrin, and chlordane, for example, resisted degradation under both flooded and nonflooded conditions (Castro and Yoshida, 1971).

The herbicides 2,4-D, 2,4,5-T, and picloram degraded fairly rapidly under both water regimes but only in nonsterile soils, a finding attributed to microbial participation (Yoshida and Castro, 1975). Of interest here is the rapid breakdown of 2,4,5-T, although according to earlier reports (Alexander, 1965) an additional chlorine attached to its benzene ring rendered it more resistant than 2,4-D to biological degradation.

4.3.2. Organophosphorus Insecticides

Hydrolysis, at ester linkages in particular, constitutes the major means of decomposition of several organophosphorus pesticides in soil and water systems. This hydrolysis can be chemical, biological, or both. Distinguishing between chemical and biological roles in such hydrolytic reactions has been difficult. Consequently, hydrolysis of chemically unstable organophosphates in natural ecosystems was attributed essentially to chemical action. But more recently, explicit evidence has been provided for microbially mediated hydrolysis of at least two important members of this group, diazinon and parathion, in tropical flooded soils and in isolated cultures of bacteria.

4.3.2.1. Diazinon

Diazinon, a widely used insecticide in rice culture, is chemically stable at neutral and alkaline pH and is readily hydrolyzed under acid conditions as in acid soils (Sethunathan and MacRae, 1969). The degradation of diazinon via hydrolysis proceeded fairly rapidly in nonsterile soils with near-neutral pH under flooded conditions (Sethunathan and MacRae, 1969). But its hydrolysis product with the pyrimidine ring persisted, and consequently only 0.4–0.7% of ring-^{14}C in diazinon was recovered as $^{14}CO_2$ from 50-day flooded soils (Sethunathan and Yoshida, 1969), due to the inhibition of oxygenase-mediated ring cleavage reactions under predominantly anaerobic conditions (Williams, 1977).

The behavior of diazinon in flooded soils previously treated with diazinon provided further insight into the role of microorganisms in its degradation. Diazinon persisted for only 15 days in a tropical flooded field soil that had been treated previously with the insecticide and over 60 days in a flooded soil with no previous history of diazinon application (Sethunathan, 1972). Likewise, diazinon disappeared completely within 5 days of its incubation with water from diazinon-treated rice fields. More in-depth studies showed that populations of microorganisms capable of hydrolyzing diazinon increased upon its repeated additions to rice fields. A *Flavobacterium* sp., isolated from diazinon-treated rice field soils, readily hydrolyzed diazinon and then mineralized the pyrimidinyl moiety to carbon dioxide in a mineral salts medium supplemented with the insecticide (Sethunathan and Yoshida, 1973*b*). Undoubtedly, microorganisms accelerated the hydrolysis of diazinon in flooded rice paddies, although according to an earlier concept (Kearney and Helling, 1969), diazinon was first hydrolyzed chemically and later microorganisms attacked the products of chemical decomposition.

Soil microorganisms implicated in diazinon degradation can be classified into three categories (see Sethunathan, 1972) with respect to their ability to degrade diazinon:

1. As sole carbon source (*Flavobacterium* sp.).
2. By cometabolism (*Arthrobacter* sp., *Corynebacterium* sp., *Pseudomonas melophthora*, *Streptomyces* sp., and *Trichoderma viride*).
3. By synergism (*Arthrobacter* sp. + *Streptomyces* sp.).

4.3.2.2. Parathion

Parathion and its methyl analog are probably the most widely used organophosphorus insecticides in agriculture. Among the organophosphates, parathion is perhaps the most resistant to chemical hydrolysis, especially in acidic and neutral conditions; but under alkaline conditions it is readily hydrolyzed (Faust and Gomaa, 1972). Sorption-catalyzed hydrolysis of parathion has been demonstrated in soil samples from Israel, but at very slow rates (Saltzman *et al.*, 1974; Yaron, 1975).

Parathion is relatively short-lived in most environments despite its resistance to chemical hydrolysis, simply because microbial degradation constitutes the major means of detoxication of parathion-polluted environments (Sethunathan *et al.*, 1977). The first established pathway for microbially mediated metabolism of parathion was via nitro group reduction to aminoparathion, but recent evidence suggests significant biological hydrolysis of parathion to *p*-nitrophenol and diethylthiophosphoric acid in natural ecosystems such as flooded soils, lake sediments, and water, especially after repeated additions (Sudhakar-Barik and Sethunathan, 1978*a*).

The degradation of parathion in four Philippine soils proceeded more rapidly under flooded than under upland conditions (Sethunathan and Yoshida, 1973*c*). The principal pathway of parathion after the first addition to a flooded soil was nitro group reduction. But after a second addition, substantial hydrolysis of parathion occurred in addition to nitro group reduction, while after the third addition the pathway shifted essentially to hydrolysis (Sudhakar-Barik *et al.*, 1979). The degradation pattern for all successive additions of parathion followed first-order kinetics, but kinetic constants indicated that hydrolysis proceeded at a faster rate than nitro group reduction. The population of parathion-hydrolyzing microorganisms increased considerably after repeated additions of the insecticide. Furthermore, parathion was converted to aminoparathion in a flooded soil not exposed to *p*-nitrophenol previously; but, in a flooded soil pretreated twice with *p*-nitrophenol, parathion was readily hydrolyzed (Fig. 4.1). The hydrolysis of

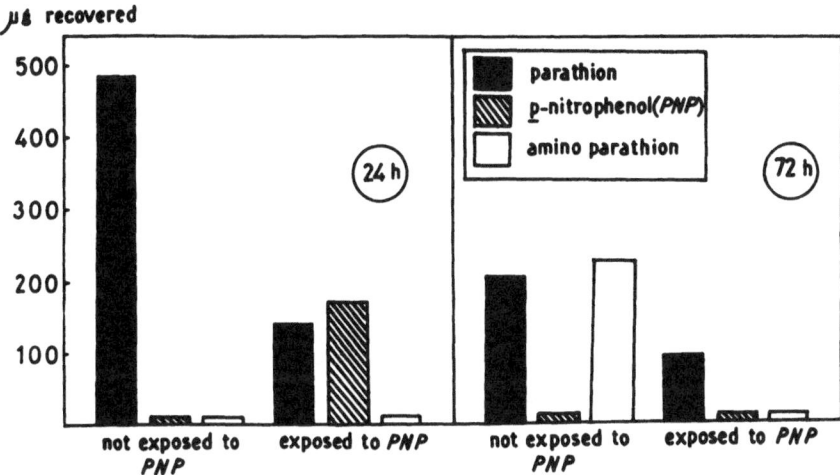

Figure 4.1.   Shift in the degradation pathway of parathion from nitro group reduction to hydrolysis in a flooded soil previously exposed to *p*-nitrophenol.

parathion, mediated by a constitutive enzyme, is not an energy-yielding reaction, and proliferation of parathion-hydrolyzing microorganisms actually occurred during the metabolism of *p*-nitrophenol.

The first direct evidence for microbial hydrolysis of parathion was obtained when the resting and growing cells and the cell-free suspension of *Flavobacterium* sp., isolated from diazinon-treated rice fields, showed an exceptional capacity to hydrolyze parathion, but its hydrolysis product, *p*-nitrophenol, persisted (Sethunathan and Yoshida, 1973*b*). In yet another study, *Pseudomonas* sp., also isolated from a flooded soil but amended with parathion, not only hydrolyzed parathion but also metabolized *p*-nitrophenol to form nitrite and carbon dioxide (Siddaramappa *et al.*, 1973; Sudhakar-Barik *et al.*, 1976). Even *m*-nitrophenol, known for its resistance to biodegradation, was metabolized by *Corynebacterium* sp. of flooded soil origin. These observations, together with the extreme instability of various nitrophenols in flooded soils (Sudhakar-Barik and Sethunathan, 1978*b*), certainly show that flooded soils harbor microorganisms, essentially bacteria, capable of hydrolyzing parathion and metabolizing related nitrophenols.

In most reported studies with flooded soils, pesticides were applied to the soils at the time of flooding and then monitored for their disappearance. In this system, pesticides are exposed to aerobic conditions for a week or more after flooding before anaerobiosis sets in. But in transplanted rice cultures pesticides are applied to the standing crop several days after soil submergence, when the soil is already in a reduced state. The persistence of parathion in the soils was influenced by the period of submergence prior to the addition of the insecticide (Wahid, 1978). Thus, parathion applied to soils preflooded for 10 and 20 days disappeared more rapidly than parathion added to soils at the time of flooding. The more the soil was reduced by presubmergence at the time of the addition of parathion, the more rapid was its degradation via nitro group reduction.

In equilibration studies (Wahid *et al.*, 1980), instantaneous surface-catalyzed degradation of parathion to aminoparathion occurred when the insecticide was shaken, even for less than 5 sec, with soils reduced by prior incubation under flooding (Fig. 4.2). Aminoparathion was further converted by dealkylation to desethyl aminoparathion in the acid sulfate soils, but not in other soils. Based on persistence data with irradiated, autoclaved, and sodium-azide-treated soils, parathion degradation in prereduced soils appeared to be mediated by soil enzymes and/or other heat-labile substances produced by soil anaerobiosis.

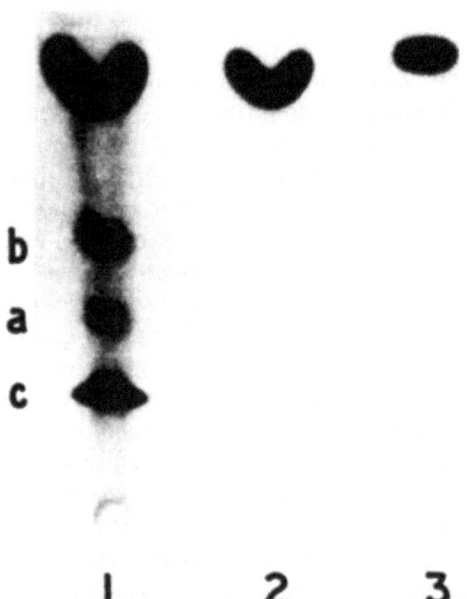

Figure 4.2. Radioautograph of parathion and its degradation products formed within 5 sec of equilibration with anaerobic *Pokkali* (acid sulfate) soil. (1) Anaerobic soil; (2) aerobic soil; (3) standard parathion; (a) aminoparathion; (b) desethyl aminoparathion; (c) unidentified product (Wahid *et al.*, 1980).

4.3.2.3. Other Organophosphates

Methyl parathion and fenitrothion, related to parathion with a common P–O–C linkage and a nitro substituent, were converted to their respective amino analogs in a flooded soil (Adhya *et al.*, 1981*a*). Particularly interesting was the nitro group reduction of both insecticides even after repeated additions vis-à-vis the shift from nitro group reduction to hydrolysis reported for parathion. The relative importance of biological hydrolysis of methyl parathion and fenitrothion in soil and water systems is yet to be established, although in at least one instance these two insecticides were hydrolyzed with ease by a *Flavobacterium* sp. (Adhya *et al.*, 1981*b*), the bacterium that hydrolyzed diazinon and parathion (Sethunathan and Yoshida, 1973*b*).

4.3.3. Carbamate Insecticides

The use of carbamate pesticides in tropical agriculture is very recent. For instance, in recent years the tremendous buildup of brown planthoppers *(Nilaparvata lugens)* in rice has led to the extensive and intensive use of the *N*-methylcarbamates carbofuran and carbaryl, by far the most effective insecticides for controlling this pest. Despite increasing use of these insecticides, our knowledge of their metabolic fate in tropical environments is rather limited.

Similar to several organophosphorus pesticides, carbofuran (Fullmer, 1977) and carbaryl (Aly and El-Dib, 1972) are susceptible to chemical hydrolysis under alkaline conditions. But in neutral soils and in acid soils capable of attaining near-neutral pH after incubation under flooding—a condition that hastens their degradation—degradation of these insecticides is both chemical and biological. Thus, heat treatment of the flooded soils prior to their incubation with insecticides increased the persistence of both carbofuran (Venkateswarlu *et al.*, 1977) and carbaryl (Venkateswarlu *et al.*, 1980), although appreciable loss of these insecticides occurred also from heat-sterilized soils, possibly by chemical means. Recent studies indicate that flooded soils harbor microorganisms (bacteria and actinomycetes) capable of degrading carbofuran and carbaryl (Venkateswarlu, 1979). Of special mention is the metabolism of both carbofuran and carbaryl in a yeast-extract-supplemented mineral medium by a *Pseudomonas* sp., isolated from a flooded soil amended with carbofuran (Venkateswarlu *et al.*, 1980). Yet the microbial involvement in carbofuran degradation has not been very convincing because no significant proliferation of carbofuran-degrading microorganisms occurred upon repeated additions of carbofuran to flooded soils (Siddaramappa *et al.*, 1978; Venkateswarlu and Sethunathan, 1978; Siddaramappa and Seiber, 1979). In fact, chemical degradation may be more important in the loss of carbofuran in situations where diurnal fluctuations in the pH of the flood water of rice fields ranged from 7.0 to as high as 9.5 (Seiber et al., 1978; Siddaramappa et al., 1978). For carbaryl, evidence for microbial degradation was more conclusive when a strain of Achromobacter sp. utilized it as a sole carbon source with concomitant formation of 1-naphthol, hydroquinone, catechol, and pyruvate (Sud et al., 1972).

Carbofuran phenol, the major product of carbofuran metabolism in flooded soils, accumulated under continued anaerobiosis (Venkateswarlu and Sethunathan, 1979). Concomitantly, evolution of $^{14}CO_2$ from the aromatic ring in carbofuran was almost negligible, accounting for less than 0.9% of the ring-^{14}C even after 40 days of flooding as compared to 27% released from the carbonyl-^{14}C (Venkateswarlu and Sethunathan, 1979).

Another insecticide, Baygon, was converted to 2-isopropyl phenol by a soil bacterium, Pseudomonas sp. (Gupta et al., 1975).

4.3.4. Fungicides

Information on the fate of relatively few fungicides in tropical areas is available, although their use is far less extensive than that of insecticides.

A widely used carboxanilide fungicide, carboxin, was converted to sulfoxide in all five soils under nonflooded conditions, but further degradation to aminophenol, ammonium, and nitrite occurred only in two soils (Balasubramanya, 1977). Under flooded conditions, the reaction ceased at the sulfoxide stage. The degradation of carboxin to sulfoxide proceeded in both sterile and nonsterile soils and past sulfoxide only in nonsterile soils. However, a strain of Pseudomonas sp., isolated by the soil perfusion technique, converted carboxin to sulfoxide, sulfone, 2-(vinylsulfonyl) acetanilide, 2-(2-hydroxyethylsulfonyl) acetic acid, aminophenol, ammonium, and nitrite in that order (Balasubramanya et al., 1980). Likewise, oxycarboxin was decomposed by the same bacterium first to 2-(vinylsulfonyl) acetanilide and thereafter by the same pathways as for carboxin.

A soil bacterium, Pseudomonas fragi, decomposed dexon through cometabolism to several products; the major product was identified as N,N-dimethyl-p-phenylenediamine (DMPDA); dexon applied to a nonflooded soil disappeared in 60 days, and DMPDA was the major product (Karanth and Vasantharajan, 1973; Karanth et al., 1974).

In aerobic soils, thiram was converted to dimethylamine, carbon disulfide, and an unidentified divalent sulfur compound (Raghu et al., 1974, 1975). The unidentified compound was subsequently characterized as copper dimethyl dithiocarbamate ($CuDDC_2$) (Kumarasamy and Raghu, 1976). DDC-α-aminobutyric acid was the major product of its metabolism by a strain of Pseudomonas sp. The breakdown products of thiram, particularly $CuDDC_2$, were highly fungitoxic, and this would explain, at least in part, the prolonged fungitoxicity of thiram despite its instability in soil. Also, ziram was decomposed by a soil bacterium essentially to water-soluble metabolites, which were not identified (Raghu *et al.*, 1976).

4.4. FACTORS INFLUENCING PERSISTENCE OF PESTICIDES

Soil properties known to influence the microbial activities and thereby the persistence of pesticides in tropical areas include moisture, organic matter content, redox status, acidity, temperature, sorption–desorption, and mineral constituents. Also, there is evidence that the persistence of a pesticide is altered significantly in the presence of another pesticide.

4.4.1. Soil Moisture

Soil moisture has a profound and direct effect on the proliferation of microorganisms and their activities. Water that competes for adsorption sites with pesticides determines the amount of pesticides available for microbial attack. Moreover, the aeration of the soil is closely linked with its moisture levels. Following heavy rain or flooding as in rice culture, the bulk of the soil is reduced and anaerobic (obligate or facultative) microorganisms become predominant. It is now well known that soil flooding accelerates the degradation of at least some persistent pesticides as discussed under Section 4.3.1. The order of persistence of pesticides in aerobic systems generally follows the order: chlorinated hydrocarbons > organophosphtes = carbamates (Kearney *et al.*, 1969). But this generalization may not always be applicable to anaerobic systems because of the susceptibility of several, if not all, chlorinated hydrocarbon pesticides to anaerobic biodegradation, with persistence curves as low as or lower than those of selected organophosphate and carbamate pesticides (Fig. 4.3). For instance, HCH, a chlorinated hydrocarbon, almost completely disappeared within 20 days of its application to microbially active soils under flooded conditions (Siddaramappa and Sethunathan, 1975), but degradation of carbofuran, a carbamate, in these soils was relatively slow during the same period (Venkateswarlu *et al.*, 1977). This emphasizes an urgent need for a systematic evaluation of the persistence curves of more pesticides from different groups under both aerobic and anaerobic conditions before generalizations on pesticide stability in the environment are made.

In many tropical areas characterized by intermittent heavy rain and dry seasons, soils are subjected to alternate periods of flooding and drying with concomitant increases in the activities of anaerobic and aerobic microorganisms, respectively. Such alternate reduction and oxidation cycles in the soil could provide a favorable environment for more extensive destruction of organic com-

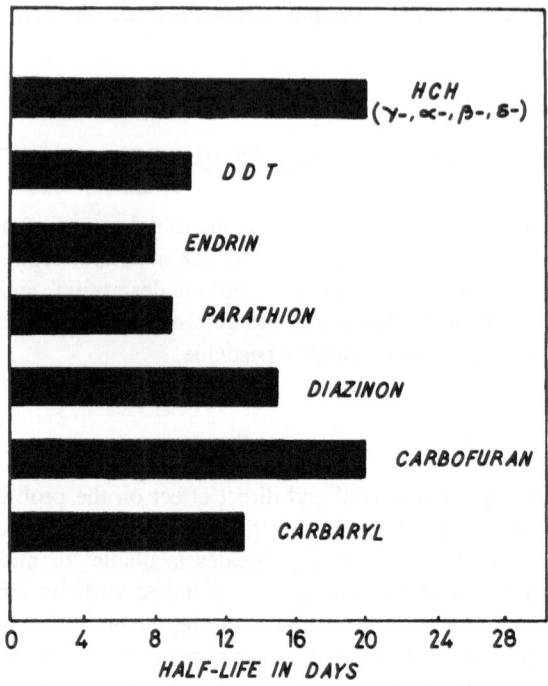

Figure 4.3.   Half-life (days) of selected pesticides in flooded soils (adapted from Sethunathan and Siddaramappa, 1978).

pounds than in either system alone. This is especially true for molecules possessing ring moieties since ring cleavage reaction requires oxygen. Diazinon was hydrolyzed in flooded soil, but the ring portion of its hydrolysis product was cleaved only under aerobic conditions following anaerobiosis (Sethunathan, 1972). Likewise, anaerobic degradation of parathion in a flooded soil led to the formation of aminoparathion and possibly other easily soil-bound residues (Katan *et al.*, 1976). *p*-Nitrophenol, formed readily after two or three additions of parathion to flooded soil, was converted to soil-bound residues under continued anaerobiosis, in contrast to its almost complete mineralization to CO_2 under aerobic conditions (Sudhakar-Barik and Sethunathan, 1978*b*). In flooded soils, conversion of DDT to DDD occurred rapidly, but DDD persisted. Probably more complete destruction of DDT past DDD can be accomplished in a system where anaerobiosis is followed by aerobiosis, as demonstrated in the extensive degradation of DDT past DDD to *p*-chlorophenylacetic acid, formed by cleavage of one of the aromatic rings by *Hydrogenomonas* sp. (Pfaender and Alexander,

1972). In recent years, there has been serious concern over the significant formation of soil-bound residues from soil-applied pesticides, especially under anaerobic conditions. The practical feasibility of accelerating the complete destruction of soil-bound residues of pesticides by returning the anaerobic system to aerobic conditions or vice versa merits intensive study.

4.4.2. Organic Matter

The importance of organic matter, native or added, in influencing the persistence of pesticides in the environment is well established. Microbial activity in a soil is very intimately associated with its organic matter content. Most tropical soils have low organic matter content due to its rapid mineralization. The addition of organic materials—a common practice to raise fertility, especially of tropical soils—increases the microbial activity and in turn accelerates the degradation of several pesticides. The higher the organic matter content in the soil, the more rapid was the degradation of chlorinated hydrocarbon insecticides, DDT, endrin, heptachlor, and four isomers (α, β, δ, γ) of HCH in flooded Philippine soils (Castro and Yoshida, 1974). The addition of organic sources such as rice straw and cellulose to flooded soils with low organic matter content further accelerated the degradation of these insecticides, but the stimulatory effect of added organic matter was less pronounced in soils with high native organic matter content. Similarly, degradation of β- and γ-HCH (Siddaramappa and Sethunathan, 1975), endrin (Gowda and Sethunathan, 1977), and carbofuran (Venkateswarlu and Sethunathan, 1979) in flooded soils proceeded much faster in the presence of rice straw than in its absence. The effect of added organic matter on the degradation of parathion in flooded soils was not always stimulatory and was governed by the pathway of its degradation (Sethunathan, 1973; Rajaram and Sethunathan, 1975). Thus the addition of organic sources to flooded soils stimulated the nitro group reduction of parathion, but its hydrolysis in a flooded soil that was inoculated with a parathion-hydrolyzing enrichment culture was almost completely inhibited by organic matter amendment. The factor inhibiting parathion hydrolysis was a water-soluble and low-molecular-weight substance(s) formed during anaerobic decomposition of organic matter in flooded soil (Rajaram and Sethunathan, 1976; Rajaram *et al.*, 1978), possibly aliphatic and/or phenolic acids which accumulate in flooded soils amended with organic matter.

4.4.3. Redox Conditions

The redox status of a soil as an important parameter in the environmental fate of pesticides was demonstrated very recently. The redox potentials of most soils especially rich in native organic matter content drop within a few days after flooding, and this drop is further accentuated in the presence of added organic sources.

The extent of degradation of β- and γ-HCH in different soils was related to the redox potentials attained by the soils following flooding (Siddaramappa and Sethunathan, 1975). The degradation of these isomers occurred only in microbially active soils capable of attaining potentials of -40 to -100 mV within a few days after flooding; degradation of β-HCH proceeded at a potential lower than that required for γ-HCH degradation. These observations are in substantial agreement with the reported molecular orbital calculations for the isomers of HCH (Block and Newland, 1975). Likewise, endrin degradation was favored by a potential of < -120 mV (Gowda and Sethunathan, 1976). Also, free oxygen, potassium nitrate, and manganese oxide, all known for their exceptional capacity to stabilize the potentials at high levels even under flooded conditions, retarded the degradation of γ-HCH in flooded soils (Yoshida and Castro, 1970). This would explain the relatively long persistence of this and related chlorinated hydrocarbon insecticides in aerobic nonflooded soils. Low potentials would certainly favor the activity and proliferation of *Clostridium* sp. and other anaerobes implicated in the degradation of HCH and related pesticides. However, ring cleavage reactions are remarkably slow or virtually stopped at low redox potentials.

4.4.4. Soil Acidity

The degradation of some pesticides, organophosphates and carbamates in particular, is affected by the pH of the soil. Although most organosphosphates undergo chemical hydrolysis under alkaline conditions, diazinon showed extreme chemical instability in acid soils (Sethunathan and MacRae, 1969). Carbamates are also rapidly hydrolyzed under alkaline conditions, as reported for carbofuran in natural ecosystems (Seiber *et al.*, 1978), whereas carbofuran persisted in acid soils (Venkateswarlu *et al.*, 1977). The persistence of organochlorine insecticides is seldom affected by soil pH. However, HCH and DDT decomposed much faster in alkaline soils (pH 9.5) than in soils with lower pH (Chawla and Chopra, 1967). In addition to the direct effects on the organic molecules, the pH may also have indirect influence on their persistence, because of its effect on microbial activities and sorption–desorption. The degradation of HCH isomers was slow in an acid sulfate soil with extremely low pH even under flooded conditions, a finding attributed to low microbial activity (Siddaramappa and Sethunathan, 1975).

4.4.5. Soil Temperature

Temperature is probably an important factor affecting the persistence of pesticides in the soil, especially in the tropics. High temperatures exist in the tropics and should favor pesticide loss through volatilization and increased microbial activity. Unfortunately, much less is known on the relationship of temperature to pesticide behavior in the tropical environments than in the temperate zone. In one instance, however, γ-HCH was shown to undergo more rapid decomposition in a flooded soil at 35°C than at 25°C (Yoshida and Castro, 1970), possibly due to increased microbial activity and a rapid decrease in the redox potential at the higher temperature (Cho and Ponnamperuma, 1971). Clearly, pesticides may undergo more rapid decomposition in a tropical soil than in a temperate soil.

4.4.6. Sorption–Desorption

Sorption–desorption by the soils largely determine the amount of pesticides available for losses through biodegradation and transport phenomena. Organic matter was the most important single factor responsible for the sorption of parathion (Wahid and Sethunathan, 1978) and three isomers (α, β, and γ) of HCH (Wahid and Sethunathan, 1979a). In soils oxidized with H_2O_2, clay and free iron oxides were implicated in sorption. Up to a 2% organic matter level, sorption of parathion was a result of an interaction between organic and inorganic surfaces; beyond a 2% organic matter level, the role of inorganic soil constituents was apparently masked, a finding attributed to "organic masking" of the inorganic surfaces. Soils prereduced by flooding sorbed less lindane than the aerobic soil, while desorption was not affected by soil anaerobiosis (Wahid and Sethunathan, 1980).

4.4.7. Mineral Constituents

Direct metabolism does not always account for widespread occurrence of reductive dechlorination of DDT to DDD in anaerobic environments since this reaction readily occurred even in oxygen-free sterile systems containing ferrous compounds (Glass, 1972; Parr and Smith, 1974). Glass (1972) proposed a mechanism for conversion of DDT to DDD whereby electrons furnished by the reduced organic substrate were transferred to DDT molecule via ferrous ion, thus initiating a free radical reaction. The addition of ferrous sulfate to a flooded soil rich in organic matter content led to more extensive metabolism of yet another insecticide, parathion, with the formation of six breakdown products including its amino analog in amended soil and only three products in unamended soil; but this effect was noticed also with other sulfate salts, viz., $MgSO_4$, $MnSO_4$, and K_2SO_4 (Rao and Sethunathan, 1979). Indeed sulfate rather than ferrous ion was implicated in the extensive metabolism of parathion in flooded soils.

More in-depth studies with acid sulfate soils confirmed the role of sulfate in parathion metabolism (Wahid and Sethunathan, 1979b). Parathion was rapidly converted to aminoparathion in acid sulfate soil and in soils with low sulfate

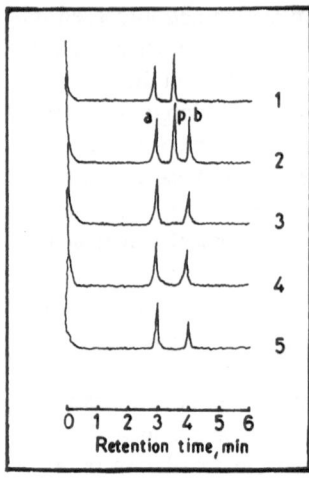

Figure 4.4. Gas chromatograms of the products of reactions between (1) parathion and anaerobic soil with low sulfate content; (2) parathion and anaerobic acid sulfate soil *(Pokkali)*; (3) aminoparathion and anaerobic *Pokkali* soil; (4) aminoparathion and sodium iodide; (5) aminoparathion and hydrogen sulfide. (a) Aminoparathion; (p) parathion; (b) desethyl aminoparathion (Wahid and Sethunathan, 1979*b*).

content under flooded conditions. But aminoparathion was further dealkylated to desethyl aminoparathion in acid sulfate soil, and not in other soils with low sulfate content. Moreover, the interaction between aminoparathion and hydrogen sulfide, and not between parathion and hydrogen sulfide, also yielded desethyl aminoparathion (Fig. 4.4). Clearly, hydrogen sulfide, the end product of sulfate metabolism in anaerobic environments, catalyzed the dealkylation of aminoparathion as follows:

$$C_2H_5O \underset{C_2H_5O}{\overset{\overset{\displaystyle S}{\|}}{\diagup}} P-O-\!\!\!\!\!\!\bigcirc\!\!\!\!-NO_2 \xrightarrow[\text{reduction}]{\text{surface-catalyzed}} C_2H_5O \underset{C_2H_5O}{\overset{\overset{\displaystyle S}{\|}}{\diagup}} P-O-\!\!\!\!\!\!\bigcirc\!\!\!\!-NH_2$$

$$\xrightarrow[\text{dealkylation}]{H_2S} C_2H_5O \underset{HO}{\overset{\overset{\displaystyle S}{\|}}{\diagup}} P-O-\!\!\!\!\!\!\bigcirc\!\!\!\!-NH_2$$

Likewise, our most recent studies (T. K. Adhya *et al.*, unpublished data) show that methyl aminoparathion and aminofenitrothion, formed from methyl parathion and fenitrothion, respectively, undergo dealkylation in flooded acid sulfate soils or upon reaction with hydrogen sulfide. Also, there is evidence that addition of sulfate accelerates the degradation of γ-HCH in flooded soil (Yoshida and Castro, 1970) and by a *Clostridium* sp. (Sethunathan *et al.*, 1969), but the mechanism is not clear. Interestingly, hydrogen sulfide has been implicated in the environmental transport of mercury when the interaction between hydrogen sulfide and mercury-containing sediment led to the evolution of volatile dimethyl mercury (Craig and Bartlett, 1978). Evidently, apart from the direct involvement of anaerobic microorganisms chemical transformations of pesticides and heavy metals, mediated by the microbial byproducts of anaerobic decomposition of inorganic soil components, can be common and widespread in anaerobic eco-systems such as lakes or estuarine sediments and flooded soils.

4.4.8. Pesticide Combinations

In recent years, it has been a common practice to apply different groups of pesticides either simultaneously or in rotation for effecting broad-spectrum con-trol of a variety of pests (e.g., insects, weeds, microbial pathogens) attacking a single crop, a practice leading to combined residues in the environment. More-over, commercial formulations of pesticide combinations (for example, Sevidol, containing carbaryl and HCH) are used increasingly in agriculture. But most studies are restricted to the overall disappearance of pesticides applied alone and not in combination. Recently, however, significant interactions between pesti-cides applied in combination, in terms of their persistence in soils and toxicity to crops and insects, have been demonstrated (Liang and Lichtenstein, 1974; Kaufman, 1977).

Parathion is generally short-lived in tropical flooded soils when applied singly. But benomyl, applied at a concentration as low as 5 ppm in combination with parathion, significantly increased the persistence of parathion (Fig. 4.5) by

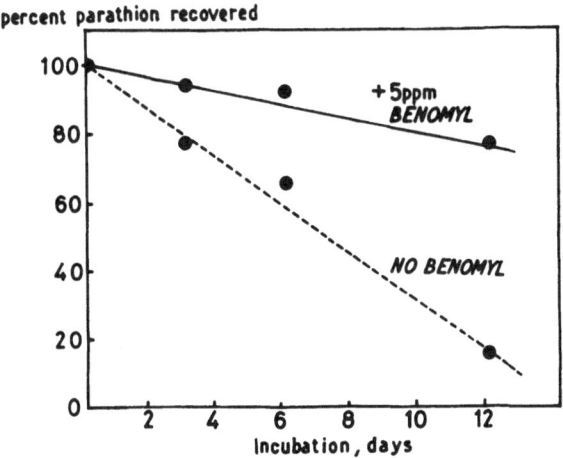

Figure 4.5. Relative persistence of parathion in unamended and benomyl-amended soil under flooded conditions (Sudhakar-Barik and Sethunathan, 1979).

inhibiting microbially mediated reactions of both nitro group reduction and hydrolysis (Sudhakar-Barik and Sethunathan, 1979). The persistence of parathion was not altered in the simultaneous presence of even 100 ppm of either HCH or 2,4-D.

The impact of pesticide combinations, vis-à-vis single applications, on microbial activities involved in pesticide degradation and biochemical transformations of importance to soil fertility merits more intensive study, particularly because the environment is subjected to pressure from more than one pesticide. From the standpoint of economical and efficient use of pesticides, especially in tropical agriculture, use of appropriate combinations could provide a potential means of increasing the persistence of readily biodegradable and short-lived pesticides, as clearly demonstrated with benomyl–parathion interaction. However, caution is warranted in such controlled persistence studies, since increased persistence of generally short-lived but highly toxic pesticides, such as several organophosphorous insecticides, under the impact of combinations may generate new problems of environmental pollution.

4.5. CONCLUSION

There is concern over environmental safety with recent increases in the number and quantity of synthetic pesticides, particularly the persistent chlorinated hydrocarbons, being introduced into tropical areas of intensive agriculture. There are considerable gaps in our knowledge of pesticide behavior and transport under more realistic field conditions in the tropics. Despite increasing use of inorganic fertilizers, little is known on the interaction between fertilizers and pesticides in the soil environment. Pesticide loss via volatilization, photodecomposition, and microbial degradation may be considerable under tropical conditions, but field measurements of the relative proportions of the pesticides lost due to these forces are not available. The extent of chemically catalyzed reactions in the environment merits more intensive study in the light of recent demonstration of the involvement of hydrogen sulfide in the transformation of parathion and mercury. Microbial degradation is by far the most powerful means of detoxifying many pesticides in the environment. But seeding the polluted environments with microorganisms capable of degrading pesticides is of questionable value owing to the inherent problems in the establishment of introduced microorganisms and possibly other side effects. Alternatively, selective stimulation of indigenous soil microflora with pesticide-degrading capabilities by suitable cultural practices, for example, flooding and organic matter amendment, provides a more effective and practical means of decontaminating pesticide-polluted environments.

REFERENCES

Adhya, T. K., Sudhakar-Barik, and Sethunathan, N., 1981*a*, Stability of selected organophosphorus insecticides in anaerobic soils, *J. Agric. Food Chem.* **29**:90.

Adhya, T. K., Sudhakar-Barik, and Sethunathan, N., 1981*b*, Hydrolysis of selected organophosphorus insecticides by two bacteria isolated from flooded soils, *J. Appl. Bacteriol.* **50**:167.

Adhya, T. K., Sudhakar-Barik, and Sethunathan, N., 1981*c*, Fate of fenitrothion, methyl parathion and parathion in anoxic sulfur-containing soil systems, *Pestic. Biochem. Physiol.* **16**:14.

Agnihothrudu, V., and Mithyantha, M. S., 1978, *Pesticide Residues: A Review of Indian Work*, Rallis India Limited, Bangalore, India.

Alexander, M., 1965, Biodegradation: Problems of molecular recalcitrance and microbial fallibility, *Adv. Appl. Microbiol.* **7**:35.

Aly, O. M., and El-Dib, M. A., 1972, Studies of the persistence of some carbamate insecticides in the aquatic environment, *Adv. Chem. Ser.* **111**:210.

Anonymous, 1966, *Annual Report of the International Rice Research Institute*, Los Banos, Philippines, p. 198.

Anonymous, 1979*a*, A status report of R & D work done in India, in: *Indo-US Workshop on Biodegradable Pesticides*, p. 69, Department of Science and Technology, New Delhi.

Anonymous, 1979*b*, *Pestic. Inf. (India)* **5**(2):29.

Aquino, G. B., and Pathak, M. D., 1976, Enhanced absorption and persistence of carbofuran and chlordimeform in rice plant on root zone application under flooded conditions, *J. Econ. Entomol.* **69**:686.

Audus, L. J., 1951, The biological detoxification of hormone herbicides in soil, *Plant Soil* **3**:170.

Balasubramanya, R. H., 1977, Microbial metabolism and behaviour in soil of two carboxanilide fungicides, p. 206, Ph.D. thesis, University of Agricultural Sciences, Bangalore, India.

Balasubramanya, R. H., Patil, R. B., Bhat, M. V., and Nagendrappa, G., 1980, Degradation of carboxin (Vitavax) and oxycarboxin (Plantvax) by *Pseudomonas aeruginosa* isolated from soil, *J. Environ. Sci. Health* **15B**:485.

Beland, F. A., Farwell, S. O., Robocker, A. E., and Geer, R. D., 1976, Electrochemical reduction and anaerobic degradation of lindane, *J. Agric. Food Chem.* **24**:753.

Bindra, O. S., and Kalra, R. L., 1973, *Progress and Problems in Pesticide-Residue Analysis*, p. 336, Punjab Agricultural University, Ludhiana, and Indian Council of Agricultural Research, New Delhi, India.

Block, A. M., and Newland, L. W., 1975, Molecular orbital calculations for the isomers of 1,2,3,4,5,6-hexachlorocyclohexane, in: *Environmental Quality and Safety*, Supplement II. *Pesticides* (F. Coulston, N. Y. Albany, and F. Korte, eds.), p. 569, Georg Thieme, Stuttgart.

Castro, T. F., and Yoshida, T., 1971, Degradation of organochlorine insecticides in flooded soils in the Philippines, *J. Agric. Food Chem.* **19**:1168.

Castro, T. F., and Yoshida, T., 1974, Effect of organic matter on the biodegradation of some organochlorine insecticides in submerged soils, *Soil Sci. Plant Nutr. (Tokyo)* **20**:363.

Chawla, R. P., and Chopra, S. L., 1967, Persistence of residues of DDT and BHC in normal and alkali soils, *J. Res. Punjab Agric. Univ.* **4**:96.

Cho, D. Y., and Ponnamperuma, F. N., 1971, Influence of soil temperature on the chemical kinetics of flooded soils and the growth of rice, *Soil Sci.* **112**:184.

Craig, P. J., and Bartlett, P. D., 1978, The role of hydrogen sulphide in environmental transport of mercury, *Nature (London)* **275**:635.

Faust, S. D., and Gomaa, H. M., 1972, Chemical hydrolysis of some organic phosphorus and carbamate pesticides in aquatic environments, *Environ. Lett.* **3**:171.

Fullmer, O. H., 1977, Report on Carbofuran, FMC Corporation, Agricultural Chemical Division, Richmond, California.

Glass, B. L., 1972, Relation between the degradation of DDT and iron redox system in soils, *J. Agric. Food Chem.* **20**:324.

Gowda, T. K. S., and Sethunathan, N., 1976, Persistence of endrin in Indian rice soils under flooded conditions, *J. Agric. Food Chem.* **24**:750.

Gowda, T. K. S., and Sethunathan, N., 1977, Endrin decomposition in soils as influenced by aerobic and anaerobic conditions, *Soil Sci.* **124**:5.

Gupta, K. G., Sud, R. K., Aggarwal, P. K., and Aggarwal, J. C., 1975, Effect of baygon on some soil biological processes and its degradation by *Pseudomonas* sp., *Plant Soil* **42**:317.

Haider, K., Jagnow, G., and Rohr, R., 1976, Anaerober Abbau von γ-Hexachlorocyclohexan durch eine bakterielle Microflora des Bodens und des Kuhpansens, *Landwirtsch. Forsch.* **32**(II):147.

Heritage, A. D., and MacRae, I. C., 1977, Identification of intermediates formed during the degradation of hexachlorocyclohexanes by *Clostridium sphenoides*, *Appl. Environ. Microbiol.* **33**:1295.

Heritage, A. D., and MacRae, I. C., 1979, Degradation of hexachlorocyclohexanes and structurally related substances by *Clostridium sphenoides*, *Aust. J. Biol. Sci.* **32**:493.

Jagnow, G., Haider, K., and Ellwardt, P. Chr., 1977, Anaerobic dechlorination and degradation of hexachlorocyclohexane isomers by anaerobic and facultative anaerobic bacteria, *Arch. Microbiol.* **115**:285.

Karanth, N. G. K., and Vasantharajan, V. N., 1973, Persistence and effect of dexon on soil respiration, *Soil Biol. Biochem.* **5**:679.

Karanth, N. G. K., Bhat, S. G., Vaidyanathan, C. S., and Vasantharajan, V. N., 1974, Conversion of dexon (*p*-dimethylaminobenzene diazo sodium sulfonate) to *N,N*-dimethyl-*p*-phenylene diamine by *Pseudomonas fragi* Bk 9, *Appl. Microbiol.* **27**:43.

Katan, J., Fuhremann, T. W., and Lichtenstein, E. P., 1976, Binding of ^{14}C-parathion in soil: A reassessment of pesticide persistence, *Science* **193**:891.

Kaufman, D. D., 1977, Biodegradation and persistence of several acetamide, acylanilide, azide, carbamate and organophosphate combinations, *Soil Biol. Biochem.* **9**:49.

Kearney, P. C., and Helling, C. S., 1969, Reactions of pesticides in soils, *Residue Rev.* **25**:25.

Kearney, P. C., Nash, R. G., and Isensee, A. R., 1969, Persistence of pesticide residues in soils, in: *Chemical Fallout: Current Research on Persistent Pesticides* (M. W. Miller and G. G. Berg, eds.), p. 531, C. C. Thomas, Springfield, Illinois.

Kulshreshtha, J. P., Anjaneyulu, A., and Padmanabhan, S. Y., 1974, The disastrous brown planthopper attack in Kerala, *Ind. Farming* **24**:5.

Kumarasamy, R., and Raghu, K., 1976, Copper dimethyldithiocarbamate, a degradation product of thiram in soil, *Chemosphere* **5**:107.

Liang, T. T., and Lichtenstein, E. P., 1974, Synergism of insecticides by herbicides: Effect of environmental factors, *Science* **186**:1128.

MacRae, I. C., Raghu, K., and Castro, T. F., 1967, Persistence and biodegradation of four common isomers of benzenehexachloride in submerged soils, *J. Agric. Food Chem.* **15**:911.

MacRae, I. C., Raghu, K., and Bautista, E. M., 1969, Anaerobic degradation of the insecticide lindane by *Clostridium* sp., *Nature (London)* **221**:859.

Matsumura, F., Khanvilkar, V. G., Patil, K. C., and Boush, G. M., 1971, Metabolism of endrin by certain soil microorganisms, *J. Agric. Food Chem.* **19**:27.

Ohisa, N., and Yamaguchi, M., 1978a, Gamma-BHC degradation accompanied by the growth of *Clostridium rectum* isolated from paddy field soil, *Agric. Biol. Chem.* **42**:1819.

Ohisa, N., and Yamaguchi, M., 1978b, Degradation of gamma-BHC in flooded soils enriched with peptone, *Agric. Biol. Chem.* **42**:1983.

Parr, J. F., and Smith, S., 1974, Degradation of DDT in an everglades muck as affected by lime, ferrous ion and anaerobiosis, *Soil Sci.* **118**:45.

Patil, K. C., Matsumura, F., and Boush, G. M., 1970, Degradation of endrin, aldrin, and DDT by soil microorganisms, *Appl. Microbiol.* **19**:879.

Pfaender, F. K., and Alexander, M., 1972, Extensive microbial degradation of DDT *in vitro* and DDT metabolism in natural communities, *J. Agric. Food Chem.* **20**:842.

Raghu, K., and MacRae, I. C., 1966, Biodegradation of the gamma-isomer of benzenehexachloride in submerged soils, *Science* **154**:263.

Raghu, K., Murthy, N. B. K., and Kumarasamy, R., 1974, Degradation of thiram in soils, in: *Proceedings of the Department of Atomic Energy Symposium on Use of Radiations and Radioisotopes in Studies of Plant Productivity*, p. 874, Bhabha Atomic Research Centre, Bombay.

Raghu, K., Murthy, N. B. K., Kumarasamy, R., Sudha-Rao, R., and Sane, P. V., 1975, Fate and persistence of thiram in plants and soils, in: *Origin and Fate of Chemical Residues in Food, Agriculture and Fisheries*, p. 137, International Atomic Energy Agency, Vienna.

Raghu, K., Kumarasamy, R., Sudha-Rao, R., Murthy, N. B. K., and Sane, P. V., 1976, Metabolism of labelled ziram in groundnut plants and its microbiological degradation, in: *Trace Contaminants of Agriculture, Fisheries and Food in Developing Countries*, p. 37, International Atomic Energy Agency, Vienna.

Rajaram, K. P., and Sethunathan, N., 1975, Effect of organic sources on the degradation of parathion in flooded alluvial soil, *Soil Sci.* **119**:296.

Rajaram, K. P., and Sethunathan, N., 1976, A factor inhibiting parathion hydrolysis in organic matter-amended soil under flooded conditions, *Plant Soil* **44**:683.

Rajaram, K. P., Rao, Y. R., and Sethunathan, N., 1978, Inhibition of biological hydrolysis of parathion in rice straw-amended flooded soil and its reversal by nitrogen compounds and aerobic conditions, *Pestic. Sci.* **9**:155.

Rao, Y. R., and Sethunathan, N., 1979, Effect of ferrous sulfate on the degradation of parathion in flooded soil, *J. Environ. Sci. Health* **14B**:335.

Saltzman, S., Yaron, B., and Mingelgrin, U., 1974, The surface-catalyzed hydrolysis of parathion on kaolinites, *Soil Sci. Soc. Am. Proc.* **38**:231.

Seiber, J. N., Catahan, M. P., and Berril, C. R., 1978, Loss of carbofuran from rice paddy water: Chemical and physical factors, *J. Environ. Sci. Health* **13B**:131.

Sethunathan, N., 1972, Diazinon degradation in submerged soil and rice-paddy water, *Adv. Chem. Ser.* **111**:244.

Sethunathan, N., 1973, Organic matter and parathion degradation in flooded soil, *Soil Biol. Biochem.* **5**:641.

Sethunathan, N., and MacRae, I. C., 1969, Persistence and biodegradation of diazinon in submerged soils, *J. Agric. Food Chem.* **17**:221.

Sethunathan, N., and Siddaramappa, R., 1978, Microbial degradation of pesticides in rice soils, in: *Soils and Rice* (F. N. Ponnamperuma, ed.), p. 479, International Rice Research Institute, Los Banos, Philippines.

Sethunathan, N., and Yoshida, T., 1969, Fate of diazinon in submerged soil: Accumulation of hydrolysis product, *J. Agric. Food Chem.* **17**:1192.

Sethunathan, N., and Yoshida, T., 1973*a*, Degradation of chlorinated hydrocarbons by *Clostridium* sp. isolated from lindane-amended flooded soil, *Plant Soil* **38**:663.

Sethunathan, N., and Yoshida, T., 1973*b*, A *Flavobacterium* sp. that degrades diazinon and parathion, *Can. J. Microbiol.* **19**:873.

Sethunathan, N., and Yoshida, T., 1973*c*, Parathion degradation in submerged rice soils in the Philippines, *J. Agric. Food Chem.* **21**:504.

Sethunathan, N., Bautista, E. M., and Yoshida, T., 1969, Degradation of benzenehexachloride by a soil bacterium, *Can. J. Microbiol.* **15**:1349.

Sethunathan, N., Caballa, S., and Pathak, M. D., 1971, Absorptin and translocation of diazinon by rice plants from submerged soils and paddy water and the persistence of residues in plant tissues, *J. Econ. Entomol.* **64**:571.

Sethunathan, N., Siddaramappa, R., Rajaram, K. P., Barik, S., and Wahid, P. A., 1977, Parathion: Residues in soil and water, *Residue Rev.* **68**:91.

Siddaramappa, R., and Seiber, J. N., 1979, Persistence of carbofuran in flooded rice soils and water, *Progr. Water Technol.* **11**:103.

Siddaramappa, R., and Sethunathan N., 1975, Persistence of gamma-BHC and beta-BHC in Indian rice soils under flooded conditions, *Pestic. Sci.* **6**:395.

Siddaramappa, R., and Sethunathan, N., 1976, Volatilization of lindane from water in soil-free and flooded soil sytems, *J. Environ. Sci. Health* **11B**:119.

Siddaramappa, R., and Watanabe, I., 1979, Evidence for vapor loss of C-14-Carbofuran from rice plants, *Bull. Environ. Contam. Toxicol.* **23**:544.

Siddaramappa, R., Rajaram, K. P., and Sethunathan, N., 1973, Degradation of parathion by bacteria isolated from flooded soil, *Appl. Microbiol.* **26**:846.

Siddaramappa, R., Tirol, A. C., Seiber, J. N., Heinrichs, E. A., and Watanabe, I., 1978, The degradation of carbofuran in paddy water and flooded soil of untreated and retreated rice fields, *J. Environ. Sci. Health* **13B**:369.

Sud, R. K., Sud, A. K., and Gupta, K. G., 1972, Degradation of sevin (1-napthyl *N*-methyl carbamate) by *Achromobacter* sp., *Arch. Microbiol.* **87**:353.

Sudhakar-Barik, and Sethunathan, N., 1978*a*, Biological hydrolysis of parathion in natural ecosystems, *J. Environ. Qual.* **7**:346.

Sudhakar-Barik, and Sethunathan, N., 1978*b*, Metabolism of nitrophenols in flooded soils, *J. Environ. Qual.* **7**:349.

Sudhakar-Barik, and Sethunathan, N., 1979, Persistence of parathion increased by benomyl in flooded soil, *Progr. Water Technol.* **11**:113.

Sudhakar-Barik, Siddaramappa, R., and Sethunathan, N., 1976, Metabolism of nitrophenols by bacteria isolated from parathion-amended flooded soil, *Antonie van Leeuwenhoek: J. Microbiol. Serol.* **42**:461.

Sudhakar-Barik, Wahid, P. A., Ramakrishna, C., and Sethunathan, N., 1979, A change in the degradation pathway of parathion after repeated applications to flooded soil, *J. Agric. Food Chem.* **27**:1391.

Talekar, N. S., Sun, L.-T., Lee, E.-M., and Chen, J.-S., 1977, Persistence of some insecticides in subtropical soil, *J. Agric. Food Chem.* **25**:349.

Tomizawa, C., 1977, Past and present status of residues of pesticides manufactured in Japan, *Jpn. Pestic. Inf.* **30**:5.

Tsukano, Y., and Kobayashi, A., 1972, Formation of γ-BTC in flooded rice field soils treated with γ-BHC, *Agric. Biol. Chem.* **36**:166.

Venkateswarlu, K., 1979, Microbial degradation of carbamate insecticides in rice soils, p. 127, Ph.D. thesis, Utkal University, Bhubaneswar, India.

Venkateswarlu, K., and Sethunathan, N., 1978, Degradation of carbofuran in rice soils as influenced by repeated application and exposure to aerobic conditions following anaerobiosis, *J. Agric. Food Chem.* **26**:1148.

Venkateswarlu, K., and Sethunathan, N., 1979, Metabolism of carbofuran in rice straw-amended and unamended rice soils, *J. Environ. Qual.* **8**:365.

Venkateswarlu, K., Gowda, T. K. S., and Sethunathan, N., 1977, Persistence and biodegradation of carbofuran in flooded soils, *J. Agric. Food Chem.* **25**:553.

Venkateswarlu, K., Chendrayan, K., and Sethunathan, N., 1980, Persistence and biodegradation of carbaryl in soils, *J. Environ. Sci. Health* **15B**:421.

Wahid, P. A., 1978, Behaviour of pesticides in soils, p. 139, Ph.D. thesis, Utkal University, Bhubaneswar, India.

Wahid, P. A., and Sethunathan, N., 1978, Sorption–desorption of parathion in soils, *J. Agric. Food Chem.* **26**:101.

Wahid, P. A., and Sethunathan, N., 1979a, Sorption–desorption of α, β and γ-isomers of hexa-chlorocyclohexane in soils, *J. Agric. Food Chem.* **27**:1050.

Wahid, P. A., and Sethunathan, N., 1979b, Involvement of hydrogen sulphide in the degradation of parathion in flooded acid sulphate soil, *Nature (London)* **282**:401.

Wahid, P. A., and Sethunathan, N., 1980, Sorption–desorption of lindane by anaerobic soils, *J. Agric. Food Chem.* **28**:623.

Wahid, P. A., Ramakrishna, C., and Sethunathan, N., 1980, Instantaneous degradation of parathion in anaerobic soils, *J. Environ. Qual.* **9**:127.

Williams, P. P., 1977, Metabolism of synthetic organic pesticides by anaerobic microorganisms, *Residue Rev.* **66**:63.

Yaron, B., 1975, Chemical conversion of parathion on soil surfaces, *Soil Sci. Soc. Am. Proc.* **39**:639.

Yoshida, T., and Castro, T. F., 1970, Degradation of gamma-BHC in rice soils, *Soil Sci. Soc. Am. Proc.* **34**:440.

Yoshida, T., and Castro, T. F., 1975, Degradation of 2,4-D, 2,4,5-T and picloram in two Philippine soils, *Soil Sci. Plant Nutr. (Tokyo)* **21**:397.

5

Persistence and Biodegradation of Herbicides

Floyd M. Ashton

5.1. INTRODUCTION

The destruction of herbicides applied to the environment by man is essential to their sustained use. Without such a mechanism, they would ultimately accumulate to levels that would be phytotoxic to most higher plants. Ideally a given herbicide should persist just long enough to control the target weeds and then be rapidly degraded to its constituent atoms. The accomplishment of this ideal situation can only be a goal; however, it must be approximated for a truly successful practice. If the period of persistence is too short, weed control will be inadequate and other control measures must be utilized. If the period of persistence is too long, injury to susceptible plants subsequently planted or long-term environmental pollution can occur. Based on our present knowledge, the latter situation does not appear to be a problem with the herbicides currently used; however, it must be an area of continuing investigation.

Herbicides are inactivated in the environment by biological, chemical, and physical means. This inactivation usually involves degradation of the molecule; however, certain intact herbicide molecules can also be made nonphytotoxic by binding tightly to other substances. The means and rate of inactivation depend upon the nature of the herbicide molecule and the environmental conditions. In general, biodegradation is dominant, but certain herbicides undergo chemical change or physical modification more readily. A limited number of herbicides

Floyd M. Ashton • Department of Botany, University of California, Davis, California 95616.

undergo molecular changes in nature that result in a compound that is more phytotoxic than the parent molecule, i.e., 2,4-DB → 2,4-D.

Essentially all herbicides used today are organic molecules that have been synthesized by man. Regardless of the fact that they are presumably new to nature, most of them undergo relatively rapid biodegradation in the environment. The mechanisms by which they are biodegraded in nature are similar to that of organic molecules which occur naturally in the environment.

Figure 5.1, prepared by Sheets and Kaufman (1970), illustrates the great diversity of processes that lead to the detoxification, degradation, and disappearance of herbicides from the site of application. Details of several of these processes will be discussed later.

Most herbicides have a relatively low toxicity to mammals including man. The Environmental Protection Agency (EPA) has established four categories of toxicity for pesticides in its Toxicology Guidelines (Table 5.1) (in addition to oral LD_{50}, the EPA also uses dermal LD_{50}, inhalation LC_{50}, eye effects, and skin irritation values for establishing these categories; however, only the oral LD_{50} is considered in the following presentation): I = 50 mg/kg or less, II = 50 through 500 mg/kg, III = 500 through 5000 mg/kg, and IV = 5000 mg/kg or greater. Class I is the most toxic, and Class IV is the least toxic. Although all herbicides should be handled with care to minimize human exposure, most herbicides are in Class III and IV and present little hazard. The oral LD_{50}, in

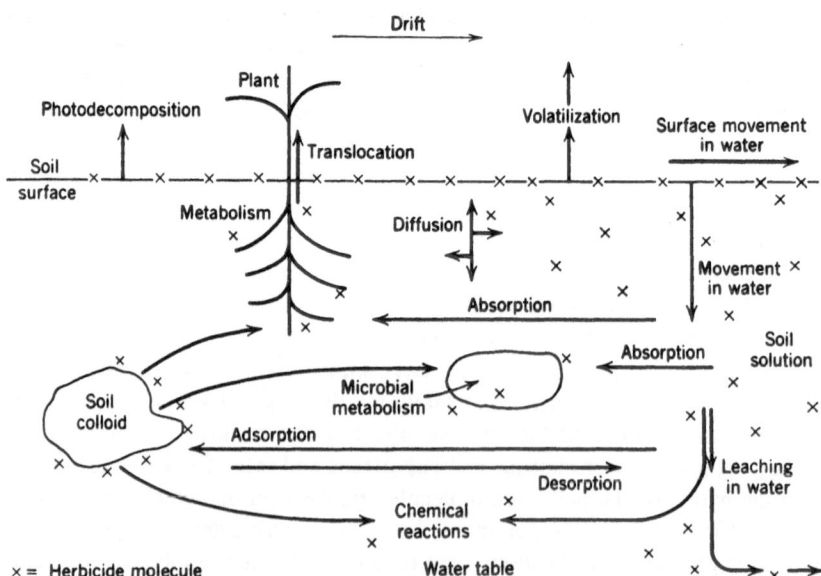

Figure 5.1. Diagrammatical sketch of the interrelations of the processes that lead to detoxication, degradation, and disappearance of herbicides (from Sheets and Kaufman, 1970).

Table 5.1. Categories of Toxicity for Precautionary Labeling in the Federal Insecticide, Fungicide, and Rodenticide Act[a,b]

Toxicity category	Signal word	Oral LD$_{50}$ (mg/kg)	Dermal LD$_{50}$ (mg/kg)	Inhalation LC$_{50}$ Dust or mist (mg/liter)	Inhalation LC$_{50}$ Gas or vapor (ppm)	Eye effects	Skin irritation
I	DANGER POISON[c] (fatal)	50 or less	200 or less	2 or less	200 or less	Irreversible corneal opacity at 7 days	Severe irritation or damage at 72 hr
II	WARNING (may be fatal)	50 through 500	200 through 2000	2 through 20	200 through 2000	Corneal opacity reversible within 7 days, or irritation persisting for 7 days	Moderate irritation at 72 hr
III	CAUTION	500 through 5000	2,000–20,000	20–200	2,000–20,000	No corneal opacity, irritation reversible within 7 days	Mild or slight irritation at 72 hr
IV	CAUTION	5000 or greater	20,000 or greater	200 or greater	20,000 or greater	No irritation	No irritation at 72 hr

[a] Adapted from EPA toxicology guidelines.
[b] All labels must state: "Keep Out of Reach of Children."
[c] Skull and crossbones must appear near word POISON.

mg/kg, of moderately toxic herbicides are as follows: paraquat (150), bromoxynil (250), diallate (395), diquat (400–440), 2,4,5-T (300), and 2,4-D (300–1000). These should be handled with unusual care. The three very toxic herbicides are dinoseb (5–60), endothall (38–51), and acrolein (46). These herbicides should be handled very, very carefully. The LD_{50} values given are from the *Herbicide Handbook* of the Weed Science Society of America (Anonymous, 1974).

During the past few years the safety of the use of 2,4,5-T and silvex has been under review by the EPA. This appears to be primarily related to the presence of a contaminant formed during the high-temperature synthesis of the intermediate 2,4,5-trichlorophenol from 1,2,4,5-tetrachlorobenzene (Crosby *et al.*, 1971; Woolson *et al.*, 1972). The contaminant 2,3,7,8-tetrachlorodibenzo-*p*-dioxin (TCDD) is a very toxic, embryotoxic, and teratogenic compound (Higgenbotham *et al.*, 1968; Sparschu *et al.*, 1971). However, oral doses of 2,4,5-T containing 0.5 ppm of TCDD given to rats (24 mg 2,4,5-T/kg, 6–15 days of pregnancy) and rabbits (40 mg 2,4,5-T/Kg, 6–18 days of pregnancy) produced no evidence of teratogenicity or embryotoxicity (Emerson *et al.*, 1971). In another study, doses of 2,4,5-T containing 0.1 ppm of TCDD given to mice (20 mg 2,4,5-T/kg/day) was established as the no-effect level (Roll, 1971). However, Roll also reported that doses of 35–130 mg 2,4,5-T/kg administered from 6 to 15 days of pregnancy produced an increase in cleft palates and embryotoxic effects. Current manufacturing methods can result in TCDD level less than 0.1 ppm in 2,4,5-T or silvex (Warren, 1979). Until recently TCDD had not been detected in nature (Crosby, 1976); however, within the past year, using refined methods, TCDD has been detected in trace amounts in nature (Warren, 1979). It has also been shown that TCDD and other dioxins are produced in trace amounts in the burning of wood, petroleum, etc. (L. E. Warren, personal communication, 1979). While TCDD is quite stable in soil or water, in the presence of organic hydrogendonors (i.e., solvents, alcohol) it is subject to rapid photodecomposition by dechlorination (Crosby *et al.*, 1971; Plimmer *et al.*, 1973). The low levels of TCDD currently present in carefully manufactured 2,4,5-T and silvex, the extremely low levels found in the environment, and the production of TCDD by burning of natural substances would suggest that the use of these materials is safe. However, in spite of these facts there is a continuing organized effort to prohibit their use in the United States; therefore, in the long run, their continued use remains obscure. TCDD is not produced during the manufacture of the phenoxy-type herbicides not using 2,4,5-trichlorophenol as an intermediate, i.e., 2,4-D.

5.2. PERSISTENCE

The persistence of a herbicide at the site of application depends upon a number of factors in addition to biodegradation, as illustrated in Fig. 5.1. Some

Table 5.2. Persistence of Biological Activity at the Usual Rate of Herbicide Application in Moist–Fertile Soils under Field Conditions and Summer Temperatures in a Temperate Climate

1 Month or less[a] (temporary effects)	1–3 Months[b] (early season control)	3–12 Months[c] (full season control)	Over 12 months[d] (total vegetation control)
Acrolein	Bentazon	Alachlor	Arsenic
Amitrole	Butachlor	Ametryn	Borate
AMS	Butylate	Atrazine	Bromacil
Barban	CDAA	Benefin	Chlorate
Cacodylic acid	CDEC	Bensulide	Fenac
Chloroxuron	Chloramben	Bromoxynil	Picloram
Dalapon	Chlorpropham	Chlorobromuron	Tebuthiuron
2,4-D	Cycloate	Cyprazine	Terbacil
2,4-DB	Diallate	DCPA	2,3,6-TBA
Dinoseb (DNBP)	2,4-DEP	Dicamba	
Diquat[2]	Diphenamid	Dichlobenil	
DSMA	EPTC	Dinitramine	
Endothall	Mecoprop	Diuron	
Fluorodifen	Naptalam	Fenuron	
Glyphosate	Pebulate	Fluometuron	
Metham	PCP	Isopropalin	
Methyl bromide	Propachlor	Linuron	
MCPA	Pyrazon	Metabromuron	
MH	Siduron	Metribuzin	
Molinate	Silvex	Monolinuron	
MSMA	TCA	Monuron	
Nitrofen	Triallate	Napropamide	
Paraquat[2]	2,4,5-T	Nitralin	
Phenmedipham	Vernolate	Norea	
Propanil		Oryzalin	
Propham		Prometryn	
		Pronamide	
		Propazine	
		Simazine	
		Terbutol	
		Terbutryn	
		Trifluralin	

[a] These are approximate values and will vary somewhat as the seven factors discussed in the text vary.
[b] Although diquat and paraquat molecules may remain unchanged in soils for long periods of time, they are adsorbed so tightly to many soils that they become biologically inactive.
[c] At higher rates of application, some of these chemicals may persist at biologically active levels for more than 12 months.
[d] At lower rates of application, some of these chemicals may persist at biologically active levels for less than 12 months.

small amount may be lost by spray drift; it may be subject to photodecomposition in the air as well as on exposed surfaces, including plants and soil surfaces. Some may be lost by leaching or runoff of surface water. Herbicides with a high vapor pressure are lost by volatilization unless incorporated into the soil. Under good agricultural practices, the above losses are minimal. Except for post-emergence applications where the applied herbicide is primarily received by plant foliage, the soil is the major recipient, reservoir, and site of degradation. Even with postemergence applications, the soil is a major site of degradation after the plant dies and disintegrates. Therefore, persistence in the soil has been the major environmental site investigated. The persistence in the soil of the most commonly used herbicides is presented in Table 5.2 (Klingman and Ashton, 1975).

Table 5.2 shows the persistence from a single application of a herbicide. A given herbicide is rarely applied more frequently than once a year to the same site. However, it may be applied to the same site annually over an extended period of time. The question then arises as to whether it will accumulate with annual applications to the same site. Theoretical curves showing maximum residues from annual applications of herbicides, which disappear at the rate of 80% and 50% per year, were prepared by Sheets and Kaufman (1970) (see Fig. 5.2 and 5.3). Even at the relatively slow rate of 50% loss per year, the residue level in the soil approaches a maximum of two times the annual rate of application. Similar curves have been developed by other research workers (Hiltbold, 1974; Kearney *et al.*, 1969; Sheets and Harris, 1965). Comprehensive treatments of the quantitative aspects of decomposition and accumulation (Hamaker, 1972)

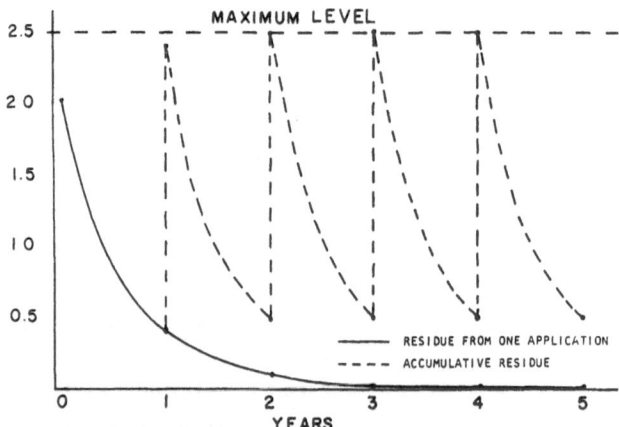

Figure 5.2. Theoretical curves showing the accumulative residue from annual applications of 2 lb/A and that remaining after a single application at the same rate for a herbicide that disappears at a rate of 80% per year (from Sheets and Kaufman, 1970).

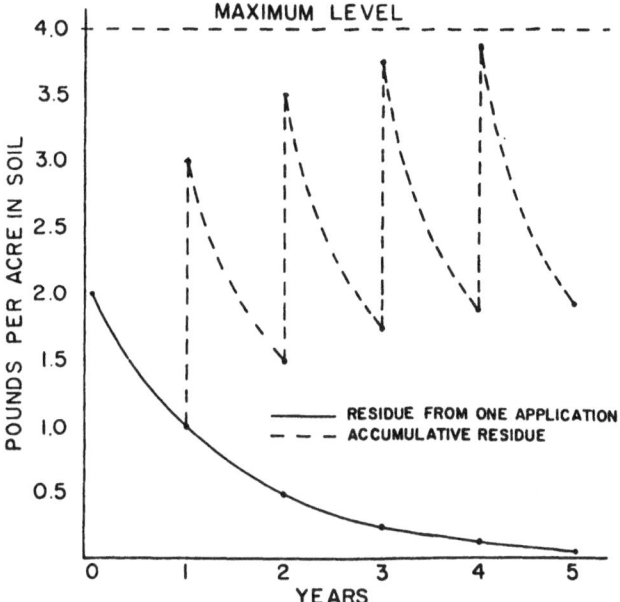

Figure 5.3. Theoretical curves showing the accumulative residue from annual applications of 2 lb/A and that remaining after a single application at the same rate for a herbicide that disappears at a rate of 50% per year (from Sheets and Kaufman, 1970).

and a review on persistence of pesticides in soil (Hiltbold, 1974) have been published. Hamaker (1966) and others have developed equations and computer models to predict the persistence of pesticides in soils.

5.3. DEGRADATION

Herbicides are degraded in the soil by biological and nonbiological means, probably almost always working in conjunction (Skipper and Volk, 1972; Zimdahl *et al.*, 1970). It would appear that distinguishing between these two basically different processes would be relatively simple; however, this is not necessarily the case. In fact, recent reviews have suggested that it is quite difficult (Crosby, 1976; Kaufman, 1974; Kaufman and Kearney, 1976) to distinguish between these two modes of degradation in most cases. Commonly used methods of sterilization also cause nonbiological changes in soils. Although comparisons between autoclaved and nonsterile soils have frequently been used, they are inadequate. Sterilization of soil by autoclaving produces chemical and physical changes in the soil that may alter the degradation of organic molecules by nonbiological means. This also appears to be true for methyl bromide fumigation. Sterilization by gamma irradiation is considered to be less destructive to the chemical and physical characteristics of soils than any other method. Fumigation and specific microbial inhibitors have also been used. Microbial enrichment techniques as well as isolation and identification of the microorganisms responsible for the degradation of the herbicide can also provide valuable information.

5.3.1. Biodegradation

This discussion of the biodegradation of herbicides will be primarily limited to microbe-induced changes in the soil, the major site of herbicide biodegradation in the environment. Previous presentations in this seminar have covered other aspects of the biodegradation of pesticides. The microbial degradation of pesticides has already been described in Chapter 3. However, insecticides have been used as examples. The other significant site of biodegradation, the higher plant, has been previously described in Chapter 2, and the biodegradation of pesticides by animals has been reviewed in Chapter 1. The ingestion of herbicides by nonsoil animals under natural conditions is limited and usually restricted to grazing animals. Several reviews have been published on the biodegradation of herbicides (Ashton and Crafts, 1973; Casida and Lykken, 1969; Frank, 1970; Frear and Shimabukuro, 1970; Hamaker, 1972; Kaufman, 1974; Kaufman and Kearney, 1976; Kearney, 1970; Kearney and Kaufman, 1975; Meikle, 1972). *Herbicides: Chemistry, Degradation, and Mode of Action* (Kearney and Kaufman, 1975) is probably the most comprehensive and presents detailed information on the degradation of many herbicides by plants, animals, and microorganisms.

The rate of microbial degradation of herbicides under field conditions depends upon a number of interacting environmental conditions. In general, the conditions that promote the growth of the microorganisms responsible for the degradation accelerate the rate, and those that inhibit the growth of these microorganisms reduce the rate. These soil factors include temperature, pH, cation exchange capacity, fertility, structure, type, moisture content, organic matter, O_2, and CO_2, as well as numerous other parameters.

Microorganisms degrade herbicides by a number of biochemical reactions, including oxidation, reduction, hydrolysis, hydroxylation, decarboxylation, deamination, dehalogenation, dethioaction, dealkylation, dealkyoxylation, dealkythiolation, and conjugation with normal metabolites, usually sugars, amino acids, or peptides (i.e., glutathione) (Kaufman, 1974; Kaufman and Kearney, 1976; Kaufman *et al.*, 1976; Kearney and Kaufman, 1975; Sheets and Kaufman, 1970). Specific pathways of degradation and the intermediates formed by the biodegradation of herbicides have been presented in numerous reviews (Ashton and Crafts, 1973; Frear and Shimabukuro, 1970; Hamaker, 1972; Kaufman,

1974; Kaufman and Kearney, 1970, 1976; Miekle, 1972; Plimmer, *et al.*, 1973). Classes of microorganisms reported to degrade herbicides include algae, actinomycetes, bacteria, and fungi. Specific microorganisms found to degrade particular herbicides have been cataloged (Audus, 1960, 1964; Kaufman, 1974; Kaufman and Kearney, 1970, 1976; Loos, 1975). There is evidence that some herbicides may be degraded in the soil by extracellular enzymes (Bartha *et al.*, 1968; Burge, 1972, 1973; Kaufman *et al.*, 1971).

A particularly interesting phenomenon of microbial degradation of herbicides that has practical significance is that of enrichment. Enrichment is an increase in the number and/or activity of the microorganisms capable of metabolizing a particular herbicide following the addition of that herbicide to the soil. When a herbicide that is subject to microbial degradation is first applied to a soil, a lag period is usually observed before degradation proceeds at a significant rate (see Fig. 5.4). This is followed by a period of relatively rapid degradation. Subsequent applications of the identical herbicide to the same soil results in an immediate rapid degradation of the herbicide with little if any lag period. Enrichment could reduce the efficacy of repeated applications of herbicide. This phenomenon is most readily demonstrated by the soil perfusion technique or other laboratory test systems, and has been shown for 2,4-D (Audus, 1960), dalapon (Kaufman, 1964), chlorpropham (Kaufman and Kearney, 1965), and others. Several studies also suggest that enrichment occurs under field conditions with 2,4,-D, 2,4,5-T, endothal, and dalapon, but not with simazine or linuron (Kaufman and Kearney, 1976). Kaufman and Kearney (1976) state that they are unaware of any data indicating that enriched populations have survived longer

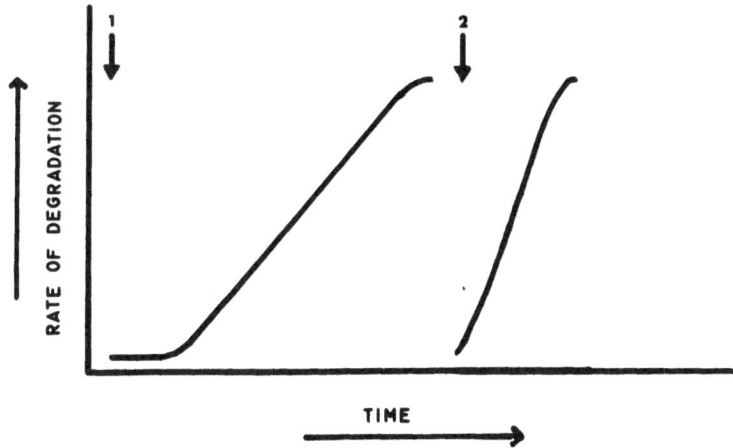

Figure 5.4. Enrichment of microbial flora with subsequent applications of a herbicide resulting in a decrease in the time required for initiation of degradation and an acceleration of the rate of degradation: (1) first application, (2) second application.

than 1 year following the last application. This suggests that enrichment should not reduce the efficacy of a herbicide applied to the same site only one time each year.

Audus (1964) suggested that the mechanism of enrichment could result from mutation or inducible enzyme formation but favored the latter hypotheses. The induction of enzyme formation in microorganisms has been proposed for several herbicides (Kaufman and Kearney, 1976). The proliferation of the population of microorganisms responsible for the degradation of a given herbicide by either mechanism is also an important aspect of enrichment.

It is well known that the adsorption of herbicides to soil components reduces their phytotoxicy. Higher rates of application are often required to produce adequate weed control in soils containing high amounts of clay (mainly kaolinite and montmorillonite) or moderate amounts of organic matter. Many herbicides are totally ineffective at reasonable rates in soils with high amounts of organic matter, i.e., peat and muck soils. Adsorption of herbicides to soil components can also reduce their biodegradation. Perhaps the best example of this is diquat. It has been demonstrated that diquat is readily degraded in solution culture but is not degraded when adsorbed to the clay montmorillonite (Weber and Coble, 1968). Diquat, a postemergence herbicide, is essentially nonphytotoxic in most soils; some phytotoxicity can be shown in very sandy soils.

5.3.2. Nonbiodegradation

Although biodegradation is the major topic of this book, dealing briefly with nonbiological degradation, an integral part of the persistence of herbicides in the environment, is also appropriate. Recent books and reviews deal with the nonbiological degradation of organic molecules (Armstrong and Konrad, 1974; Crosby, 1976; Goring and Hamaker, 1972; Guenzi, 1974).

The nonbiological degradation of herbicides occurs in the air, water, and soil. They are altered by both chemical and physical processes. They are subject to oxidation, reduction, hydrolysis, epoxidation, nucleophilic displacement, and free-radical-induced reactions as well as photodecomposition which occurs in the air, water, and exposed surfaces, including soil and plant surfaces. Initial degradative reactions may occur by nonbiological processes and further degradation carried out by biological means, or vice versa.

5.4. MAN'S ACTIVITIES

Man can alter the persistence and degradation of herbicides in the environment. His major methods are proper herbicide selection, correct application rate selection, effective application, and manipulation of controllable environmental factors to obtain maximum efficacy and minimal persistence beyond the required period of weed control. Burnside (1974) has prepared an excellent review on the prevention and detoxification of pesticide residues in soils. He suggests that the following steps can minimize pesticide residues in soils: (1) use an integrated pest control system, (2) use alternative pest control methods, (3) improve efficacy, (4) select pesticides with short residual properties, and (5) rotate pesticides and crops.

Most introductory textbooks of weed science stress several methods of weed control, i.e., mechanical, crop competition, crop rotation, biological, fire, and chemical control (Klingman and Ashton, 1975). These are the approaches to integrated pest management (IPM) and alternate pest control methods of weed science. Often the best and most economical way to control weeds is a combination of two or more of these methods. Since most herbicides are used to reduce the weed competition to the desired plant and excessive rates often injure the desired plant, minimal rates are mandatory. In row crops like orchards and vineyards, the amount of herbicide required can be further reduced by using a band or strip treatment rather than treatment of the entire area. The weeds in the areas between the bands can be controlled by cultivation. Rotation of crops has several advantages in weed control including different cultural practices, crop competition aspects, crop–weed associations, and rotation of herbicides that can prevent an increase in the population of a tolerant weed and accumulation of a single herbicide and/or its degradation products. Rotation of herbicides should also be used in monoculture for this same reason.

In general, long-term herbicidal residues have not been a problem in environmental pollution. However, even short-term residues can be a problem with crop failure, errors in application, or unpredicted changes in land use when it is desirable to plant a susceptible species. Under these conditions, man can occasionally utilize certain methods to effectively reduce herbicide residues. Although each situation requires specific methods, the following approaches may be considered. Physical or chemical methods should be more rapid than biological methods. In general, chemical methods have not been effective under field conditions (Burnside, 1974). Physical methods such as adsorption by activated charcoal, dilution by tillage, and leaching with water have been effective with certain herbicides. Total removal of the contaminated soil has been useful for small areas when the herbicide is limited to the surface few centimeters of soil. However, under many conditions biological methods are the most practical. The primary biological method is the use of a tolerant plant species to absorb and degrade the herbicide, i.e., maize for simazine or atrazine. The promotion of the growth of soil microorganisms can be helpful. The inoculation of the site with microorganisms which have been shown to degrade the herbicide is a technique that appears promising but has had little utilization. However, the degradation of DDT by this means has been studied with some success (Kearney, *et al.*, 1969). The addition of large amounts of plant residues and/or animal manure has also been useful; this probably not only increases microbial activity but may also adsorb some of the herbicide. Combinations of these treatments should be considered.

5.5. CONCLUSION

The persistence and degradation of herbicides in the environment have been reviewed and key references cited. In general, we know the approximate period of persistence of most herbicides in the soil based on their phytotoxicity to higher plants. This information has been primarily developed by empirical testing and field observations. Future research should stress model systems under controlled environmental conditions and the development of mathematical equations or computer models. The use of physical models should also allow us to study techniques that have the potential of acclerating herbicide degradation more efficiently than field investigations. Of course, any model system must ultimately be field tested to prove its worth in the real world. More attention should be given to the persistence of herbicide degradation products in the environment. Although investigations appear to be limited, the author is unaware of any evidence that suggests that any herbicide or its degradation products undergo bioaccumulation. However, the potential for bioaccumulation exists and should be subjected to further study.

There are some situations where we wish to increase the persistence of a herbicide. For example, some herbicides are degraded too rapidly to give season-long weed control. The use of controlled-release formulations has been investigated to increase the period of effectiveness of such herbicides (Cardarelli, 1976); however, acceptance of this technique has not been widely adapted. A nonphytotoxic chemical, *p*-chlorophenyl-*N*-methylcarbamate, has been shown to approximately double the period of weed control with chlorpropham (E. K. Plant, personal communication, 1979). It appears to block the effect of the degradative enzyme(s) of several microorganisms but does not alter their growth. It delays the initiation of degradation but does not alter the rate once degradation has started. EPA approval for this use in the United States is expected soon.

Future research on the biodegradation of herbicides should also include (1) identification of higher plants and microorganisms that rapidly degrade specific herbicides and develop techniques for their use in the field, (2) search for suitable nonphytotoxic substrates that will promote the growth and activity of these degradative microorganisms, (3) study of the mechanisms of degradative enzyme induction in higher plants and microorganisms, (4) investigation of the environmental impact and mammalian toxicity of the metabolites of herbicides, and (5) additional research on biochemical pathways of herbicide degradation in higher plants, microorganisms, and animals.

REFERENCES

Anonymous, 1974, *Herbicide Handbook,* 3rd ed., Weed Science Society of America, Urbana, Ill.

Armstrong, D. E., and Konrad, J. G., 1974, Nonbiological degradation of pesticides, in: *Pesticides in Soil and Water* (W. D. Guenz, ed.), pp. 123–131, Soil Science Society of America, Madison, Wisc.

Ashton, F. M., and Crafts, A. S., 1973, *Mode of Action of Herbicides,* John Wiley, New York.

Audus, L. J., 1960, Microbiological breakdown of herbicides in soils, in: *Herbicides in the Soil* (E. K. Woodford and G. R. Sager, eds.), pp. 1–19, Blackwell, Oxford.

Audus, L. J., 1964, Herbicide behavior in the soil, II. Interaction with soil micro-organisms, in: *The Physiology and Biochemistry of Herbicides* (L. J. Audus, ed.), pp. 163–206, Academic Press, New York.

Bartha, R., Linke, H. A. B., and Pramer, D., 1968, Pesticide transformations: Production of chloroazobenzenes from chloroanilines, *Science* **161:**582.

Burge, W. D., 1972, Microbiol population hydrolyzing propanil and accumulation of 3,4-dichloroaniline and 3,3′,4,4′-tetrachloroazobenzine in soils, *Soil Biol. Biochem.* **4:**379.

Burge, W. D., 1973, Transformations of propanil-derived 3,4-dichloroaniline in soil to 3,3′,4,4′-tetrachloroazobenzene as related to soil peroxidases, *Proc. Soil Sci. Soc. Am.* **37:**392.

Burnside, O. C., 1974, Prevention and detoxification of pesticide residues in soils, in: *Pesticides and Soil and Water* (W. D. Guenzi, ed.), pp. 387–412, Soil Science Society of America, Madison, Wisc.

Cardarelli, N., 1976, *Controlled Release Pesticide Formulations,* CRC Press, Cleveland.

Casida, J. E. and Lykken, L., 1969, Metabolism of organic pesticide chemicals in higher plants, *Annu. Rev. Plant Physiol.* **20:**607.

Crosby, D. G., 1976, Nonbiological degradation of herbicides in the soil, in: *Herbicides: Physiology, Biochemistry, and Ecology,* Vol. II (L. J. Audus, ed.), pp. 65–97, Academic Press, New York.

Crosby, D. G., Wong, A. S., Plimmer, J. R., and Woolson, E. A., 1971, Photodecomposition of chlorinated dibenzo-*p*-dioxins, *Science* **173:**748.

Emerson, J. L., Thompson, D. J., Strebing, R. J., Gerbig, C. G., and Robinson, V. B., 1971, Teratogenic studies on 2,4,5-trichlorophenoxyacetic acid in the rat and rabbit, *Food Cosmet. Toxicol.* **9:**395.

Frank, P. A., 1970, Degradation and effects of herbicides in water, in: *FAO International Conference on Weed Control* (T. J. Holstun, Jr., ed.), pp. 539–559, Weed Science Society of America, Urbana, Ill.

Frear, D. S., and Shimabukuro, R. H., 1970, Metabolism and effects of herbicides in plants, in: *FAO International Conference on Weed Control* (T. J. Holstun, Jr., ed.), pp. 560–578, Weed Science Society of America, Urbana, Ill.

Goring, C. A. I., and Hamaker, J. W. (eds.), 1972, *Organic Chemicals in the Soil Environment,* 2 vols., Marcel Dekker, New York.

Guenzi, W. D., 1974, *Pesticides in Soil and Water,* Soil Science Society of America, Madison, Wisc.

Hamaker, J. W., 1966, Mathematical prediction of cummulative levels of pesticides in soil, in: *Organic Pesticides in the Environment* (R. F. Gould, ed.), American Chemical Society, Washington, D.C.

Hamaker, J. W., 1972, Decomposition: Quantitative aspects, in: *Organic Chemicals in the Soil Environment* (C. A. I. Goring and J. W. Hamaker, eds.), pp. 253–340, Marcel Dekker, New York.

Higgenbotham, G. R., Huang, A., Firestone, D., Verrett, J., Ress, J., and Campbell, A. D., 1968, Chemicals and toxicological evaluations of isolated and synthetic chloro derivatives of dibenzo-*p*-dioxin, *Nature (London)* **220**:702.

Hiltbold, A. E., 1974, Persistence of pesticides in soil, in: *Pesticides in Soil and Water* (W. D. Guenzi, ed.), pp. 203–222, Soil Science Society of America, Madison, Wisconsin.

Kaufman, D. D., 1964, Microbiol degradation of 2,2-dichloropropionic acid in five soils, *Can. J. Microbiol.* **10**:843.

Kaufman, D. D., 1974, Degradation of pesticides by soil microorganisms, in: *Pesticides in Soil and Water* (W. D. Guenzi, ed.), Soil Science Society of America, Madison, Wisconsin.

Kaufman, D. D., and Kearney, P. C., 1965, Microbial degradation of isopropyl-*N*-3-chlorophenylcarbamate and 2-chloroethyl-*N*-3-chlorophenylcarbamate, *Appl. Microbiol.* **13**:443.

Kaufman, D. D., and Kearney, P. C., 1970, Microbial degradation of triazine herbicides, *Residue Rev.* **32**:235.

Kaufman, D. D., and Kearney, P. C., 1976, Microbial transformation in soil, in: *Herbicides: Physiology, Biochemistry, and Ecology*, Vol. II (L. J. Audus, ed.), pp. 29–64, Academic Press, New York.

Kaufman, P. C., Blake, J., and Miller, D. E., 1971, Methylcarbamate affects acylanilide residues in soil, *J. Agric. Food Chem.* **19**:204.

Kaufman, D. D., Still, G. G., Paulson, G. D., and Bandal, S. K. (eds.), 1976, *Bound and Conjugated Pesticide Residues*, ACS Symposium Series 29, American Chemical Society, Washington, D.C.

Kearney, P. C., 1970, Herbicides in the environment, in: *FAO International Conference on Weed Control* (T. J. Holstun, Jr., ed.), pp. 496–512, Weed Science Society of America, Urbana, Ill.

Kearney, P. C., and Kaufman, D. D., 1975, *Herbicides: Chemistry, Degradation, and Mode of Action* 2 vols. (P. C. Kearney and D. D. Kaufman, eds.), Marcel Dekker, New York.

Kearney, P. C., Nash, R. G., and Isensee, A. R., 1969, Persistence of pesticide residues in soils, in: *Chemical Fallout* (M. W. Miller and G. G. Berg, eds.), C. C. Thomas, Springfield, Ill.

Klingman, G. C., and Ashton, F. M., 1975, *Weed Science: Principles and Practices*, John Wiley, New York.

Loss, M. A., 1975, Phenoxyalkonic acids, in: *Herbicides: Chemistry, Degradation, and Mode of Action* (P. C. Kearney and D. D. Kaufman, eds.), pp. 1–128, Marcel Dekker, New York.

Meikle, R. W., 1972, Decomposition: Qualitative relationships, in: *Organic Chemicals in the Soil Environment* (C. A. I. Goring and J. W. Hamaker, eds.), pp. 145–251, Marcel Dekker, New York.

Plimmer, J. R., Crosby, D. G., Wong, A. S., and Klingebiel, U. I., 1973, Photochemistry of dibenzo-*p*-dioxins, *Adv. Chem. Ser.* **120**:44.

Roll, R., 1971, Studies of the tetragoenic effects of 2,4,5-T in mice, *Food Cosmet. Toxicol.* **9**:671.

Sheets, T. J., and Harris, C. I., 1965, Herbicide residues in soils and their phytotoxicities to crops grown in rotations, *Residue Rev.* **11**:119.

Sheets, T. J., and Kaufman, D. D., 1970, Degradation and effects of herbicides in soils, in: *FAO International Conference on Weed Control* (T. J. Holstun, Jr., ed.), pp. 513–538, Weed Science Society of America, Urbana, Ill.

Skipper, H. D., and Volk, V. V., 1972, Biological and chemical degradation of atrazine in three Oregon soils, *Weed Sci.* **20**:344.

Sparschu, G. L., Dunn, F. L., and Rowe, V. K., 1971, Study of the teratogenicity of 2,3,7,8-tetrachlorodibenzo-*p*-dioxin in the rat, *Food Cosmet. Toxicol.* **9**:405.

Weber, J. B., and Coble, H. D., 1968, Microbiol decomposition of diquat adsorbed on montmorillonite and kaolinite clays, *J. Agric. Food Chem.* **16**:475.

Woolson, E. A., Thomas, R. F., and Ensor, P. D. J., 1972, Survey of polychlorodibenzo-*p*-dioxin in selected pesticides, *J. Agric. Food. Chem.* **20**:351.

Zimdahl, R. L., Freed, V. H., Montgomery, M. L., and Furtick, W. R., 1970, The degradation of triazine and uracil herbicides in soil, *Weed Res.* **10**:18.

6

Biodegradation of Agricultural Fungicides

Hugh D. Sisler

6.1. INTRODUCTION

Most natural organic matter decomposes rapidly to CO_2 and water under conditions favorable for biodegradation. However, when unfavorable conditions prevail, such as anaerobic environments, extreme pH, or very low temperature, natural organic matter persists for very long periods and material such as wood and even whole animal bodies is conserved for centuries (Kaars Sijpesteijn et al., 1977). While the rate of degradation of many organic pesticides is similar to that of natural materials, the situation with pesticides is more complicated because some molecules or their metabolites may persist even under the most favorable conditions for biological attack. A vast number of different situations prevail in respect to pesticide degradation in the environment. We should strive to develop pesticides which degrade as readily as natural products; however, even if this goal is attained, pesticide molecules or their metabolites may still persist under conditions unfavorable for biodegradation. Biodegradability, therefore, must be defined in terms of the environment to which a pesticide is subjected.

In the following sections some of the properties and degradation products of a few of the more important agricultrual fungicides will be discussed. The

Hugh D. Sisler ● Department of Botany, University of Maryland, College Park, Maryland 20742. This is contribution No. 5638, Publication No. A2599, from the University of Maryland Agricultural Experiment Station.

treatment is by no means exhaustive, but it is hoped that it will give a useful overview of the subject.

6.2. TOXICITY OF FUNGICIDES TO NONTARGET ORGANISMS

Apart from mercury compounds, cycloheximide, and a few other compounds of minor significance, fungicides have a low mammalian toxicity (Table 6.1). The acute oral LD_{50} value of several important fungicides such as Bordeaux mixture, thiram, and triphenyltin hydroxide lies between 100 and 1000 mg/kg; however, the value for most fungicides is greater than 1000 mg/kg. In view of the low application rates and minor significance of cycloheximide and the discontinued or severely restricted use of mercury compounds in many countries, the fungicides used in agriculture do not constitute a serious problem as acute toxicity hazards to mammals. With the realization that fungicides, their contaminants, or their degradation products may have obscure or delayed toxic effects on humans and other organisms or enter into food chains and become greatly concentrated, we have become more concerned about the fate of fungicides in the environment. In fact, the need to know the degradation characteristics as well as the biological effects of new and existing agricultural fungicides is now widely recognized.

Table 6.1. Fungicides Grouped According to Acute Oral Mammalian Toxicity $(LD_{50})(mg/kg)$[a]

1–50	1000 or greater
Cycloheximide (2.5)[b]	Anilazine
Mercuric chloride (7–9)	Benomyl
Phenylmercury salts (5–70)	Captafol
Methyl mercury salts (16–32)	Captan
Ethyl mercury salts (16–28)	Carboxin
	Chloroneb
50–100	Chlorothalonil
Cadmium chloride (88)	Dichlone
Diazoben (60)	Dodine
	Ferbam
100–1000	Folpet
Bordeaux mixture (300)	Glyodin
Triphenyltin hydroxide (108–209)	Maneb
Thiram (375–865)	Thiabendazole
Sodium pentachlorophenate (210)	Zineb
	Ziram

[a] Values for mercury compounds from Ulfvarson (1969); all others from the United States Department of Agriculture guidelines (1974).
[b] Value(s) in parentheses: LD_{50} of fungicide(s).

With regard to toxicity to nontarget organisms other than man, fungicides such as elemental sulfur, dinocap, and benomyl have deleterious effects on certain predacious mites and insects and may interfere with the biological control of some insect pests (Brown, 1978). Frequent application of fungicides of relatively low toxicity can lead to accumulations in soil which affect earthworm populations. The use of copper fungicides in English orchards over a number of years has resulted in levels as high as 2000 ppm in the surface layer of soil and has lead to the disappearance of earthworms (Brown, 1978). Frequent applications of benzimidazole fungicides in orchards results in temporary reduction of earthworm populations (Stringer and Lyons, 1974). There are, however, beneficial nontarget effects of fungicides. Benzimidazole fungicides, for example, may aid in the control of parasitic mites (Upham and Delp, 1973) and nematodes (Miller, 1969).

6.3. STABILITY OF FUNGICIDES

There is considerable literature on this subject, but wide gaps in our knowledge still exist, particularly in respect to the ultimate fate of certain degradation products. Although stability of organic fungicides or their metabolites is not

Table 6.2. Stability of Various Fungicides in Nonsterile Soil

Fungicide	Half-life (days)	Comments	Reference
Benomyl	90–365	Based on total benzimidazole residues following application of 2.3–5.6 kg/ha	Baude *et al.* (1974)
Captan	3–4	Application rate—100 ppm, initial soil pH, 6.4	Burchfield (1959)
	>65	Application rate—1000 ppm, initial pH 5.7	Munnecke (1958)
Chloroneb	30–90	Application rate—2.25 kg/ha	Rhodes *et al.* (1971)
PCNB	117–1059	Based on field samples	Beck and Hansen (1974)
	>21	Flooded (anaerobic soil)	Ko and Farley (1969)
Thiram	>40	Not detectable after 40 days at application rates of 250 ppm, more persistent at higher concentrations	Munnecke and Mickail (1967)
Triphenyl tin acetate	140	Based on $^{14}CO_2$ released from 5–10 ppm aromatic-labeled fungicide	Barnes *et al.* (1973)

generally recognized as a factor leading to environmental problems, this may reflect, in part, a lack of knowledge in this area.

Few organic fungicides are highly stable under a wide variety of conditions. Only hexachlorobenzene, which is used in minor quantities for seed treatment, appears to rival the more stable chlorinated hydrocarbon insecticides in persistence. The half-life of several fungicides in nonsterile soil is given in Table 6.2. The important soil fungicide pentachloronitrobenzene (PCNB) is quite stable and may persist in the soil for several years. Maximum persistence of other fungicides listed in Table 6.2 is considerably less than that of PCNB; however, benzimidazole residues of benomyl have a half-life in soil of a year under certain conditions.

In the following section, consideration will be given to the degradation characteristics of several types of agricultural fungicides.

6.4. BIODEGRADATION OF SELECTED FUNGICIDES

6.4.1. Triphenyltins

Certain organometallic compounds of mercury and tin are potent fungicides. The organic mercuries were introduced in 1915 (Ulfvarson, 1969) and proved to be highly valuable for seed treatments; however, toxicity to various forms of animal life led to discontinued or severely restricted use of these compounds as agricultural fungicides in many countries.

Organic tin compounds have come into widespread use as fungicides during the past 20 years. The principal compounds used for disease control are triphenyltin derivatives (Fig. 6.1). Degradation of triphenyltin chloride on sugar beet leaves proceeds via the di- and monophenyl derivatives by a process which may be spontaneous rather than biological (Kaars Sijpesteijn *et al.*, 1977). Breakdown in the soil likewise involves release of the aromatic groups and subsequent degradation of these, a process which is probably due solely to the action of

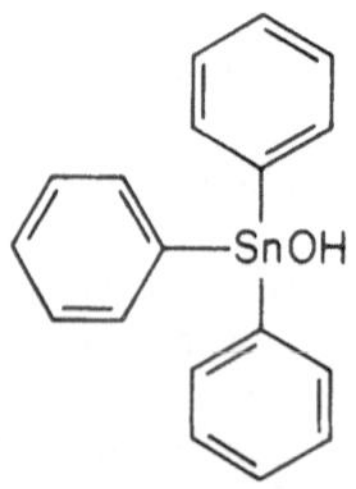

Figure 6.1. Structure of the fungicide triphenyltin hydroxide.

microorganism (Barnes *et al.*, 1971, 1973). Studies made with 5 and 10 ppm of ^{14}C-aromatic-labeled triphenyltin acetate in soil showed that the half-life was about 140 days based on $^{14}CO_2$ evolution; only traces of $^{14}CO_2$ were evolved from heat-sterilized soil (Barnes *et al.*, 1971, 1973). These and other studies indicate a slow conversion of ^{14}C phenyl groups of triphenyltin to CO_2 (Kaufman, 1977). There remains, however, the need for better characterization of inter- mediate breakdown products. Although inorganic tin, the anticipated end product of degradation, is essentially devoid of biological activity (Kaars Sijpesteijn *et al.*, 1969), the fate of the tin is of interest since it is subject to biological methylation and may enter a food chain as highly toxic methyl tin derivatives (Ridley *et al.*, 1977).

6.4.2. PCNB (Terraclor, Quintozene)

PCNB is used as a seed and soil treatment to control several soil-borne fungal pathogens. It is sometimes used at rates as high as 200 lb/acre, but the usual application rates are much lower (Sharvelle, 1961). Disease control in soil may persist for as long as 1 year following application, although it is not known whether the parent compound accounts for the long residual activity (Ko and Farley, 1969). PCNB (Fig. 6.2) is known to persist for long periods in the soil. Half-lives ranging from 117 to 1059 days were estimated on the basis of field samples collected in Denmark (Beck and Hansen, 1974). A half-life of 4.7–9.7 months at 25°C is reported for PCNB in three soil types added to flasks (Wang and Broadbent, 1973). Nevertheless, under certain conditions the fungicide is degraded quite rapidly. Flooding of soil or exclusion of oxygen markedly en-

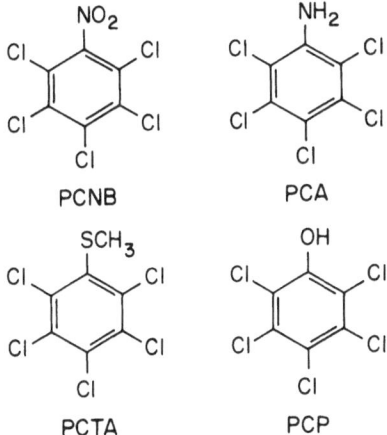

Figure 6.2. Structures of PCNB, PCA, PCTA, and PCP.

hances microbial degradation of PCNB (Ko and Farley, 1969; Wang and Broadbent, 1973). In moist, nonsterilized soil, 82% of the PCNB persists after 3 weeks whereas less than 1% remains in submerged soil (Ko and Farley, 1969). The major metabolite of PCNB in soil is pentachloroaniline (PCA) (Fig. 6.2), the formation of which is favored by reducing conditions (Ko and Farley 1969). Murthy and Kaufman (1978) demonstrated that [^{14}C]-PCNB is converted to [^{14}C]-PCA and [^{14}C]pentachlorothioanisole ([^{14}C]-PCTA) in flooded soils. After 40 days the products recovered in hexane consisted of 13% PCNB, 86% PCA, and 0.5% PCTA. Although pentachlorophenol (PCP) was detected, no ^{14}CO$_2$ was evolved, indicating a high resistance of the metabolites to complete degradation. PCA appears to be a very stable compound in soils (Ko and Farley, 1969). Little loss of this metabolite from aerobic soils occurred even after a period of nearly 2 years (D. D. Kaufman, personal communication).

A variety of fungi and actinomycetes in pure culture convert PCNB to PCA and PCTA (Chacko et al., 1966; Nakanishi and Oku, 1969). On the other hand, some microorganisms oxidize PCA to PCNB (Kaufman, 1977), a factor which may account for the long persistence of PCNB in aerated soils (Kaars Sijpesteijn, et al., 1977; Kaufman, 1977). Plants take up PCNB from the soil. The metabolites PCA and PCTA are found in the tissues (Gorbach and Wagner, 1967; Kuchar et al., 1969), but whether these metabolites are formed from PCNB in the tissue or are taken up from the soil, or both, remains an interesting question.

The ultimate fate of PCA and PCTA is of interest. Murthy and Kaufman (1978) regard them as end products of PCNB degradation in the soil and assume that they remain as residues unless absorbed by plants. Conversion to PCP and further breakdown of this metabolite would seem to be the only pathway for further degradation (Murthy and Kaufman, 1978).

Soils treated with technical PCNB, which contains impurities of pentachlorobenzene, hexachlorobenzene, and tetrachloronitrobenzene, can be expected to contain appreciable residues of the parent compound and of these impurities as well as PCA and PCTA for at least 2–3 years (Beck and Hansen, 1974). It would seem desirable, therefore, to have substitutes for PCNB which are more readily degradable.

6.4.3. Dithiocarbamates

Dithiocarbamates constitute the most important class of organic fungicides used for plant disease control on a worldwide basis (EBDC, Fungicide Assessment Team, 1977). Two major groups within this class, the monoalkyl and the dialkyl derivatives, are recognized in accordance with differing modes of action and degradation pathways (Kaars Sijpesteijn et al., 1977; Kaars Sijpesteijn and van der Kerk, 1954). The former group, drived from primary amines, possess a reactive hydrogen on the nitrogen atom(s) and as a consequence yield conversion products which differ in many respects from those of dialkyldithiocarbamates (Kaars Sijpesteijn *et al.*, 1977). With the exception of the soil fungicide sodium methyldithiocarbamate, the practical monoalkyldithiocarbamate fungicides are derivatives of ethylenediamine, whereas dialkyldithiocarbamate fungicides are derivatives of dimethylamine.

6.4.3.1. Monoalkyldithiocarbamates

Fungicides in this group include maneb, zineb (Fig. 2.3), and the closely related derivatives mancozeb and metriam (Kaars Sijpesteijn *et al.*, 1977). The water-soluble compound nabam, disodium ethylenebisdithiocarbamate (Fig. 6.3), is not used as a practical fungicide, but has served as a useful model for studying the action and degradation of ethylenebisdithiocarbamate (EBDC) fungicides.

Metabolism of bisdithiocarbamates by plants and microorganisms has been recently reviewed (Kaars Sijpesteijn *et al.*, 1977). Degradation in soil is discussed by Kaufman (1977), and nonbiological conversions are discussed by Woodcock (1977).

EBDC fungicides are relatively unstable compounds which are transformed to a variety of products mainly by chemical processes, but with significant

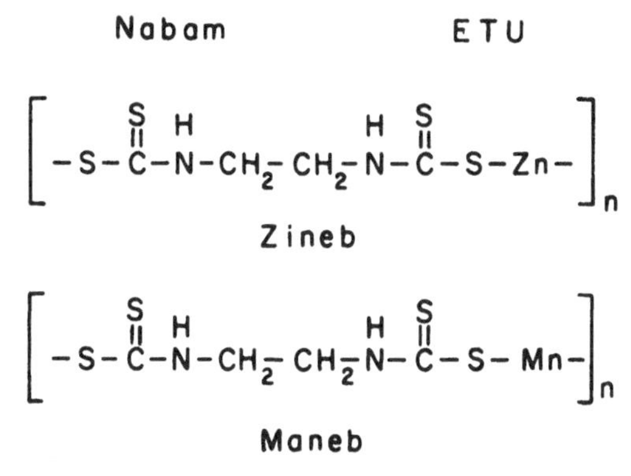

Figure 6.3. Structures of some ethylene bisdithiocarbamates and ETU.

biological involvement. Nabam, for example, is extremely unstable in aqueous solutions and is transformed to the following products: ethylenethiourea (ETU), 5,6-dihydro-3H-imidazo(2,1-c)-1,2,4-dithiazole-3-thione (DIDT), polymeric ethylenethiuram disulfide, ethylenediamine, ethylenediisothiocyanate, elemental sulfur, CS_2, and H_2S (Kaars Sijpesteijn et al., 1977). Zineb and maneb yield the same decomposition products in aqueous solution as nabam, but at a slower rate (Kaars Sijpesteijn et al., 1977).

ETU (Fig. 6.3), an impurity found in technical EBDC fungicides (Woodcock, 1977), is also a major degradation product of these fungicides in various environments (Anomymous, 1977) and is a product about which there has been much concern because of its potential hazard to man (Fishbein, 1977). Although ETU forms by chemical degradation of EDBC fungicides, microorganisms accelerate formation from the intermediate breakdown product DIDT. Bacteria and fungi as well as crude enzyme preparations from these organisms convert DIDT to ETU; however, these microorganisms do not degrade ETU (Vonk, 1975).

Soil degradation products of nabam include ETU, DIDT, CS_2, H_2S, and COS (Kaufman, 1977; Kaufman and Fletcher, 1973; Moje et al., 1964; Munnecke, 1972). ETU is degraded rapidly in nonsterile soil; 200 ppm is converted to ethyleneurea in 8 days (Kaufman and Fletcher, 1973). A similar but slower conversion of ETU occurs in autoclaved soil; however, further degradation of ethyleneurea with evolution of CO_2 occurs only in nonsterile soil (Kaufman and Fletcher, 1973). Microorganisms therefore are apparently involved not only in hastening conversion of ETU to ethyleneurea, but also in degrading the latter. Hydation and Jaffé's base are also metabolites of ETU found in soil (Kaufman and Fletcher, 1973).

Ethyleneurea and 2-imidazoline are metabolites of ETU in plants (Hoagland and Frear, 1976; Vonk, 1975). In cucumbers, the conversion of ETU to these products is rapid; the products are subject to further degradation (Kaars Sijpesteijn et al., 1977).

Although ETU is subject to rapid degradation by light and microorganisms, the compound is reasonably stable in the absence of these agents. Formation of ETU from EBDC residues on food crops may be accentuated by heating during processing (Anomymous, 1977; Newsome, 1976). Every effort should therefore be made to reduce these residues to the lowest possible level before processing.

6.4.3.2. Dialkyldithiocarbamates

Agricultural fungicides in this group include the water-insoluble derivatives, zinc dimethyldithiocarbamate (ziram), ferric dimethyldithiocarbamate (ferbam), and the oxidation product tetramethylthiuram disulfide (thiram). Sodium dimethyldithiocarbamate (NaDDC), a fungitoxic water-soluble salt, has no practical agricultural application but is frequently used in mode of action or transformation

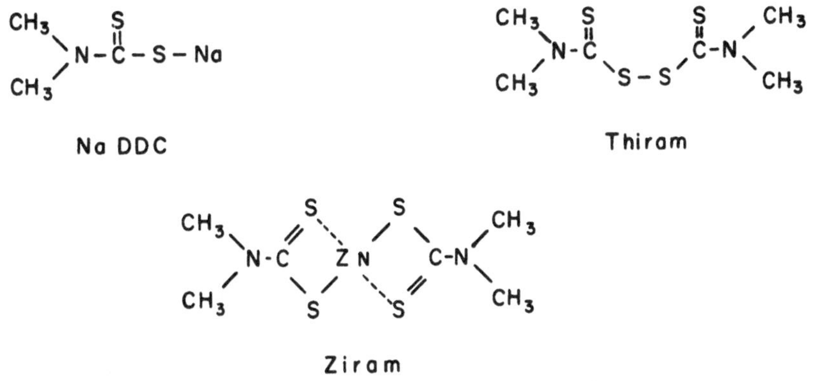

Figure 6.4. Structures of some dialkyldithiocarbamates.

studies. The structures of ziram, thiram, and NaDDC are shown in Fig. 6.4. Dialkyldithiocarbamates are easily oxidized to thiram disulfides (Thorne and Ludwig, 1962), and the latter are readily reduced to dialkyldithiocarbamates by glutathione (Johnston, 1953) and by fungal cells (Goksøyr, 1955).

Dimethyldithiocarbamates are readily decomposed to CS_2 and dimethylamine under acidic conditions (Thorne and Ludwig, 1962). The decomposition of thiram to these products by microorganisms (Kaars Sijpesteijn *et al.*, 1977; Sisler and Cox, 1954) probably takes place after reduction to dimethyldithiocarbamate. Breakdown of the latter to CS_2 and dimethylamine may be brought about by acids produced by the organisms; however, the involvement of enzymatic mechanisms cannot be excluded.

DDC ions taken up by plants are readily converted into three fungitoxic conjugates, two of which have been identified as DDC-β-glucoside and DDC-alanine (Fig. 6.5). The third derivative has not been identified. A fourth metabolite, thiazolidine-2-thione-4-carboxylic acid (TTCA), is a nonfungitoxic com-

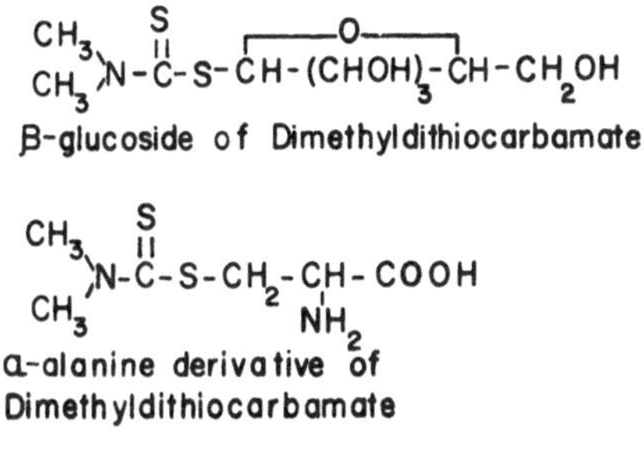

β-glucoside of Dimethyldithiocarbamate

α-alanine derivative of
Dimethyldithiocarbamate

Figure 6.5. Plant metabolites of dimethyldithiocarbamates.

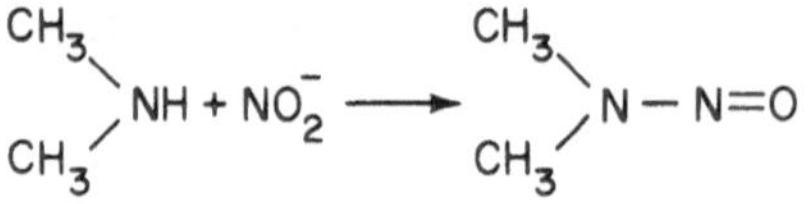

Figure 6.6. Reaction of dimethylamine with nitrite to form dimethylnitrosamine.

pound formed nonenzymatically from DDC-alanine by loss of dimethylamine (Kaars Sijpesteijn *et al.*, 1977). The alanine and glucoside conjugates of DDC as well as TTCA are also found in rice plants sprayed with ziram (Kumarasamy and Raghu, 1976). Other unidentified metabolites of dialkyldithiocarbamates are reported to occur in plants; there is evidence that ^{35}S from these fungicides enters sulfur amino acids and becomes incorporated into proteins (Kaars Sijpesteijn *et al.*, 1977). Degradation of the DDC conjugates and the fate of the products in plants have not been fully resolved (Kaars Sijpesteijn *et al.*, 1977).

In contrast to the conjugation products formed by higher plants, fungi and bacteria form α-aminobuyteric and α-ketobuyteric acid conjugates of DDC (Kaars Sijpesteijn *et al.*, 1963, 1977).

The rate of breakdown of thiram in soil is dependent on the concentration applied (Munnecke and Mickail, 1967). In soils treated with 250 ppm thiram, degradation is fairly rapid and the fungicide is undetectable after 49 days or less. However, in soils treated with 1000 ppm, degradation is very slow and much of the fungicide remains after 64 days. Breakdown is more rapid in unsterilized soil than in sterilized soil, indicating a role of microorganisms in the degradation (Munnecke and Mickail, 1967). The effect of concentration on decomposition rate probably reflects in part an inhibition of microbial activity.

A pathway of thiram degradation in the soil proposed by Raghu *et al.* (1975) includes the microbial metabolites α-aminobuyteric acid and α-ketobuyteric acid conjugates of DDC and other products such as dimethylamine, dimethylnitrosamine, CS_2, elemental sulfur, methionine, ammonia, and formaldehyde.

Dimethylnitrosamine is formed from thiram in the presence of nitrate or nitrite in acidic soil under flooded conditions (Ayanaba *et al.*, 1973), probably from the breakdown product dimethylamine (Fig. 6.6). Whether nitrosamine formation constitutes a hazard of any consequence in the practical use of thiram and other dialkyldithiocarbamates remains an important question in need of further study.

6.4.4. Substituted Phthalimides

The substituted phthalimide fungicides captan, folpet, and captafol (Fig. 6.7) are important surface protectants used to control a broad spectrum of plant pathogenic fungi. These fungicides are decomposed by light (Serra, 1964; Woodcock, 1977) and are readily hydrolyzed when dissolved in aqueous solutions under neutral or alkaline conditions (Siegel and Sisler, 1968; Wolfe *et al.*, 1976).

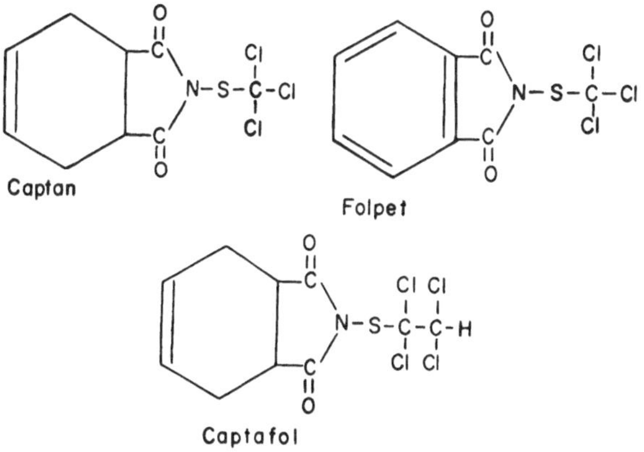

Figure 6.7. Structures of substituted phthalimide fungicides.

The half-time decomposition value for captan in buffer of pH 7.0 at 28–29°C is about 2.5 hr (Burchfield, 1959; Wolfe *et al.*, 1976). Folpet decomposes more rapidly than captan (Wolfe *et al.*, 1976). Half-time decomposition values recorded for this fungicide in buffered nutrient solutions at pH 6.5 and 3.5 at 30°C were 40 min and 350 min, respectively (Siegel and Sisler, 1968).

Hydrolysis of captan yields, in addition to tetrahydrophthalimide, products such as chloride, elemental sulfur, H_2S, and CO_2 that are naturally occurring and constitute no environmental hazard (Wolfe *et al.*, 1976). Similar hydrolysis products would also be anticipated for folpet and captafol.

Captan remained essentially unchanged for 65 days in both sterilized and unsterilized soils of pH 5.7 when applied at relatively high concentrations (Munnecke, 1958). A half-life of more than 70 days for captan in soil was recorded by Domsch (1958); however, Burchfield (1959) found a half-life of only 3–4 days in soil at an initial pH of 6.4. Stability in soil is apparently determined by such factors as rate of solubilization, pH, and temperature. There is a lack of information concerning the role of microorganisms in the degradation of the phthalimide fungicides in the soil. Captan has a broad antimicrobial spectrum, and therefore its application at high rates would probably lead to inhibition of both fungal and bacterial growth and thus to the suppression biodegradation processes.

Various studies with captan and folpet have shown that these compounds are rapidly decomposed in direct reactions with fungal cell components (Lukens and Sisler, 1958; Owens and Blaak, 1960; Richmond and Somers, 1966; Siegel, 1970). Degradation primarily involves direct reaction of the fungicides with thiol constitutents of cells (Engst and Raab, 1973; Lukens and Sisler, 1958; Owens and Blaak, 1960; Siegel and Sisler, 1968). Phthalimide is a major breakdown

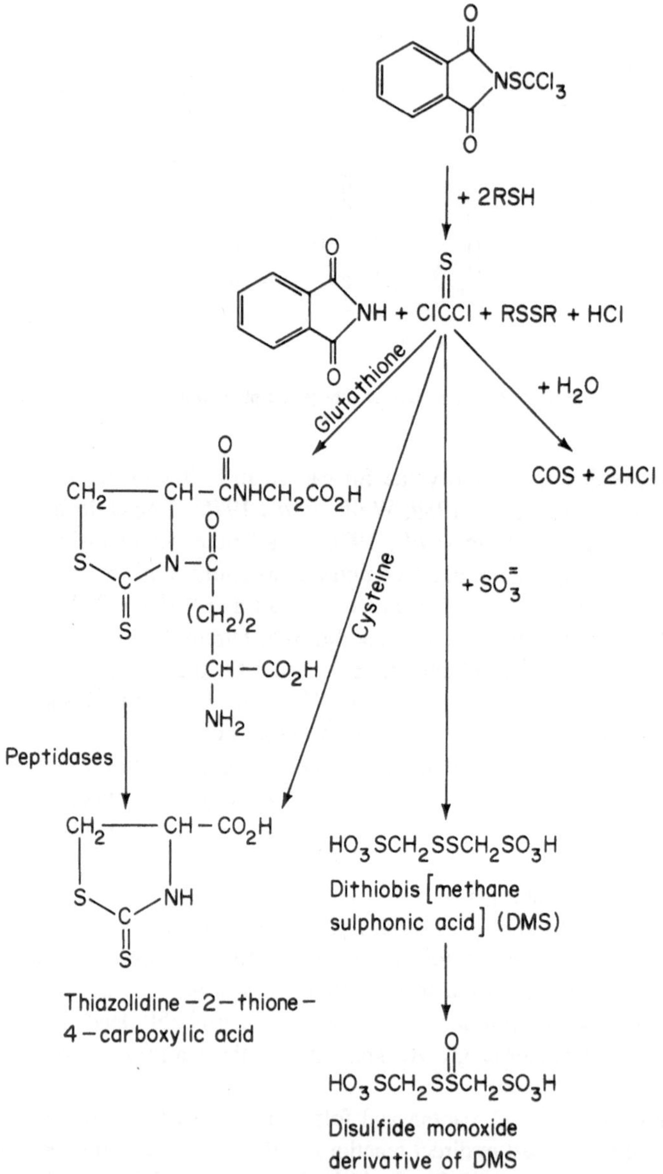

Figure 6.8. Degradation pathways of substituted phthalimide fungicides in biological systems.

product of folpet (Fig. 6.8), while much of the fungicide sulfur is released as volatile products, including carbonyl sulfide (Siegel and Sisler, 1968), presumed to arise from the hydrolysis of the intermediate breakdown product thiophosgene (Somers *et al.*, 1967). A number of products formed in the reaction of folpet with cell components contain sulfur derived from the fungicide (Siegel, 1970). One of these is probably the thiazolidine thione derivative of glutathione (Richmond and Somers, 1968).

TTCA is a major metabolite found in the urine of rats fed captan (DeBaun *et al.*, 1974). It is apparently formed directly in the reaction of thiophosgene with cysteine (DeBaun *et al.*, 1974; Lukens and Sisler, 1958) or in an analogous reaction with reduced glutathione (Fig. 6.8) followed by the action of peptidases. Other animal metabolites include a salt of dithiobis(methane sulfonic acid) and the disulfide monoxide derivative of dithiobis(methane sulfonic acid) (Fig. 6.8), tetrahydrophthalimide, and tetrahydrophthalic acid (DeBaun *et al.*, 1974; Engst and Raab, 1973; Lukens and Sisler, 1958).

Although captan and related phthalimide fungicides are easily degraded by chemical, photochemical, and biological processes, there is little information concerning the ultimate fate of degradation products such as the phthalimide moiety or thiazolidinethione derivatives.

6.4.5. Chloroneb

Chloroneb (1,4-dichloro-2,5-dimethoxybenzene) is a narrow-spectrum fungicide used primarily for seed treatment or soil application to control soil-borne pathogens such as *Pythium* and *Rhizoctonia*, It is slightly systemic in plants, accumulating primarily in the roots and lower portion of the stem (Fielding and Rhodes, 1967).

A half-life in soil of 3–6 months was determined for chloroneb at an application rate 2.25 kg/ha (Rhodes *et al.*, 1971). About 90% of the residue recovered from soil was chloroneb. The remainder was unidentified but was not 2,5-dichloro-4-methoxyphenol, 2,5-dichlorohydroquinone, or 2,5-dichloroquinone.

Bean plants, (Rhodes *et al.*, 1971; Thorne, 1973), various fungi (Hock and Sisler, 1969; Wiese and Vargas, 1973), and animals (Gutenmann and Lisk, 1969; Rhodes and Pease, 1971) demethylate chloroneb to 2,5-dichloro-4-methoxyphenol (Fig. 6.9). Conversion is relatively slow in bean plants. After 12 days the plants contain about equal amounts of chloroneb and DCMP, which account for 95% of the chloroneb taken up. More recent work (Thorne, 1973) indicates that most of the DCMP in bean plants actually exists as the β-D-glucoside (Fig. 6.9). Conjugates of DCMP are also reported as metabolites in animals (Gutenmann and Lisk, 1969; Rhodes and Pease, 1971).

Wiese and Vargas (1973) demonstrated that some fungi convert chloroneb

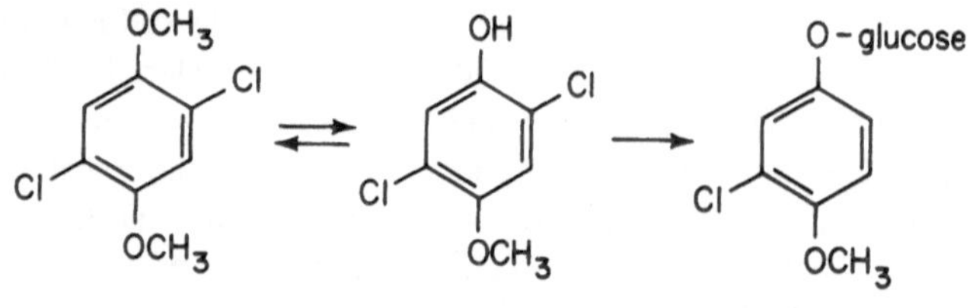

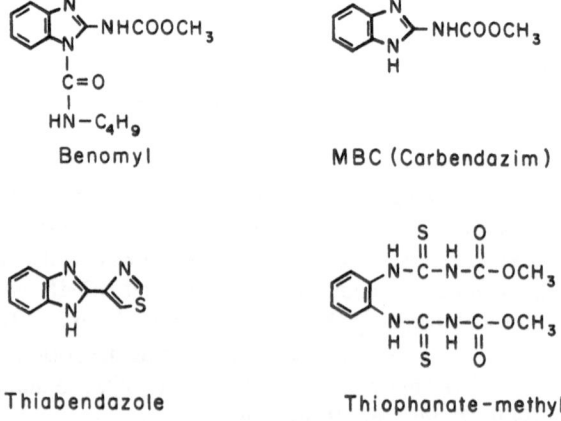

Figure 6.9. Pathway of biotransformation of chloroneb.

to DCMP whereas others convert DCMP to chloroneb. Certain fungi were capable of carrying out the conversion in either direction (Fig. 6.9). Thus, microbial resynthesis of chloroneb from the degradation product DCMP may account in part for the long-term effectiveness of chloroneb in soil.

6.4.6. Benzimidazoles

Benzimidazole fungicides have assumed major significance as crop protectants within the past decade. The most important compounds of this group are benomyl (Benlate), methyl-1-(butylcarbamoyl)-2-benzimidazole carbamate; carbendazim (MBC), methyl-2-benzimidazole carbamate; Mertec), 2-(4'thiazolyl)-benzimidazole; and thiophanate-methyl, 1,2 bis(3-methoxycarbonylthioureido) benzene (Fig. 6.10). Although the latter compound is not a benzimidazole, it undergoes conversion to MBC, through which antifungal activity is mediated (Selling *et al.*, 1970). MBC is also a conversion product of benomyl and is regarded as the component responsible for fungitoxicity (Clemons and Sisler,

Benomyl

MBC (Carbendazim)

Thiabendazole

Thiophanate-methyl

Figure 6.10. Benzimidazole fungicides and thiophanate-methyl.

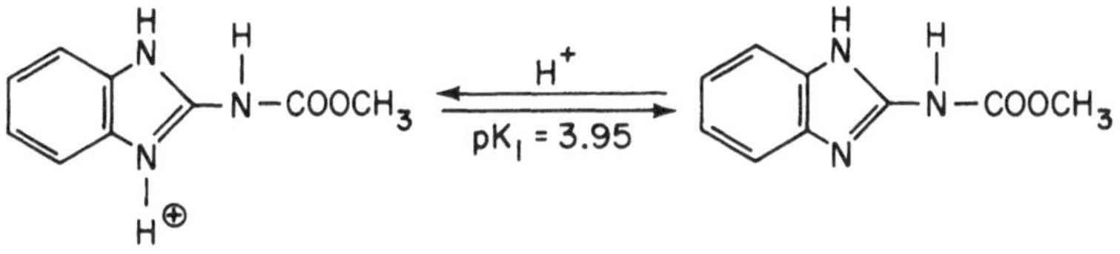

Figure 6.11. Interconversion of the protonated and neutral forms of MBC.

1969). This discussion will focus on the biodegradation of benomyl and MBC, but limited consideration will also be given to other derivatives.

While MBC may be applied as a fungicide, field performance may vary from that obtained when it is generated on or in the plant from a parent compound such as benomyl or thiophanate-methyl. The differences are due to such factors as retention, tissue penetration, and redistribution. For example, when benomyl and MBC are applied to foliage the former penetrates more readily and redistributes better in plant tissue than the latter (Upham and Delp, 1973).

Benzimidazoles may exist in the biological pH range as neutral derivatives or as protonated derivatives (Fig. 6.11), which are much more water soluble than the neutral forms (Erwin, 1977).

Benomyl rapidly converts to MBC in aqueous solutions (Clemons and Sisler, 1969) and in various types of soils (Baude *et al.*, 1974). MBC, however, is resistant to degradation and remains as the major soil metabolite together with lesser amounts of 2-aminobenzimidazole after several months. Baude *et al.* (1974) found a half-life of total benzimidazole residues following benomyl application of 3–6 months on turf and 6–12 months on bare soil. These rates of disappearance are similar to those observed for MBC in soil by Aharonson and Kafkafi (1975) and Janutolo and Stipes (1978).

The fungicide thiophanate-methyl also undergoes rapid transformation to MBC in soil. Transformation is four times as rapid in soil at pH 7.4 as in soil at 5.6 (Fleeker *et al.*, 1974). The rate of conversion is reduced by steam treatment, indicating the involvement of microoranisms in the transformation process. A relatively high stability of MBC in soil was also noted in these studies. Soil incubated for 51 days with [2-^{14}C(ring)]-MBC and [methyl-^{14}C]-MBC released less than 1% and 16%, respectively, of the applied ^{14}C as ^{14}CO$_2$. Recovery of ^{14}C from [2-^{14}C]-MBC-treated soils after 43 days was 53–78%, nearly all of which was in MBC (Fleeker *et al.*, 1974). The slow release of ^{14}C from the benzimidazole ring indicates that it is quite resistant to complete biodegradation. It would be interesting to know the course of benzimidazole ring degradation in soil and whether the rate of breakdown is hastened in soil where benzimidazole fungicides have been used for several years.

Information concerning microbial degradation of benomyl or MBC is very limited. Helwig (1972) reported degradation of benomyl to nonfungitoxic compounds by bacteria and fungi. Mixed cultures of bacteria were reported to degrade ring-labeled MBC; 2-aminobenzimidazole (2AB) was identified as one of the metabolites, and $^{14}CO_2$ was evolved, indicating benzimidazole ring cleavage (Fuchs and Bollen, 1975). Methyl-5-hydroxy-2-benzimidazole carbamate (5-hydroxy-MBC, Fig. 6.12) has been identified as a transformation product of MBC in cultures of the fungi *Pellicularia sasakii, Alternaria mali* (Yasuda *et al.*, 1973), and *Aspergillis nidulans* (Davidse, 1976). To my knowledge, this compound has not been reported as a soil metabolite of benomyl, MBC, or thiophanate-methyl. One avenue of loss of MBC from soil might be the leaching of this hydroxylated derivative.

Principal residues following benomyl application to plant foliage are benomyl and MBC (Baude *et al.*, 1973). Due to its instability in aqueous solutions (Clemons and Sisler, 1969), benomyl does not persist for long in plant tissues (Fuchs *et al.*, 1972; Peterson and Edgington, 1969; Sims *et al.*, 1969). MBC, on the other hand, is quite stable in plant tissues. Fifty-two days after application of [^{14}C]-MBC to roots of pea plants, 78% of the label remaining in the plant tissue was in MBC (Siegel and Zabbia, 1972). The metabolites present were not identified except for traces of 2AB. Degradation of MBC was more rapid in strawberry plants than in pea plants, but except for 2AB the metabolites were not characterized fully (Siegel, 1973). The benzimidazole nucleus is quite stable in plants (Siegel, 1973); however, there is evidence for slow degradation. Solel *et al.* (1973) reported that about 1.5% of ^{14}C in ring-labeled MBC applied to melon plants was released as $^{14}CO_2$ in 14 days.

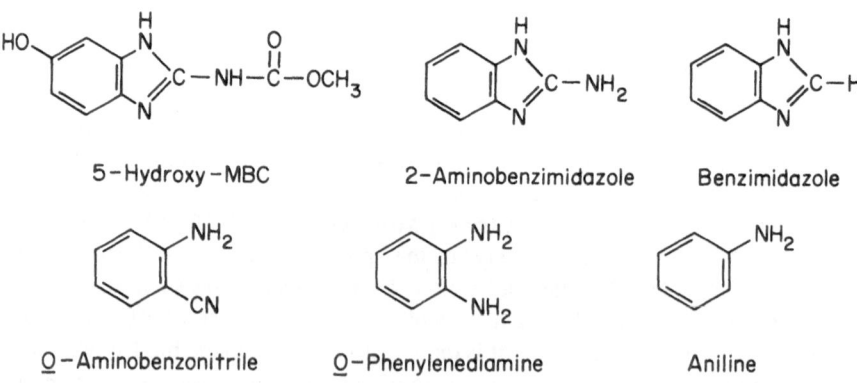

5-Hydroxy-MBC   2-Aminobenzimidazole   Benzimidazole

O-Aminobenzonitrile   O-Phenylenediamine   Aniline

Figure 6.12.   Degradation products of MBC.

A variety of metabolites (Fig. 6.12) were found in melon plants exposed for 2 months to 20 μg/ml of benomyl in the nutrient solution. The plants contained the following metabolites in the relative proportions indicated: MBC (free and conjugated), 53.5%; 2AB (free and conjugated), 27.5%; benzimidazole, 8.8%; *o*-aminobenzonitrile, 8.4%; and aniline, 1.8% (Rouchaud *et al.*, 1974). Photochemical reactions may be involved in the formation of the last two compounds (Rouchaud *et al.*, 1974). More recent studies demonstrated the conversion of benzimidazole and 2AB in melon plants to aniline, *o*-aminobenzonitrile, and *o*-phenylenediamine (Rouchaud *et al.*, 1977*a*). The degradation products of benomyl found in melon plants were also found in carrot, strawberry, and apple tissue (Rouchaud *et al.*, 1977*b*). The pathway of conversion in plant tissue appears to be

$$
\text{Benomyl} \rightarrow \text{MBC} \rightarrow \text{2AB} \rightarrow \text{benzimidazole} \rightarrow \left\{ \begin{array}{l} \text{aniline} \\ o\text{-phenylenediamine} \\ o\text{-aminobenzonitrile} \end{array} \right.
$$

Benomyl and MBC are metabolized by animals to 5-hydroxy-MBC, which is eliminated in the urine and feces as glucuronide and/or sulfate conjugates (Gardiner *et al.*, 1974). More than 99% of a single oral dose of benomyl was eliminated in a rat and dog in 24 hr. On the other hand, mice, sheep, and rats dosed orally with benomyl are reported to excrete not only 5-hydroxy-MBC but also significant quantities of MBC, 2AB, and 5-hydroxy-2-aminobenzimidazole. In all three species about 20% of the administered dose was excreted as conjugates of hydroxylated derivatives (Douch, 1973).

A recent summary of literature of TBZ metabolism in animals shows that 5-hydroxy-TBZ or its sulfate or glucuronide derivatives are the major metabolites excreted (Paulson, 1977). Benzimidazole metabolites of thiophanate-methyl in animals are similar to those reported for benomyl (Douch, 1973); however, a number of nonbenzimidazole metabolites are also present (Paulson, 1977).

6.5. EFFECT OF FUNGICIDES ON PESTICIDE DEGRADATION

Fungicides may affect degradation of other pesticides by inhibiting growth of microorganisms or the action of enzymes involved in the degradation process. Kaufman (1972) demonstrated, for example, that PCNB or a combination of DDT and captan increases soil persistence of the herbicide chlorpropham. Degradation of the fungicide dibutyl *N*-methyl-*N*-phenylphosphoramidate by the fungus *Pyricularia oryzae* is markedly inhibited by another synergistic fungicide, diisopropyl *S*-benzylphosphorothiolate (Kitazin) (Uesugi and Sisler, 1978). The latter compound apparently inhibits a hydroxylase or *N*-demethylase involved in the metabolism of the former.

Several fungicides such as imazalil, triadimefon, triforine, and fenarimol strongly inhibit sterol C-14 demethylation, possibly by interfering with a cytochrome P-450 mixed-function oxidase (Ragsdale, 1977). Although these fungicides are probably not general inhibitors of this type of activity (Ragsdale, 1977), the possibility that they may interfere with the oxidative metabolism of other pesticides should not be overlooked.

6.6. SUMMARY AND CONCLUSIONS

With a few minor exceptions, agricultural fungicides do not pose a serious acute toxicity hazard to mammals and most other forms of animals life. On the other hand, obscure or delayed toxic effects of chemicals are not always recognized; therefore exposure to these compounds should be held to the minimum possible levels.

Most organic fungicides do not remain for long periods in the environment, since they are readily degraded by chemical, photochemical, or biological processes. There are notable exceptions, however, such as PCNB, which may persist in some soils for 3 or more years. Metabolites of fungicides sometimes persist for much longer periods than the parent compound. PCNB, for example, is rapidly reduced in anaerobic soils to PCA, a compound which remains largely undegraded after 2 or more years. Benomyl is rapidly converted to carbendazim and other residues in soils which may have a half-life as long as 1 year. The ultimate fate of many organic fungicide degradation products has not been fully determined. More information is needed concerning the fate of such residues as the phthalimide moiety of captan and related compounds, the benzimidazole moiety of benomyl and related fungicides, and PCA derived from PCNB.

Environmental factors can have a marked effect on the biodegradation of fungicides. Compounds which readily degrade in soils under favorable conditions for microbiological activity may persist for very long periods in unfavorable environments such as extreme pH, very low temperatures, or anaerobic conditions.

Interaction of a fungicide or its breakdown products with other substances under certain conditions can lead to the formation of hazardous or otherwise undesirable products. An example is the formation of dimethylnitrosomine from thiram or its breakdown products in acidic soils under flooded condtions.

It should be expected that systemic fungicides would be more resistant to biodegradation than surface protectants since the effectiveness of the latter is more dependent on stability in plant tissue than that of the former, but there are undoubtedly exceptions to this generalization.

From the environmental point of view it is desirable to have agricultural fungicides that rapidly biodegrade to harmless natural products. However, this expectation may not be wholly consistent with the objectives of fungicide application, which require that the compounds be present for a certain period to achieve the desired effect. Meeting acceptable standards for both goals is the challenge which must be met, and this will require, among other things, full knowledge of the rates and pathways of fungicide degradation.

REFERENCES

Aharonson, N., and Kafkafi, U., 1975, Absorption, mobility and persistence of thiabendazole and methyl 2-benzimidazole-carbamate in soils, *J. Agric. Food Chem.* **23**:720.

Anonymous, 1977, Ethylenethiourea, *Pure Appl. Chem.* **49**:675.

Ayanaba, A., Verstraete, W., and Alexander, M., 1973, Formation of dimethylnitrosamine, a carcinogen and mutage, in soils treated with nitrogen compounds, *Soil Sci. Soc. Am. Proc.* **37**:565.

Barnes, R. D., Bull, A. T., and Poller, R. C., 1971, Behavior of triphenyltin acetate in soil, *Chem. Ind. (London)*, p. 204.

Barnes, R. D., Bull, A. T., and Poller, R. C., 1973, Studies on the persistence of the organotin fungicide fentin acetate (triphenyltin acetate) in the soil and on surfaces exposed to light, *Pestic. Sci.* **4**:305.

Baude, F. J., Gardiner, J. A., and Han, J. C. Y., 1973, Characterization of residues on plants following foliar spray applications of benomyl, *J. Agric. Food Chem.* **21**:1084.

Baude, F. J., Pease, H. L., and Holt, R. F., 1974, Fate of benomyl on field soil and turf, *J. Agric. Food Chem.* **22**:413.

Beck, J., and Hansen, K. E., 1974, The degradation of quintozene, pentachlorobenzene, hexachlorobenzene and pentachloraniline in soil, *Pestic. Sci.* **5**:41.

Brown, A. W. A., 1978, *Ecology of Pesticides*, Wiley, New York.

Burchfield, H. P., 1959, Comparative stabilities of dyrene, 1-fluoro-2,4-dinitrobenzene, dichlone and captan in a silt loam soil, *Contrib. Boyce Thompson Inst.* **20**:205.

Chacko, C. I., Lockwood, J. L., and Zabik, M., 1966, Chlorinated hydrocarbon pesticides: Degradation by microbes, *Science* **154**:893.

Clemons, G. P., and Sisler, H. D., 1969, Formation of a fungitoxic derivative from Benlate, *Phytopathology* **59**:705.

Davidse, L. C., 1976, Metabolic conversion of methyl benzimidazol-2-yl carbamate (MBC) in *Aspergillus nidulans*, *Pestic. Biochem. Physiol.* **6**:538.

DeBaun, J. R., Miaullis, J. B., Knarr, J., Mihailovski, A., and Menn, J. J., 1974, The fate of N-trichloro[^{14}C]methylthio-4-cyclohexene-1,2-dicarboximide ([^{14}C]captan) in the rat, *Xenobiotica* **4**:101.

Domsch, K. H., 1958, Die Wirkung von Bodenfungiciden. II. Wirkungsdauer, *Z. Pflanzenkr. Pflanzenschutz* **65**:651.

Douch, P. G. C., 1973, The metabolism of benomyl fungicide in mammals, *Xenobiotica* **3**:367.

EBDC, Fungicide Assessment Team, U.S. Department of Agriculture, 1977, Assessment of ethy-lenebisdithiocarbamate (EBDC) fungicide uses in agriculture. I. An analysis of uses and their relationship to exposure, U.S. Department of Agriculture, Washington, D.C.

Engst, R., and Raab, M., 1973, Zum Metabolismus fungizider phthalimid-Derivate in lebensmittelchemischtoxikologischer Sicht, *Nahrung* **17**:731.

Erwin, D. C., 1977, Control of vascular pathogens, in: *Antifungal Compounds*, Vol. 1 (M. R. Siegel and H. D. Sisler, eds.), pp. 163–224, Marcel Dekker, New York.

Fielding, M. J., and Rhodes, R. C., 1967, Studies with C^{14}-labeled chloroneb fungicides in plants, *Cotton Dis. Counc. Proc.* **27**:56.

Fishbein, L., 1977, Toxicological aspects of fungicides, in: *Antifungal Compounds*, Vol. 1 (M. R. Siegel and H. D. Sisler, eds.), pp. 537–598, Marcel Dekker, New York.

Fleeker, J. R., Lacy, H. M., Schultz, I. R., and Houkom, E. C., 1974, Persistence and metabolism of thiophanate-methyl in soil, *J. Agric. Food Chem.* **22**:592.

Fuchs, A., and Bollen, G. J., 1975, Benomyl after seven years, in: *Systemic Fungicides* (H. Lyr and C. Polter, eds.), pp. 121–136, Akademie-Verlag, Berlin.

Fuchs, A., Van den Berg, G. A., and Davidse, L. C., 1972, A comparison of benomyl and thiophanates with respect to some chemical and systemic fungitoxic characteristics, *Pestic. Biochem. Physiol.* **2**:192.

Gardiner, J. A., Kirkland, J. J., Klopping, H. L., and Sherman, H., 1974, Fate of benomyl in animals, *J. Agric. Food Chem.* **22**:419.

Goksøyr, J., 1955, The effect of some dithiocarbamyl compounds on the metabolism of fungi, *Physiol. Plant.* **8**:719.

Gorbach, S., and Wagner, U., 1967, Pentachloronitrobenzene residues in potatoes, *J. Agric. Food Chem.* **15**:654.

Gutenmann, W. H., and Lisk, D. J., 1969, Metabolic studies with chloroneb fungicide in a lactating cow, *J. Agric. Food Chem.* **17**:1008.

Helwig, A., 1972, Microbial breakdown of the fungicide benomyl, *Soil Biol. Biochem.* **4**:377.

Hoagland, R. E., and Frear, D. S., 1976, Behavior and fate of ethylenethiourea in plants, *J. Agric. Food Chem.* **24**:129.

Hock, W. K., and Sisler, H. D., 1969, Metabolism of chloroneb by *Rhizoctonia solani* and other fungi, *J. Agric. Food Chem.* **17**:123.

Janutolo, D. B., and Stipes, R. J., 1978, Benzimidazole fungitoxicants in Virginia soils: Movement, disappearance and effect on microorganisms, *Va. Wat. Res. Cent. Bull. No.* **113**.

Johnston, C. D., 1953, The *in vitro* reaction between tetraethylithiuram disulfide (Antabuse) and glutathione, *Arch. Biochem. Biophys.* **44**:249.

Kaars Sijpesteijn, A., and van der Kerk, G. J. M., 1954, Investigations on organic fungicides. VIII. The biochemical mode of action of bisdithiocarbamates and diisothiocyanates, *Biochim. Biophys. Acta* **13**:545.

Kaars Sijpesteijn, A., Dekhuijzen, H. M., Kaslander, J., Pluijger, C. W., and van der Kerk, G. J. M., 1963, Metabolism of sodium dimethyldithiocarbamate by plants and microorganisms, *Meded. Landbouwhogesch. Gent.* **28**:597.

Kaars Sijpesteijn, A., Luijten, J. G. A., and van der Ker, G. J. M., 1969, Organometallic fungicides, in: *Fungicides*, Vol. 2 (D. C. Torgeson, ed.), pp. 331–366, Academic Press, New York.

Kaars Sijpesteijn, A., Dekhuijzen, H. M., and Vonk, J. W., 1977, Biological conversion of fungicides in plants and microorganism, in: *Antifungal Compounds*, Vol. 2 (M. R. Siegel and H. D. Sisler, eds.), pp. 91–147, Marcel Dekker, New York.

Kaufman, D. D., 1972, Degradation of pesticide combinations, *Pestic. Chem.* **6**:175.

Kaufman, D. D., 1977, Soil-fungicide interactions, in: *Antifungal Compounds*, Vol. 2 (M. R. Siegel and H. D. Sisler, eds.), pp. 1–49, Marcel Dekker, New York.

Kaufman, D. D., and Fletcher, C. L., 1973, Ethylenethiourea degradation in soil, Abstracts of the Second International Congress on Plant Pathology, Minneapolis.

Ko, W. H., and Farley, J. D., 1969, Conversion of pentachloronitrobenzene to pentachloroaniline in soil and the effect of these compounds on soil microorganisms, *Phytopathology* **59**:64.

Kuchar, E. J., Geenty, F. O., Griffith, W. P., and Thomas, R. J., 1969, Analytical studies of metabolism of terrachlor in beagle dogs, rats and plants, *J. Agric. Food Chem.* **17**:1237.

Kumarasamy, R., and Raghu, W., 1976, Conversion of the fungicide, ziram, in rice plants, *Agric. Biol. Chem.* **40**:297.

Lukens, R. J., and Sisler, H. D., 1958, Chemical reactions involved in the fungitoxicity of captan, *Phytopathology* **48**:235.

Miller, P. M., 1969, Benomyl and thiabendazole suppress root invasion by larvae of *Heterodera tobacum, Phytopathology* **59**:1040.

Moje, W., Munnecke, D. E., and Richardson, L. T., 1964, Carbonyl sulphide, a volatile fungitoxicant from nabam in soil, *Nature (London)* **202**:831.

Munnecke, D. E., 1958, The persistence of nonvoliatile diffusable fungicides in soil, *Phytopathology* **48**:581.

Munnecke, D. E., 1972, Factors affecting the efficacy of fungicides in soil, *Annu. Rev. Phytopathology* **10**:375.

Munnecke, D. E., and Mickail, K. Y., 1967, Thiram persistence in soil and control of damping-off caused by *Pythium ultimum, Phytopathology* **57**:969.

Murthy, N. B. K., and Kaufman, D. D., 1978, Degradation of pentachloronitrobenzene (PCNB) in anaerobic soils, *J. Agric. Food Chem.* **26**:1151.

Nakanishi, T., and Oku, H., 1969, Metabolism and accumulation of pentachloronitrobenzene by phytopathogenic fungi in relation to selective toxicity, *Phytopathology* **59**:1761.

Newsome, W. H., 1976, Residues of four ethylenebis (dithiocarbamates) and their decomposition products on field-sprayed tomatoes, *J. Agric. Food Chem.* **24**:999.

Owens, R. G., and Blaak, G., 1960, Chemistry of the reactions of dichlone and captan with thiols, *Contrib. Boyce Thompson Inst.* **20**:475.

Paulson, G. D., 1977, Biological conversions of fungicides in animals, in: *Antifungal Compounds,* Vol. 2 (M. R. Siegel and H. D. Sisler, eds.), pp. 149–208, Marcel Dekker, New York.

Peterson, C. A., and Edgington, L. V., 1969, Quantitative estimation of the fungicide benomyl using a bioautograph technique, *J. Agric. Food Chem.* **17**:898.

Raghu, K., Murthy, N. B. K., Kumarasamy, R., Rao, R. S., and Sane, P. V., 1975, Fate and persistence of thiram in plants and soil, in: *Proceedings of the Joint FAO/IAEA Division of Atomic Energy in Food and Agriculture,* pp. 137–148, International Atomic Energy Agency, Vienna.

Ragsdale, N. N., 1977, Inhibitors of lipid synthesis, in: *Antifungal Compounds,* Vol. 2 (M. R. Siegel and H. D. Sisler, eds.), pp. 333–363, Marcel Dekker, New York.

Rhodes, R. H., and Pease, H. L., 1971, Fate of chloroneb in animals, *J. Agric. Food Chem.* **19**:750.

Rhodes, R. C., Pease, H. L., and Brantley, R. K., 1971, Fate of C^{14}-labeled chloroneb in plants and soils, *J. Agric. Food Chem.* **19**:745.

Richmond, D. V., and Somers, E., 1966, Studies on the fungitoxicity of captan. IV. Reactions of captan with cell thiols, *Ann. Appl. Biol.* **57**:231.

Richmond, D. V., and Somers, E., 1968, Studies on the fungitoxicity of captan. VI. Decomposition of ^{35}S-labeled captan by *Neurospora crassa conidia, Ann. Appl. Biol.* **62**:35.

Ridley, W. P., Dizikes, L. J., and Woods, J. M., 1977, Biomethylation of toxic elements in the environment, *Science* **197**:329.

Rouchaud, J. P., Decallonne, J. R., and Meyer, J. A., 1974, Metabolic fate of methyl-2-benzimidazole carbamate in melon plants, *Phytopathology* **64**:1513.

Rouchaud, J. P., Decallonne, J. R., and Meyer, J. A., 1977a, Metabolism of benzimidazole and 2-aminobenzimidazole in melon plants, *Pestic. Sci.* **8**:31.

Rouchaud, J. P., Lhoest, G. J., Mercier, M. J., and Meyer, J. A., 1977b, Metabolism of benomyl in carrot, strawberry and apple, *Pestic. Sci.* **8**:23.

Selling, H. A., Vonk, J. W., and Kaars Sijpesteijn, A., 1970, Transformation of the systemic fungicide methyl thiophanate to 2-benzimidazole carbamic acid methyl ester, *Chem. Ind. (London)*, p. 1625.

Serra, G., 1964, Etude de la dégradation du captane du Phaltane et du Difolatan sous l'influence de la lumière, *Phytiatr. Phytopharm.* **13**:107.

Sharvelle, E. G., 1961, *The Nature and Uses of Modern Fungicides*, Burgess, Minneapolis, Minnesota.

Siegel, M. R., 1970, Reactions of certain trichloromethyl sulfenyl fungicides with low molecular weight thiols: *In vivo* studies with cells of *Saccharomyces pastorianus*, *J. Agric. Food Chem.* **18**:823.

Siegel, M. R., 1973, Distribution and metabolism of methyl-2-benzimidazole carbamate, the fungitoxic derivative of benomyl in strawberry plants, *Phytopathology* **63**:890.

Siegel, M. R., and Sisler, H. D., 1968, Fate of the phthalimide and trichloromethylthio (SCCl₃) moieties of folpet in toxic action on cells of *Saccharomyces pastorianus*, *Phytopathology* **58**:1123.

Siegel, M. R., and Zabbia, A. J., Jr., 1972, Distribution and metabolic fate of the fungicide benomyl in dwarf pea, *Phytopathology* **62**:630.

Sims, J. J., Mee, H., and Erwin, D. C., 1969, Methyl 2-benzimidazole-carbamate, a fungitoxic compound isolated from cotton plants treated with methyl 1-(butylcarbamoyl)-2-benzimidazole carbamate (benomyl), *Phytopathology* **59**:1775.

Sisler, H. D., and Cox, C. E., 1954, Effects of tetramethylthiuram disulfide on metabolism of *Fusarium roseum*, *Am. J. Bot.* **41**:338.

Solel, Z., Schooley, J. M., and Edgington, L. V., 1973, Uptake and translocation of benomyl and carbendazim (methylbenzimidazol-2yl-carbamate) in the symplast, *Pestic. Sci.* **4**:713.

Somers, E., Richmond, D. V., and Pickard, J. A., 1967, Carbonyl sulphide from the decomposition of captan, *Nature (London)* **215**:214.

Stringer, A., and Lyons, C. H., 1974, The effect of benomyl and thiophanate-methyl on earthworm populations in apple orchards, *Pestic. Sci.* **5**:189.

Thorne, G. D., 1973, Uptake and metabolism of chloroneb by *Phaseolus vulgaris*, *Pestic. Biochem. Physiol.* **3**:137.

Thorne, G. D., and Ludwig, R. A., 1962, *The Dithiocarbamates and Related Compounds*, Elsevier, Amsterdam.

Uesugi, Y., and Sisler, H. D., 1978, Metabolism of a phosphoramidate by *Pyricularia oryzae* in relation to tolerance and synergism by phosphorothiolate and isoprothiolane, *Pestic. Biochem. Physiol.* **9**:247.

Ulfvarson, U., 1969, Organic mercuries, in: *Fungicides*, Vol. 2 (D. C. Torgeson, ed.), pp. 303–329, Academic Press, New York.

United States Department of Agriculture, 1974, *Guidelines for the Chemical Control of Plant Diseases and Nematodes*, Agriculture Handbook No. 378, Washington, D.C.

Upham, P. M., and Delp, C. J., 1973, Role of benomyl in systemic control of fungi and mites on herbaceous plants, *Phytopathology* **63**:814.

Vonk, J. W., 1975, Chemical decomposition of bisdithiocarbamate fungicides and their metabolism by plants and microorganisms, Ph.D. Thesis, University of Utrecht.

Wang, C. H., and Broadbent, F. E., 1973, Effect of soil treatments on losses of two chloronitrobenzene fungicides, *J. Environ. Qual.* **2**:511.

Wiese, M. V., and Vargas, J. M., 1973, Interconversion of chloroneb and 2,5-dichloro-4-meth-oxyphenol by soil microorganisms, *Pestic. Biochem. Physiol.* 3:214.

Wolfe, N. L., Zepp, R. G., Doster, J. C., and Hollis, R. C., 1976, Captan hydrolysis, *J. Agric. Food Chem.* 24:1041.

Woodcock, D., 1977, Nonbiological conversions of fungicides, in: *Antifungal Compounds*, Vol. 2 (M. R. Siegel and H. D. Sisler, eds.), pp. 209–249, Marcel Dekker, New York.

Yasuda, Y., Hashimoto, S., and Soeda, Y., 1973, Metabolism of thiophanate-methyl by pathogenic fungi and antifungal activity of its metabolites, *Ann. Jpn. Phytopathol. Soc.* 39:49.

7

Biodegradable Insecticides
Their Application in Forestry

Carl E. Crisp

7.1. INTRODUCTION

The demand for greater output from forest lands has been matched by two other competing demands: maintaining the quality of the environment and more extensive and intensive management of the land. To manage insect pests that compete with human use of forest lands, the resource manager must rely on pesticides (NAS, 1975b). Following the best application strategies is a key part of an integrated pest management program. At the same time, undiminished effort must be made to prevent pollution of the air, land, and water beyond a level considered safe for nontarget life forms. To minimize risks, the resource manager must apply the best scientific findings available.

Pesticide applications must be done under the guidelines of legislative mandates at the federal and state levels of government (Deck, 1975). Consequently, the resource manager now has only limited insecticide tools in pest management that are registered with the U.S. Environmental Protection Agency (EPA) and approved for use (Dewey, 1979; U.S. Department of Agriculture 1976a, 1977a, 1978a).

Forest pest control and the application of chemicals to forests have been reviewed by the National Academy of Sciences (1975b) and by Hobart (1977). Pschorn-Walcher (1977) summarized the status of biological control of forest insects. This review of the literature is restricted to research and the development of insecticides and their application in forestry. Most of the references cited are

Carl E. Crisp ● Pacific Southwest Forest and Range Experiment Station, Forest Service, U.S. Department of Agriculture, Berkeley, California 94701.

from current publications, reports, and studies from the two agencies that have led the way in the application and use of biodegradable, environmentally safe pesticides for the control of major insect pests in the United States and Canada. These agencies are the Forest Service, U.S. Department of Agriculture, through its Insecticide Evaluation Research Work Unit and Field Evaluation of Chemical Insecticides Research Work Unit, both of the Pacific Southwest Forest and Range Experiment Station, Berkeley, California; and the Forestry Service, Canadian Department of Environment, through its Forest Pest Management Institute, Sault Ste. Marie, Ontario. Hundreds of cooperators in industry, government, and academic institutions in Canada and the United States have contributed to this effort. The close working relationship between the two countries was brought about by a need to resolve pest problems common to both (Honing, 1976). An example of this cooperation, which has gained official status, is the Canada–United States Spruce Budworms Program (CANUSA) (CANUSA, 1979; USDA, 1976b). The United States role in CANUSA and all other United States pest control programs is in accordance with laws and regulations (USDA, 1976b) under authority of the McSweeney–McNary Forest Research Act of May 22, 1928 (45 Stat. 699), as amended and supplemented (16 U.S.C. 581, 581a–581i, 76 Stat. 579 and 92 Stat. 365–375), and the Cooperative Forestry Assistance Act of 1978. The Forest and Rangeland Resource Planning Act supersedes the Mc-Sweeney–McNary Act.

The implementation of pesticide use, regulation, and management by the United States has a worldwide impact (NAS, 1978). What it does in legislation, regulation, management, and application is often adapted by other countries. In many Third World countries public health considerations and economic capabilities enter judgments to accept or reject new technologies.

The use of an insecticide for operational control of a pest in the United States depends on whether the EPA has registered it as an approved formulation in a prescribed application method for that particular pest (Deck, 1975). Under some conditions states can grant a local use permit. Thus, the risk–benefit analysis conducted by the EPA ultimately determines if a particular insecticide strategy can be used (NAS, 1978). Pesticide registration of a particular formulation depends on many factors not related to efficacy, e.g., carcinogenicity (NAS, 1978). Much of what is reviewed here is the result of efforts directed at sound scientific data that can be used by industry to make risk–benefit analyses and to assure that the pesticide will not result in an unreasonable adverse effect on humans or the environment (NAS, 1978). Determinations are made on a scientific basis alone (e.g., laboratory screening, small- and large-scale field tests). The quantification of unreasonable adverse effect is based in part on scientific data, but to ascertain or agree upon what constitutes an unreasonable environmental risk is almost impossible because of the widely divergent views between resource managers of pest management. The goal of forestry insecticide R&D is to provide the forest manager with a choice of registered insecticides as part of an integrated pest management program for suppression of major forest pest problems. The approach used by the Forest Service to make the transition from DDT to the present use of conventional biodegradable insecticides is the focus of this review.

To stress the importance of the environmental aspect of pesticide R&D, a former chief of the Forest Service (McGuire, 1976) has said:

> The solutions to our problems are becoming more difficult to achieve and will continue to become increasingly complex because of environmental considerations; but this is only proper. We must be responsive to the environmental impacts associated with our programs and the programs of others. We must broaden our responsibilities to include all aspects of environmental quality as it affects the health and vitality of forest stands.

7.2. NEED FOR INSECTICIDES

In the United States, native and introduced insect populations in forests at times cause considerable economic damage (NAS, 1975*b*). Most of the significant insect damage to forests is done by defoliators and bark beetles. The most important defoliators are the spruce budworm [*Choristoneura fumiferana* (Clem.)], western spruce budworm (*Choristoneura occidentalis* Freeman), Douglas fir tussock moth [*Orgyia pseudotsugata* (McDunnough)], and gypsy moth [*Lymantria dispar* (L.)]. Other defoliators are serious pests at times on specialty sites (e.g., Christmas tree farms) (NAS, 1975*b*).

The most destructive cambium–phloem-feeding insects are the bark beetles. Predominant species creating major economic losses are the western pine beetle (*Dendroctonus brevicomis* Le Conte), spruce beetle [*Dendroctonus rufipennis* (Kirby)], mountain pine beetle (*Dendroctonus ponderosae* Hopkins), and southern pine beetle (*Dendroctonus frontalis* Zimmerman). The trees lost from these cryptic insects are highly visible because of changes in coloration. Such changes are associated with impending death in trees.

Impact of forest insects is hard to assess (NAS, 1975*a,b*) and is a major part of future programs to develop technology in impact assessment of defoliators (CANUSA, 1979; USDA, 1977*b*, 1978*b*) and bark beetles. The impact of insect defoliators on growth and mortality of trees has been reviewed (Kulman, 1971). Radial growth ceases only if defoliation is complete (Rose, 1958). Partial defoliation, as associated with most coniferous insect defoliators, results in a reduction in radial growth and may cause top-kill and dieback. The major impact of insect defoliation or growth of conifer trees more closely correlates with utilization than with production of photosynthate, since stored carbohydrate is often present but not utilized in the absence of plant hormones. Usually, the greatest and first observable effects are noted in the living crown where hormones are produced (Kulman, 1971). Trees in Minnesota forests infested with jack pine budworm (*Choristoneura pinus* Freeman) have lost 55–61% of their timber volumes compared to noninfested trees. Heavy defoliation of forests in New Brunswick by spruce budworm can cause volume losses of 33–50% in 10 years. One year of light defoliation has little or no impact on long-term growth (Kulman, 1971; Fettes and Buckner, 1976).

In the forests of the northwestern United States, where the western spruce budworm is the major defoliator, the greatest damage is (1) reduction in height and radial growth, and top-killing and tree-killing in regeneration, sapling, and some pole-size stands; (2) growth reduction and top-killing in older growth stands; and (3) damage to cones and seeds (Fellin, 1980). The effect of defoliation by gypsy moth on eastern hardwood forests is a 24–37% reduction in volume— depending on the tree species (Kulman, 1971).

Defoliation as a stress factor in forests is not the same as in agriculture (NAS, 1975b). Because the rotation times for mature trees are much longer, the general effect of defoliation by most insects is usually not tree mortality but retardation of growth and in some cases lengthening of the rotation time.

The loss on commercial forest land attributable to all insects totals 1.3 billion board feet per year (Johnson and Lawrence, 1977). The total dollar value of agricultural crop losses due to insects has been estimated at 18% of the potential crop value (Pimentel *et al.*, 1978). With the use of insecticides, this loss was reduced to 13%. And for every cost unit invested in pest control, four units of profit were returned in additional agricultural products. A similar study needs to be done on losses in timber production caused by insects.

The effect of a major insect outbreak and the resulting defoliation on esthetic resources and wildlife can be both positive and negative depending on the value judgment assigned to the forest unit under management (McGuire, 1976). Spruce budworm attacks not only kill balsam fir and white spruce trees in 3–5 years of extreme defoliation but also increase the fuel load, with threat of vast fires as an aftermath to epidemics (Fettes and Buckner, 1976).

Aerial surveys presently estimate defoliator boundaries and defoliation intensities (Krebs, 1976). Results from aerial surveys show that 52.8 million hectares in Canada and the United States are infested with spruce budworm each year.

Not all infested areas surveyed will be treated chemically, because they are not all managed under extensive or intensive silvicultural practices (NAS, 1975b). As future demands for forest resources increase, a trend toward intensive management appears likely. With such management, the application of insecticides usually increases as part of the pest management program (NAS, 1975b). But this may not be true if sound prevention practices are part of the overall pest management plan. Then the use of insecticides may actually decrease. Most forests in North America are extensively managed. Intensive management should reduce the losses attributed to insects.

The major method for suppressing insect outbreaks, especially of defoliators, is by chemical means (Ciesla, 1976, 1977; Fettes and Buckner, 1976; Graham, 1975; Johnson and Lawrence, 1977; Krebs, 1976; Lyon, 1974; NAS, 1975*b;* Mrak, 1969; Pimentel *et al.,* 1978; and Sanders, 1976). Chemicals are used because no viable immediate alternative exists to suppress an outbreak (Honing, 1976; Pimentel *et al.,* 1978). The availability of insect-resistant trees has been slow to develop (Irving, 1970). Microbials have been used with some success (Morris, 1977). Biological control in forestry (Pschorn-Walcher, 1977) is a young, unproven science. And pheromone strategies for the manipulation of forest insects to control outbreaks or suppress them (Wood, 1977) remain to be realized.

Some scientists are opposed to the use of chemicals on the grounds that insects soon develop resistance to chemicals and that this approach will prove to be ineffective (Luck *et al.,* 1977). Resistance has not been a major problem, however, in forest pest management. Furthermore it remains to be proven that chemicals will provide a no-risk input into the environment. The cost of R&D in the continuing search for new chemicals (Rumker *et al.,* 1970), biologicals (Pschorn-Walcher, 1977), and pheromones (Wood, 1977) continues to escalate. Likewise, the controversy continues over which pest management strategy is best. Perhaps in the near future pest management by biological control can be upgraded to a profit-making enterprise and become competitive with insecticides.

From 1945 to 1974, a total of 35 forest insect pests were treated with insecticides over an area covering approximately 52 million hectares in the United States and considerably more in Canada. The land infested by the western spruce budworm and gypsy moth accounted for 82.4% of this area (NAS, 1975*b*). To accomplish this spray program, which was primarily for budworm, extending over 29 years, 20.4 million pounds of insecticide was used, and in Canada this figure must be considerably higher. The most widely used insecticide was DDT. Since the banning of DDT in 1972, the insecticide mass applied to forests has been approximately 15% of the pre-1968 totals (NAS, 1975*b*). More recently, the insecticides used in control programs and large experimental tests were carbaryl, mexacarbate, malathion, trichlorfon, fenitrothion, tetrachlorvinphos, aminocarb, phosphamidon, dimethoate, and propoxur.

7.3. USE OF DDT: 1945–1974

Chemical control of budworm in Canada and the United States began in the late 1940s, after DDT had been developed and military aircraft could be refitted to conduct large-scale operations (Fettes and Buckner, 1976). By 1954 several million acres were being sprayed (Ciesla, 1976) without any regard for environmental impact by current standards. In 1962, a total of 920,000 pounds of

DDT was used (Johnson and Lawrence, 1977). With the publication of *Silent Spring* (Carson, 1962), the dawning environmental movement called for a ban on DDT. The Mrak Commission documented some of the side effects associated with that insecticide (Mrak, 1969). DDT was reported to be responsible for eggshell thinning (Bitman *et al.*, 1970). But DDT was faulted primarily for its bioaccumulation in body tissues (Kenaga, 1972), although the literature may seem contradictory on this point. DDT was last used for forest pest management in the United States in 1974 (Graham *et al.*, 1975; Williams *et al.*, 1978*a*). It successfully suppressed a 600,000-acre outbreak of Douglas fir tussock moth in Washington, Oregon, and Idaho.

7.4. ALTERNATIVES TO DDT AND OTHER INSECTICIDES

Noncholinergic chemical alternatives for control of forest pests are stand management, insect-resistant stands of trees, and biological control (e.g., parasites, predators, viruses, bacteria, insect sterility, attractants, and hormones) (Holcomb, 1970; Irving, 1970). The application of these alternatives to forestry has not been without problems (Lyon, 1976). The application of unconventional chemicals such as attractants, juvenile hormones, and feeding deterrents has had great potential for many years, but the approach is still in its infancy. Costly and elaborate test procedures (Ospenson, 1977) as well as a limited market for unconventional chemicals probably are the primary reasons they have not come into wide-scale practice.

One of the most promising insect growth regulators is diflubenzuron. It affects chitin synthesis and has been extensively tested for control of Douglas fir tussock moth (Ciesla, 1977; Gillette *et al.*, 1978; Neisess *et al.*, 1976). Although it may affect nontarget arthropods (Cunningham, 1976; Shea *et al.*, 1978), careful application strategies of this insecticide at low dosages show great promise for controlling some defoliators (Ciesla, 1977; Ellis, 1978; Granett and Dunbar, 1975). Diflubenzuron is registered with EPA for application on gypsy moth and, on a conditional basis, for application on cotton.

Insecticides for management of bark beetles have been limited primarily to bark applications to individual trees to prevent attack of uninfested trees and to suppress emergence from trees already infested (Hastings and Jones, 1976; Ragenovich and Coster, 1974). Insect behavior regulators, such as pheromones, show great promise for managing bark beetles (Wood, 1977). The major advantages are environmental safety, high selectivity, extreme effectiveness in small quantities, and biodegradability. The impact of pheromones on nontarget organisms needs to be carefully studied and established, especially regarding their interference with introduced and natural parasite–predator complexes applied in biological control programs (Pschorn-Walcher, 1977). In the future, insect behavior regulators will provide alternatives to insecticides, but in the last 10 years, relatively few successes have been achieved, and the list of alternative controls remains small (NAS, 1975*b*).

A comparison of insecticide use reports (USDA, 1976*a*, 1977*a*, 1978*a*) filed with the Forest Service for the period 1975 to 1977, and the summaries in the National Academy of Sciences report on forest pest control (NAS, 1975*b*), shows that the total insecticide mass used has increased fivefold, with a corresponding increase in the application of different types of compounds. The increase in total mass was due to the shift in responsibility for suppression of the gypsy moth from the Animal and Plant Health Inspection Service, U.S. Department of Agriculture, to the Forest Service. Until 1974, the number of approved insecticides was restricted to 9. Increased use of insecticides for cone and seed insect suppression expanded the list to 27 insecticides. From 1945 to

Table 7.1. Insecticides Used in Forest Spray Programs for Control of Insect Pests by the Forest Service, U.S. Department of Agriculture, 1975–1977, by Acreage Treated

Insecticide	Acres sprayed or treated
Carbaryl	5,240,063
Fenitrothion	1,521,074
Trichlorfon	294,642
Mexacarbate	237,784
Malathion	116,820
Lindane	86,936
Acephate	73,289
DDT[a]	34,979
Toxaphene	21,241
Methoxychlor	16,000
Dimilin	14,602
Carbofuran	13,288
Aminocarb	5,910
BHC	5,688
Phorate	4,807
Dibrom	3,000
Mirex	2,226
Phosmet	1,802
Dimethoate	1,115
Crotoxyphos	900
Methomyl	450
Abate	361
Azinphosmethyl	300
Disulfoton	207
Diazinon	143

[a] Used to control plague fleas, a use permitted by law.

1974, approximately 20.4 million pounds of pesticides was used, equivalent to 0.68 million pounds per year. From 1974 to 1977, insecticides totaled 5.1 million pounds or the equivalent of 1.7 million pounds per year (Tables 7.1 and 7.2).

Insecticide use patterns as a function of total pounds used (Table 7.2) should be interpreted cautiously. The values reported are predominantly from large-scale uses but include insecticides reported on experimental-use permits. Carbaryl is the only insecticide that is registered with EPA for control of the four major

Table 7.2.   Insecticides Used by the Forest Service, U.S. Department of Agriculture, in Forest Insect Control Programs, 1975–1977, by Pounds Used

Insecticide	Pounds used
Carbaryl	4,180,878
Fenitrothion	387,851
Trichlorfon	270,074
Malathion	82,912
Acephate	38,036
DDT[a]	37,202
Mexacarbate	35,688
Crotoxyphos	19,576
Azinphosmethyl	8,633
Carbofuran	6,485
Lindane	5,677
Mirex	3,936
BHC	3,296
Dichlorphos	2,420
Dimethoate	1,766
Aminocarb	1,332
Chlordane	877
Disulfoton	855
Dimilin	592
Disyston	525
Toxaphene	500
Diazinon	394
Methomyl	263
Phorate	134
Tetrachlorvinphos	134
Chlorpyrifos	116
Pyrethrins	114
Dieldrin	50
Oxydemetonmethyl	50
Chlorpyrifos methyl	44
Dicofol	42
Methoxychlor	35

[a] Used to control plague fleas, a use permitted by law.

Lepidoptera pests: western spruce budworm, spruce budworm, gypsy moth, and Douglas fir tussock moth. Fenitrothion is used extensively in Canada. This compound is registered in the United States for spruce budworm, and most of the pounds reported were applied in Maine in 1978, but it is no longer used. Trichlorfon is registered for gypsy moth and spruce budworm, but the formulation for use on western spruce budworm is no longer available. Malathion is registered for use in spray programs for both spruce budworm and western spruce budworm, but the reproducibility of results is highly variable (Lyon *et al.*, 1968). Acephate is registered for many defoliators, including western spruce budworm, spruce budworm, and gypsy moth. Mexacarbate was last used in Maine in 1975 for control of spruce budworm and is no longer available (Graham, 1975).

7.5. INSECTICIDE EVALUATION RESEARCH

The Forest Service's Insecticide Evaluation Research Work Unit, head-quartered in Berkeley, California, is charged with developing and evaluating safe, effective chemicals for controlling destructive forest pests. Present emphasis is on defoliating insects previously suppressed with DDT. In setting up the unit, the Forest Service recognized that basic and applied chemical research for insect control had to be conducted on a broader scale and in greater depth than in the past (Moore, 1969). DDT and other chlorinated hydrocarbon insecticides could no longer be used on the forests in the United States. Thus, the unit was charged with finding suitable replacements, but the chemicals had to be selective in action, of low hazard to associated insects—especially natural enemies of the target pests—short-lived, degradable into innocuous residues in the forest, and generally harmless to the total environment (Lyon and Camp, 1972).

The unit's research from 1964 to 1979 emphasized four lines of investigation: screening and bioassay of candidate insecticides; chemistry, including synthesis, residue analysis, and metabolism; research on systemic insecticides, including time and method of application; and field testing of the most promising insecticides indicated by laboratory studies. The Forest Management Institute in Canada followed a similar approach.

Work on any particular insecticide began with laboratory screening and progressed through studies on residual life, rainfastness, and toxicity to various instars. If an insecticide was selected for further study, it was evaluated under field conditions, sometimes starting with small, individual tree studies to simulate the dynamics of an aerial application (Barry *et al.*, 1976), then progressing to environmental safety tests to determine the environmental risks to nontarget organisms (Shea, 1979), to small plot field trials to evaluate efficacy to the target pest (Hard, 1979), and to pilot control projects to determine effectiveness under operational conditions (Ciesla, 1977). Most field studies were conducted with the full cooperation of the manufacturer of the pesticide under study. Thus, the field efficacy and environmental data can be evaluated early to determine if industry is interested in expanding its current pesticide registration to include the new use or to seek registrations for a particular forestry application.

The role of industry in the development of forest insecticides differs considerably from that in agriculture. Insecticide manufacturers carry the primary responsibility for insecticide R&D (Ospenson, 1977; Peck, 1966; Rumker et al., 1970), including EPA registration (Deck, 1975). Some of the important tasks in the registration process are compliance with environmental guidelines (Kenaga, 1972), chemistry and development of tolerances (Benvenue and Kawano, 1971), interactions that produce insecticide-stimulated or insecticide-inhibited metabolism of another insecticide (Conney and Burns, 1972), and toxicology of mutagenic–teratogenic–carcinogenic actions (Durham and Williams, 1972; Mrak, 1969). In general, the protocol for evaluations follows closely that defined in the National Academy of Sciences reports (1975a–c).

Industrial R&D in insecticides is directed primarily at agricultural and public health applications rather than forestry application. Industry has limited resources to develop the forestry market, since it is a small portion of the total market. Forestry users account for less than 1% of the total insecticide use. Furthermore, many forest defoliators may be cyclical in their outbreaks or they may last 10–15 years. They may warrant spraying every year, only once or twice in 10 years, or perhaps only once during the rotation of a stand. In contrast to agriculture, where multiple applications are made every year, forestry normally has two or more applications, except in the United States, where one application per year is a more normal frequency. These limited application practices do not provide an attractive market.

If forestry is to have insecticides for use in pest management, most of the burden for the R&D effort must be the responsibility of scientists representing public resource management agencies. Thus, forestry's responsibility is secondary to industry and encompasses the following categories: toxicology, environmental chemistry (persistence, penetration, and translocation in plants; development of residue analysis methods for forest substrates; water analysis; photodegradation; phytopersistence), fish and wildlife safety, and impact on other nontarget animals (aquatic insects, vertebrate fauna, and especially impact on parasites and predators).

Before an insecticide is submitted to the EPA for registration, industrial data supporting an existing registration in agriculture is amended with the supplementary data from the forestry sponsored research. Additional studies may be conducted to answer questions about any uncertainty determined to exist by the EPA Office of Pesticide Programs (NAS, 1978).

The lack of data to support a registration application may not be due to the unavailability of an insecticide, but to the unwillingness of industry to market a particular pesticide (e.g., mexacarbate) (Graham, 1975) or to develop a for-mulation of an insecticide (e.g., trichlorforn) (Hard, 1979) for the forestry mar-ket. For these reasons, pesticide availability needs to be determined early in the R&D process to avoid unnecessary expenditure of tax-supported funds in an effort that cannot come to fruition. Thus, the philosophy of the Forest Service regarding insecticide development requires that the insecticide must be registered, or nearly so, for a major agricultural use (Lyon, 1974; McKnight, 1976). This philosophy more adequately assures future availability of the pesticide for forestry use.

Since the forestry market for insecticides is small, the problems related to a "minor use" have recently been evaluated by the National Academy of Sciences (1975*b*). Its report highlighted one of the major problems associated with the application of biodegradable pesticides in forestry:

> Forestry has depended almost entirely upon pesticides developed for use in agriculture, because it is in the minor use category with respect to the pesticide market. There is little incentive for manufacturers to develop and register formulations for minor uses, and useful, relatively safe pesticides have been taken off the market when their use in agriculture declined. The result is that many pesticides that are potentially useful in forestry are unavailable, and in some cases, there have been no alternative solutions to pest problems, while in others the alternative has been more costly with more adverse environmental effects.

The Academy recommended establishment of mechanisms that would provide a greater range of chemicals for the specific needs of minor users.

7.6. TESTING PROTOCOL

A testing protocol for the research and development of insecticides has several steps (Lyon, 1974, 1976; Lyon and Camp, 1972; Markin and Shea, 1978). Most of the field and environmental safety testing is performed for the Forest Service by the Field Evaluation of Insecticides Research Work Unit, headquartered at Davis, California. Other research centers conduct field testing on more specific and local research missions. The Forest Pest Management Institute in Canada follows a similar testing protocol. For both research groups, the incorporation of chemical control into an integrated pest management program is a massive web of legislation, regulation, chemistry, biological phenomena, and environmental awareness. The state of Maine has, for example, implemented an efficient system for managing spruce budworm, which includes budworm biology, control, impact, environmental monitoring, and detection (Burke and Hulsey, 1979).

Principal steps in the testing procedure for an insecticide have been devel-oped into a working protocol (Markin and Shea, 1978). Specific examples of the various steps have been described and should be consulted for methodological details and approaches to problem solving in these research areas: laboratory screening tests (Hastings and Jones, 1976; Robertson *et al.*, 1976; Nigam, 1978), single-tree tests (Maksymiuk and Orchard, 1974; Merkel, 1970; Sundaram and Hopewell, 1976), small-scale field tests (Hard, 1979; Markin *et al.*, 1978; Granett and Dunbar, 1975), large-scale field tests (Dewey *et al.*, 1974; Morris, 1977; Williams, 1973; Williams and Walton, 1968), supportive tests (Brewer and Markin, 1978; Markin and Wilcox, 1977; Markin, 1977), safety and environmental tests (Cunningham, 1976; Kingsbury, 1976; Shea, 1979), pilot control tests (Lyon, 1976; Ciesla, 1977; Randall, 1976; Williams *et al.*, 1978*a*), and operational tests (Randall, 1976).

7.6.1. *Laboratory Testing and Evaluation*

Laboratory evaluation is conducted to isolate those compounds that are most promising for field tests and to determine potential hazards associated with each new insecticide (Markin and Shea, 1978). Laboratory studies involve much more than basic screening of insecticides to determine relative toxicities to target insects. They have the following major goals:

- Determining difference between various methods of introducing the toxicant to the insect, e.g., contact and feeding.
- Establishing the response to sublethal dosing.
- Observing side effects that may be useful in insecticide application strategies, e.g., knockdown, hormone mimic actions, time-to-death.

Guidelines for this type of investigation have been reviewed (NAS, 1975*c*). In addition, various specific techniques have been described (Robertson, 1978*a*, 1979; Robertson and Boelter, 1979*b*; Robertson and Kimball, 1979*a*; Robertson and Rappaport, 1979; Robertson *et al.*, 1976, 1978*a*, 1979).

Once colonies of the desired insects have been established (Lyon *et al.*, 1972*a,b*; Robertson, 1979) and the techniques for assessment of toxicity evaluation have been developed, the bioassay methods can be used to evaluate many different types of toxicological parameters—topical LD_{50}, feeding LC_{50}, spray chamber aerosol LC_{50}, response of different populations to insecticides, toxicity response of different stages of development of the same insect, genetic factors, and insecticide resistance.

Screening procedures can be modified for bioassays to provide data for assessing (1) residues in field samples, (2) rainfastness of test materials, and (3) the efficacy of systemic insecticides. Large numbers of insects are required for screening and bioassay. And they must be representative of the target insect population found in the field.

Insects for laboratory work can be field-collected, but the research is restricted to those periods of the season when they are available. Most toxicology laboratories establish colonies of insects needed for conducting bioassays and screening tests. Laboratory-reared insects are acceptable if they are continually compared with field populations and found to behave similarly. Field collections are used only when the toxicological effort is short-term or rearing procedures cannot be established. Insect toxicologists have succeeded in establishing rearing procedures for gypsy moth (Singh, 1977) and spruce budworm (Lyon *et al.*, 1972*a,b*; Robertson, 1979). The procedure for spruce budworm has been adapted for fall cankerworm [*Alsophila pometaria* (Harris)] (Lyon and Brown, 1970) and Douglas fir tussock moth (Lyon and Flake, 1966).

7.6.1.1. Analytical and Statistical Procedures

Analytical and statistical techniques for evaluating results include probit analysis, the preferred method of evaluating dose response data (Russell *et al.*, 1977; Savin *et al.*, 1977). A computer program for probit analysis, POLO (Probit Or LOgit analysis), is a data-handling and statistical tool (Robertson *et al.*, 1980; Russell and Robertson, 1979). POLO has been used for several years by the Forest Service and appears to have broad acceptance.

7.6.1.2. Basic Screening for Relative Toxicity

The kinds of toxicity tests currently conducted are contact toxicities on larvae or adults by direct application to the insect or in spray chambers and feeding toxicity on foliage dosed in a spray chamber or on a spiked artificial diet. Similar procedures and tests are used by the Forest Pest Management Institute in Canada (Nigam 1977, 1978). Toxicological evaluation of this kind provides toxicity data which ultimately lead to qualified judgments about the most promising candidate materials and formulations and provide guidelines for selecting rational dosage levels and other variables in field tests (Lyon, 1976).

The possible actions of candidate chemicals are mortality (acute and latent), knockdown, sterilization, interference with growth and development, alteration of behavior, disease enhancement, synergism, and potentiation.

7.6.1.3. Topical Tests on Insects

Topical (contact) toxicity tests for a broad spectrum of the most commonly available insecticides and many experimental insecticides have been conducted against larvae of the western spruce budworm. The pyrethroids structurally related to isomers of decamethrin and cypermethrin are among the most toxic compounds to sixth-stage budworm larvae. Highly effective pyrethroids from these classes are NRDC-168S (d,*cis*-dichlorochrysanthemic acid + 3-cyano-

phenoxybenzyl alcohol-[s]), decamethrin, NRDC-156 (d,*cis*-dibromochrysan-
themic acid + 3-cyanophenoxybenzyl alcohol-[s]), NRDC-160 (± *cis* analog
of cypermethrin), bioethanomethrin, and cypermethrin. NRDC-168S, the completely resolved isomer of cypermethrin, is 3590 times more potent than DDT
(Robertson, 1978*b;* Robertson *et al.,* 1976, 1977).

The most important defoliator in Canada and Maine is spruce budworm.
Juvenile hormones are alternative agents to the use of insecticides (Lyon,
1976), but the R&D process has not been completed for any of the major
budworms. Seven juvenile hormone analogs were evaluated against the last instar
of western spruce budworm (Robertson and Kimball, 1979*a,b*). Results of tests
to determine lethal contact effectiveness showed that ZR-1622 (ethyl[2e4e]-10-
methoxy-3,7,11-trimethyl-2,4-dodecadienoate) is the most effective, but is not
likely to attain the commercial availability of methoprene. The lethal contact
effectiveness of methoprene is about twice that of malathion, carbaryl, DDT,
or acephate, while the lethal effectiveness by feeding is substantially greater than
the feeding activities of conventional insecticides (e.g., permethrin, mexacarbate,
and acephate). Since methophrene affects reproductive biology, it may be more
effective than carbaryl. Juvenile hormones have two major disadvantages which
limit their usefulness for forest protection: they break down rapidly when exposed
to sunlight (Quistad *et al.,* 1975), and they function primarily at the end of the
last larval instar—after most of the damage to trees by feeding has occurred
(Granett, 1978).

The most important defoliator in Canada and Maine is spruce budworm.
Contact toxicity tests conducted by Nigam (1978), Randall and Nigam (1966),
and Robertson *et al.* (1978*b*) show that the most toxic insecticides to budworm
larvae are cypermethrin, permethrin, fenvalerate, azamethophos, pyrethrins,
mexacarbate, and fenitrothion.

Tests against the Douglas fir tussock moth were similar to those against the
budworms (Lyon *et al.,* 1970; Page and Lyon, 1973; Robertson and Lyon,
1973*c*). Pyrethroids again headed the list of most toxic compounds (e.g., bioethanomethrin, *cis*-resmethrin and *trans*-resmethrin were very toxic to these larvae).

Southern pine beetle is another major forest pest. Topical toxicity to adults
by insecticides shows that the following are toxic: permethrin, chlorpyrifos-
methyl, stirofos, chlorpyrifos, naled, and fenitrothion (Hastings and Jones, 1976).
The halogenated pyrethroids have physical-chemical characteristics that would
seem to make them ideal candidates for thin film applications to the main trunk
of trees for protection against pine beetles. Western pine beetle adults were killed
by decamethrin, permethrin, chlorpyrifos-methyl, carbofuran, and chlorpyrifos
(Robertson and Gillette, 1978). Lyon (1971) evaluated the contact toxicity of
insecticides to the adult California five-spined ips (*Ips paraconfusus* Lanier) and
reported that the most toxic insecticides were landrin, endosulfan, lindane, malathion, and phorate.

Pine butterfly (*Neophasia menapia* Felder and Felder) is generally found throughout the ponderosa pine forests of the northwestern United States and British Columbia. Tests to determine contact toxicity to larvae showed that resmethrin, pyrethrins, chlorpyrifos-methyl, methomyl, and chlorpyrifos were effective insecticides (Lyon and Brown, 1971). Pyrethroids were toxic to two eastern hardwood defoliating insects—the spring cankerworm [*Paleacrita vernata* (Peck)] (Page *et al.*, 1974) and the elm spanworm [*Ennomos subsignarius* (Hubner)] (Robertson and Lyon, 1973a). The most toxic insecticides were ethanoresmethrin, resmethrin, pyrethrins, mexacarbate, and phoxim (Robertson and Lyon, 1973a).

A comparison of the relative contact toxicity of insecticides to two subspecies of western tent caterpillar [*Malacosoma californicum lutescens* (Neumoegen and Dyar) and *M.c. californicum* (Packard)] showed that resmethrin, ethanoresmethrin, pyrethrins, mexacarbate, and methomyl were effective (Robertson and Gillette, 1973; Page and Lyon, 1975). Results of contact toxicity tests for the forest tent caterpillar (*Malacosoma disstria* Hubner) larvae were very similar to those for the western tent caterpillar (Lyon *et al.*, 1972a).

A major pest of eastern North America which is destructive to pine reproduction is pales weevil [*Hylobius pales* (Herbst)]. Insecticides for use against this pest should be persistent within the growing seedling and toxic enough to kill feeding weevils for one year or more (Hobart, 1977). Topical tests against the adult weevil showed that fospirate, chlorpyrifos, bioethanomethrin, methomyl, and pyrethrins were effective (Robertson *et al.*, 1975).

The relative toxicities of the pyrethroids would seem to suggest that they would have promise for field testing. However, less than 1000 acres were sprayed from 1945 to 1974 with pyrethroids (NAS, 1975b).

Contact toxicity to defoliators and beetles is usually greatest with the pyrethroids. Most control programs use organophosphates and carbamates at the present time. The real potential of the pyrethroids remains to be realized in forest pest management. If the new halogenated pyrethroids can meet the challenge of environmental safety, they may have a future in forestry.

One environmental concern has been the impact of pyrethroids on aquatic biology. Permethrin applied by aircraft to small lakes at 35 g active ingredient per acre caused significant, but short-lasting, effects on zooplankton and bottom fauna. Native fish suffered essentially no mortality (Kingsbury, 1976). Some fish biologists have been concerned about the reported high toxicity of pyrethroids to fish (Mauck *et al.*, 1976). However, the results with permethrin to date are encouraging.

7.6.1.4. Feeding Toxicities

Feeding toxicities of a broad spectrum of the most commonly available insecticides and some experimental materials have been determined for some forest insect pests. According to Gillette *et al.* (1978) and Robertson (1978b) the following insecticides are toxic to western spruce budworm by feeding action: chlorpyrifos-methyl, chlorpyrifos, bioethanomethrin, diflubenzuron, permethrin, aminocarb, and mexacarbate. Similar results have been reported for feeding action to Douglas fir tussock moth larvae, where the most toxic insecticides were permethrin, diflubenzuron, bioethanomethrin, DDT, mexacarbate, carbaryl, and acephate (Gillette *et al.*, 1978). Nigam (1978) reports that the most effective insecticides to spruce budworm are decamethrin, cypermethrin, NRDC-160 (± *cis* analog of cypermethrin), chlorpyrifos-methyl, permethrin, and acephate.

The feeding toxicity of diflubenzuron to larvae of introduced sawfly [*Diprion similis* (Hartig)] was evaluated by Valovage and Kulman (1977), who dipped cut branches of white pine [*Pinus strobus* (L.)] in various concentrations of diflubenzuron. Dipping permits uniform coverage of the substrate. Concentrations greater than 25 ppm gave effective control.

7.6.1.5. Spray Chamber Tests

Application of insecticides to potted trees or directly onto insects placed in the Moellman spray chamber (Robertson *et al.*, 1979) permits assessment of toxicity under laboratory conditions. Direct, indirect, and residual toxicities of insecticide sprays to western spruce budworm were evaluated (Robertson and Rappaport, 1979). Permethrin was one of nine insecticides tested in the Moellman spray chamber. It was more toxic when sprayed directly on sixth instar larvae than when first sprayed on foliage. All other insecticides were more toxic when sprayed on foliage.

The residual toxicity of several insecticides to fourth instar Douglas fir tussock moth larvae caged on 2-year-old potted Douglas fir seedlings was determined (Robertson and Boelter, 1979*b*). Bioethanomethrin and permethrin were substantially more toxic than DDT both by contact and by ingestion. Diflubenzuron, though not as toxic as pyrethroids, was consistently more toxic than DDT.

Spray chamber tests were used to evaluate some selected insecticides for toxicity to western black-headed budworm [*Acleris gloverana* (Walsingham)]. The most toxic insecticides were chlorpyrifos-methyl, methomyl, mexacarbate, malathion, and aminocarb (Robertson, 1976). Using similar techniques, Page and Lyon (1975) investigated the effectiveness of some selected insecticides to the cottonwood leaf beetle (*Chrysomela scripta* F.) and report that mexacarbate, resmethrin, chlorpyrifos, phoxim, and propoxur were the most toxic compounds.

7.6.1.6. Toxicity Tests on Different Species and Populations

The toxicologist needs to know if significant differences in toxicity exist between species of the same genus. The response of six species of *Choristoneura* to insecticides was tested (Robertson *et al.*, 1978*b*). These results showed that extrapolating toxicity response from one species to another should be avoided. Similar results have been noted for two different populations of western black-headed budworm (Robertson *et al.*, 1973). Stock and Robertson (1979) report that in Douglas fir tussock moth, variation in sibling group responses of different populations to acephate and carbaryl were related quantitatively to esterase isozymes.

7.6.1.7. Toxicity Tests on Different Instars

The relative susceptibility of selected developmental stages—instars—to insecticide treatments provides data for gauging the correct time of application for maximum mortality under field conditions. Timing the application is critical if the insecticide is short-lived. If protecting the foliage is the purpose of insect population reduction, an early application strategy will be required. The toxicity of mexacarbate to various instars of western spruce budworm has been determined (Robertson *et al.*, 1976). Third to fifth instars and immature sixth instars were the most susceptible. Under laboratory conditions first instars were the least susceptible. Early instars of the Douglas fir tussock moth and western spruce budworm were more susceptible to diflubenzuron than the last or large instars (Gillette *et al.*, 1978). Acephate, carbaryl, and permethrin were most toxic to first instars (Robertson and Boelter, 1979*a,b*). Spray chamber treatments yielded similar results: acephate, carbaryl, and permethrin were most toxic to first instars, while diflubenzuron was most toxic to second instars. Sixth instars were least susceptible to acephate and permethrin. Yet, in California oakworm (*Phryganidia californica* Packard), the first instars were most susceptible to mexacarbate (Robertson, 1972).

7.6.1.8. Evaluation of Sublethal Dose Effects

When sublethal doses of methomyl were applied to western spruce budworm larvae, the toxicological response was that of a juvenomimetic (Smith, 1971). Sublethal doses of mexacarbate produced a similar loss in larvae weight and premature development due to modified diuresis. Reversal of cholinesterase inhibition from mexacarbate-treated mice has been demonstrated to be rapid (Lang and Miskus, 1967). The metabolism to nontoxic metabolites is also rapid (Roberts *et al.*, 1969). These results suggest that the rapid disappearance of mexacarbate, especially in doses common to sublethal studies, must contribute significantly to the diuresis.

7.6.1.9. Resistance Studies

Mexacarbate treatment in 14 generations of nondiapausing western spruce budworm larvae showed no trend toward increased tolerance (Robertson and

Lyon, 1973*a*–*c*). Generation mortality in response to pyrethrins, mexacarbate, and DDT has been investigated in depth (Robertson *et al.*, 1976). No significant change in the pattern of response to mexacarbate throughout the period of rearing to the nondiapausing colony could be established.

Development of resistance by forest insect defoliators is not expected to occur, since the frequency of application is only once or twice per 10-year period and seldom more than once per season. Genetic stress of such low magnitude is not expected to produce resistance. On the other hand, if the frequency of application increases then genetic stress may follow.

7.6.2. Bioassay Studies

Bioassays with laboratory-reared and field-collected insects are used to obtain an LD_{50} or LC_{50} that can be used to characterize other responses. Some examples of bioassays for special uses are bioassays of field-collected plant parts to determine residues (Barger, 1978; Hopewell, 1977; Markin *et al.*, 1978), rainfastness (Robertson, 1979*b*), anatomical susceptibilities (Roberts *et al.*, 1976), evaluations of insecticides for systemic activity in plants (Crisp, 1972), testing synergism (Lang, 1970; Roberts *et al.*, 1972), and juvenile hormones (Richmond, 1972). Bioassays have been used to evaluate structure–activity relationships (Look *et al.*, 1976; Miskus *et al.*, 1968) and to evaluate the impact of fungi and bacteria on insects (Lewis and Filer, 1977). Bioassays have been found useful for evaluating the toxicity of insecticide metabolites generated by various *in vivo* and *in vitro* techniques (Roberts *et al.*, 1969, 1978). Even the shelf life of insecticides can be checked with bioassays (Page and Robertson, 1976).

7.6.3. Individual Tree Evaluations

The use of single trees for insecticide efficacy tests has had mixed acceptance among forest entomologists (Lyon, 1976). In Canada, after laboratory testing, candidate insecticides are generally tested on individual trees, then on tens of thousands of acres of trees. In the United States, individual tree tests are not generally conducted before aerial tests, (Lyon, 1976). The major rationale against individual tree tests is that the statistical sample is too small, insect populations within trees and between trees are highly variable with respect to stage of development and density, and field parameters such as drop spectrum, spray volume, and coverage are difficult to simulate on individual trees. In spite of these limitations, individual tree tests have yielded a wealth of useful information. Three basic application methods used in single-tree treatments are hydraulic, aerial application to potted trees placed on airport runways, and simulated aerial spray tests.

7.6.3.1. Hydraulic Applications with Backpack Mistblower

Single trees infested with Douglas fir tussock moth larvae were sprayed with 15 insecticides at three different application rates using a backpack mistblower. Results permitted the establishment of a dosage range than could be ascertained from potted trees in greenhouse studies (Markin and Wilcox, 1977). Concentrations greater than 250 ppm were effective.

Acephate was evaluated on individual trees infested with western spruce budworm by using a gasoline-powered backpack sprayer (Brewer and O'Neal, 1977). The evaluation considered mortality inside needles and emerging buds, and the degree of defoliation. Mortality of early instars was high, and the data suggest that acephate has some type of systemic action that can protect new growth from defoliation.

Ground applications to control western spruce budworm in a tree plantation confirmed the potted-tree studies (Richmond *et al.*, 1978). Ground tests conducted in New Mexico to reduce a heavy infestation of Douglas fir tussock moth on Douglas fir and white fir trees showed that acephate treatments with concentrations of 0.5 lb active ingredient per 100 gal were effective in reducing larval populations (Linane, 1978).

7.6.3.2. Hydraulic Application with Tractor-Mounted Equipment

Tractor-mounted hydraulic equipment for application of ULV dosages to individual trees was successful (Morris, 1976) in evaluating insecticides to control cottonwood leaf beetle with malathion and chlorpyrifos. Results confirmed the laboratory findings of an earlier report (Page and Lyon, 1975).

7.6.3.3. Airport Tests

A novel application strategy using aerial application and potted trees placed at 10-ft intervals across the spray swath at an airport yielded useful information for improving aerial application techniques (Maksymiuk and Orchard, 1974). Sprayed trees were bioassayed with insect larvae to determine effectiveness of the aerial application.

7.6.3.4. Simulated Aerial Applications

Simulated aerial tests can be conducted with single trees (Hopewell and Nigam, 1974). The simulator is engineered to contain conventional aircraft spray equipment (e.g., nozzles and formulation delivery system) in a portable shelter that can be easily transported and placed over a single tree. The efficacy of acephate, phoxim, and fenitrothion was tested with the simulator and produced results comparable to those of an actual aerial application. Simulated single-tree tests can provide unique information before expensive field tests are held.

7.6.4. Field Testing

A field test is an evaluation of a candidate insecticide under actual field conditions (Hard, 1979). Aircraft are used in larger field tests. In small field tests, several doses or formulations can be evaluated to define what is optimum for a larger field experiment. Two or more independent field tests of a formulation are desirable to establish consistent statistically significant results.

A field test is conducted to obtain efficacy data for the resource manager and should be conducted if any of the following criteria are evident, according to the National Academy of Sciences (1975c):

- The insecticide is toxic or persistent.
- Potential harmful effects are indicated from initial laboratory toxicology, e.g., bioaccumulation.
- Anticipated population risk is suggested by preliminary laboratory data, e.g., pyrethroid toxicity to fish.
- Anticipated social benefit from the insecticide is suggested, e.g., to save a forest from massive defoliation during an outbreak of a defoliator.

Field tests are of two kinds—safety tests for nontarget animals and efficacy tests for target organisms (Hard, 1979; Lyon, 1976; Lyon and Camp, 1972; Markin and Shea, 1978; Shea 1977, 1979). Safety tests are conducted to determine toxic effects of insecticides on fish, birds, other wildlife, and nontarget aquatic and terrestrial insects. The insecticides are applied at two to four times the dosage levels expected to be used under operational conditions. Safety margins for wildlife can be established, and unforeseen risks associated with larger operations can be delineated. Plot size is a minimum of 160 acres. Insecticide residue analysis may be conducted as part of these tests (Roberts, 1978; Pieper and Miskus, 1967; Richmond *et al.*, 1979.)

Field experiments are directed against target insects and are tests of efficacy (Lyon and Camp, 1972; Markin and Shea, 1978). Aerial applications are used to determine spray techniques (Wernz and Markin, 1977), minimum effective dosage, and formulation and spray timing (Blais, 1979). Efficacy is measured in terms of target insect mortality and survival, foliage protection, and amount of subsequent tree damage.

Selection of candidate insecticides from the list of those tested at the laboratory level and on individual trees during supportive tests are based on the following criteria (Lyon, 1974):

- High toxicity to the target insect.
- Potential high environmental safety.

- Significant, but not persistent, residual action.
- Previous experience in the field against the target insect.
- Registered or near registration for agricultural pests.

For a summary of the results of field tests against the major forest insect pests, the review of the National Academy of Sciences is unsurpassed (NAS, 1975*b*). The report of the Committee for the Working Conference on Principles of Protocols for Evaluating Chemicals in the Environment is an excellent reference on techniques and approaches to field testing (NAS, 1975*c*).

Concomitant formulation and application of *Bacillus thuringiensis* and acephate for spruce budworm control (Morris, 1977) show great promise as a new strategy for an early application to protect new current-year foliage. Acephate would be the controlling factor in the early instars with the bacteria promoting protection in the later instars after the acephate has degraded—usually about 14 days.

Markin and Shea (1978), Brooks *et al.* (1978), and the USDA (1978*b*) have prepared summaries of small and large field tests conducted for control of Douglas fir tussock moth and western spruce budworm. Acephate is registered for use against those two species. Other promising candidates are aminocarb (pending establishment of a tolerance in western states), methomyl, permethrin, and trichlorfon (pending reestablishment of the old formulation that was available when the field testing began) (Lyon, 1974). Carbaryl was registered with the EPA in 1978 for use against the western spruce budworm and Douglas fir tussock moth. Morrison and Dimond (1978) have prepared a history and bibliography of field trials for control of spruce budworm in Maine. Carbaryl (Sevin-4-Oil), acephate, and aminocarb are the most efficacious insecticides for spruce budworm management. Diflubenzuron is effective against the Douglas fir tussock moth, but its efficacy toward spruce budworm is poor.

Larch casebearer [*Coleophora laricella* (Hubner)] is an important pest of western larch. Malathion is registered to control this insect. Aerial applications of acephate (Hard *et al.*, 1977*b;* Washburn *et al.*, 1977) were highly effective at 1.0 lb/gal per acre and are not as variable as malathion. Chemical control methods for larch casebearer may be set aside, if the recently developed biological control methods are as effective as the early indications suggest (Bergstrom, 1978).

A compendium from the Douglas fir Tussock Moth Research and Development Program (Brooks *et al.*, 1978) documents the findings of this major pest-control program. The integrated approach to R&D used by the program is an example for forest insect pest-control research. At the onset ground spraying of small plots indicated favorable results for trichlorfon, carbaryl, acephate (Markin, 1977; Brewer and Markin, 1978), diflubenzuron (Hard *et al.*, 1977*a*, 1978), and pyrethrins (stabilized). Aerial application over large plots showed that mexacarbate at 0.15 lb/acre was highly effective in suppressing the moth population

(Williams *et al.*, 1969, 1978*b*, 1979). Carbaryl, trichlorfon, mexacarbate, and bioethanomethrin were further tested (Williams, 1973). Mexacarbate, trichlorfon, and carbaryl performed satisfactorily. On the basis of additional field experiments conducted in 1974 and 1978, acephate and diflubenzuron emerged as potential candidates for a large-scale operational program. Diflubenzuron has been issued a conditional registration for use on cotton, which may open the way for registration for forestry use.

Large variations in results from field testing can often be attributed to spray physics and associated field techniques. More than one field, pilot, and operational test has failed because small details in spray physics were overlooked. The contemporary forest pesticide applications manager must take this basic science into account in aerial applications of insecticides (Roberts, 1976). The physical problems of pesticide application from the standpoint of equipment, nozzle design, and performance have been reviewed with respect to forestry applications (Akesson and Yates, 1976). Meteorological effects on the impingement of air-applied small droplets were given considerable attention (Cramer and Boyle, 1976). Small droplets less than 50 microns in diameter are the most effective on western budworm (Himel and Moore, 1967); other targets may require different sizes. Techniques and equipment for evaluating viruses and other water-soluble formulations are available (Maksymiuk and Orchard, 1974; Sundaram, 1978).

7.7. SYSTEMIC INSECTICIDES

Systemic insecticides may offer a promising new approach to insect management. They can be classified into two fundamental groups—phloem mobile or xylem mobile. Many insecticides are xylem mobile, particularly if they are soluble in water. Phloem-mobile systemic pesticides are more difficult to find, characterize, and evaluate because they must be taken into living tissue by energy-dependent, enzyme-supported mechanisms (Crisp and Look, 1979).

Systemic insecticides are useful tools for managing cryptic insects, e.g., cone and seed insects, bark beetles, shoot tip moth larvae, and twig borers (Lyon, 1974).

The status of systemic insecticides as related to translocation and molecular structure has been reviewed (Crisp, 1972) as well as the relationship of systemic insecticides to phloem transport of other xenobiotics (Crafts and Crisp, 1971).

Phloem-mobile systemic insecticides provide the most efficient means to control cryptic insects because the toxicant can translocate with the photosynthate (food) to the tissue where the target insect is feeding. Limitations to the application of this strategy are lack of knowledge concerning the basic structure–activity relationships of molecular structure to phloem transport for insecticidal materials, persistence within the living tissue for periods of time sufficient to allow the toxicant to translocate and accumulate in the photosynthate sinks (areas of new growth), selective cholinergic or other toxic mechanisms of sufficient strength to kill the insect by ingestion, and availability of candidate toxicants.

Xylem-mobile systemic insecticides can be applied by soil application (Brown and Eads, 1975), trunk injection (Brown and Eads, 1975; Merkel, 1970), trunk implantation (Brown *et al.*, 1979), or bark painting (Johnson, 1965; Moody *et al.*, 1976, 1977*a,b;* Ragenovich and Coster, 1974). Some xylem-mobile insecticides are aminocarb (Sundaram and Hopewell, 1976, 1977), dimethoate (Crafts and Crisp, 1971; Johnson, 1965), carbofuran (Solomon and Oliveria, 1977), and acephate (Sundaram and Hopewell, 1976; Sundaram *et al.*, 1977).

Trunk implantation of systemic insecticides shows promise for protecting high-value trees that produce cone crops for seed used in regeneration (Merkel, 1970.) Methamidophos, dimethoate, oxydemetonmethyl, and dicrotophos provided prophylaxis for up to 6 months or more in slash pine. Future studies in this area will make use of implants, where the unformulated, water-soluble, technical-grade insecticide is encapsulated and placed under the bark for slow release. Implant treatment strategies have been successful in suppressing Jeffrey pine needle minor [*Coleotechnites* near *milleri* (Heinrich)] (Brown *et al.*, 1979). Acephate implants provided protection for up to 6 weeks.

The persistence, distribution, and translocation of acephate in spruce trees shows that the insecticide is very xylem mobile and is degraded in approximately 14 days (Sundaram and Hopewell, 1976; Sundaram *et al.* 1977). Acephate is phloem mobile when applied to photosynthate sources (foliage) on 15-year-old Jeffrey pine trees with strong photosynthate sinks (Crisp *et al.*, 1979). Approximately 5% of the applied dose translocated through the phloem to the new growth after treatment of the previous year's foliage. Methamidophos, a metabolite of acephate, was also detected in the sinks. This observation was reported earlier in spuce trees (Sundaram *et al.*, 1977).

Acephate would seem to have the potential to protect the new growth from defoliation by the early instar western spruce budworm (Brewer and O'Neal, 1977; Richmond *et al.*, 1978). Two factors are critical if an early spray strategy is to be successful—timing of the application and spray volume. The systemic insecticide needs sufficient volume to allow cuticular penetration and absorption to occur over a thoroughly wet surface.

Aminocarb translocation was characterized in potted conifers as weakly xylem mobile (Crisp, 1972). Field studies confirm this mobility (Sundaram, 1978; Sundaram *et al.*, 1977). It is apoplastic in white spruce [*Picea glauca* (Moench)]. Aminocarb persisted in trace amounts for periods up to 64 days postspray.

The fate, persistence, and translocation of fenitrothion in conifers and some eastern hardwood species has been evaluated (Pomber *et al.*, 1973, 1974*a,b*, 1975*a,b,*1976; Prasad, 1977; Prasad and Moody, 1974, 1976). It has some xylem mobility, but its potential as a systemic seems limited. Fenitrothion accumulates in the cuticular layers of conifer needles. Additional data related to the translocation of fenitrothion can be found in reports by Hallett *et al.* (1973, 1974, 1975) and Weinberger *et al.* (1978*a–c*).

7.8.   TRENDS IN FOREST PEST MANAGEMENT

Chemical insecticides will probably always be used in forest insect pest management. Resistance to insecticides as described by Luck *et al.* (1977) is not likely to develop in forest insect pests because the genetic stress is low. Biological control and third-generation pesticides (noncholinergic) will be developed and used in forestry. As environmental risk assessment increases the cost of insecticide R&D, the search for and registration of new insecticides will most likely become prohibitive. In the future, the concepts of biological controls in the broadest sense will undoubtedly play a prominent role in integrated pest management programs and at the same time become more competitive with insecticides in the marketplace (Holcomb, 1970).

Current research emphasis in forest pest management by the CANUSA program (CANUSA, 1979; USDA, 1977*b*) shows a greater emphasis on silviculture, biological control, and third-generation insecticides than in previous programs. Future trends will probably concentrate on detecting and treating epicenters (areas that support rapid population growth of key insects) early in the outbreak (Sanders, 1976). Understanding the basic causes of epicenter development may be at the very foundation of future suppression programs. The epicenter theory, if it is valid, would be ideal for use of pheromones, epizootics, and viruses in a pest suppression program.

The application of biodegradable insecticides to forest pest management problems is based on an in-depth R&D program ranging from basic research in the laboratory and field, which provides supporting data for registration of new and some selected old insecticides for forest pests, and concomitantly, a better understanding of the ecological factors involved in forest pest management. Perhaps the biggest emphasis will be in the use and acceptance of new strategies for forest insect control, where sophisticated combinations of silvicultural, biological, and insecticide practices will be applied. Concomitantly the hazards and undue risk to the environment must not be overlooked and more recently have received major attention in the testing protocol of new insecticides in North America (Buckner *et al.*, 1976).

7.9. CONCLUSIONS

The R&D process for selecting, evaluating, and applying insecticides in forestry is a massive web of legislation, regulation, chemistry, biological phenomena, and environmental awareness. The pathway used in the R&D process employs several critical steps and attention to appropriate staging. Some of the critical steps are determination of the relative toxicity of the insecticide to the target insect, prior registration for agricultural use, small-scale field testing to determine efficacy under field conditions, large-scale field tests to more accurately define dosage and efficacy, safety tests under field conditions to evaluate the impact of the candidate insecticide on a limited number of nontarget species, and finally, an operational test to evaluate the effectiveness of an efficacious insecticide for suppression of an outbreak. The cost of each step in the pathway increases in the selection of a new insecticide. As a result, staging the tests in the order described assists in the avoidance of unsuccessful costly tests.

The state of the art is the most advanced for suppression of defoliating insect pests. Several insecticides are now registered for use against these pests: carbaryl, acephate, and trichlorfon. Diflubenzuron is emerging as a new noncholinergic-type insecticide for forestry use.

Large-scale suppression of bark beetles with insecticides does not seem feasible with today's insecticides, and suppression programs are more effective that employ an integrated pest management approach, an approach that places a major emphasis on silvicultural practices.

New pyrethroid insecticides are frequently the most toxic compounds tested at the laboratory level on most forest insect pests. Only a limited number of small-scale field tests have been conducted with the pyrethroids, and further testing needs to be done at this level.

REFERENCES

Akesson, N. B., and Yates, W. F., 1976, Physical parameters relating to pesticide application, in: *Pesticide Spray Application, Behavior, and Assessment: Workshop Proceedings* (R. B. Roberts, ed.), pp. 4–26, U.S. Department of Agriculture Forest Service General Technical Report PSW-15, Pacific Southwest Forest and Range Experiment Station, Berkeley, California.

Barger, J. H., 1978, Smaller European elm bark beetle elm bole bioassay tests, *Insecticide and Acaricide Tests* 3:142.

Barry, J. W., Tysowsky, M., Jr., Orr, G. F., Ekblad, R. B., Marsalis, R. B., and Ciesla, W. M., 1976, Impaction of Zectran particles on spruce budworm larvae a field experiment, in: *Pesticide Spray Application, Behaviour, and Assessment: Workshop Proceedings* (R. B. Roberts, ed.), pp. 40–47, U.S. Department of Agriculture Forest Service General Technical Report PSW-15, Pacific Southwest Forest and Range Experiment Station, Berkeley, California.

Barry, J. W., Ekblad, R. B., Markin, G. P., and Trostle, G. C., 1978, Methods for sampling and assessing deposits of insecticidal sprays released over forests, U.S. Department of Agriculture Technical Bulletin 1596, 162 p.

Benvenue, A., and Kawano, Y., 1971, Pesticides, pesticide residues, tolerances, and the law (U.S.A.), *Residue Rev.* **35**:103.

Bergstrom, D., 1978, Parasite gains on the larch casebearer. Forestry Research: What's New in the West? pp. 6–9, U.S. Department of Agriculture Forest Service, Fort Collins, Colorado.

Bitman, J., Cecil, H. C., and Fries, G. F., 1970, DDT-induced inhibition of avian shell gland carbonic anhydrase: A mechanism for thin eggshells, *Science* **168**:594.

Blais, J. R., 1979, Rate of defoliation of balsam fir in relation to spruce budworm attack and timing of spray application, *Can. J. For. Res.* **9**:354–361.

Brewer, J. W., and Markin, G. P., 1978, Bioassay of acephate-treated foliage of three instars of the Douglas-fir tussock moth, U.S. Department of Agriculture Forest Service Research Paper PNW-241, 7 p., Pacific Northwest Forest and Range Experiment Station, Portland, Oregon.

Brewer, J. W., and O'Neal, J., 1977, Early ground application of acephate for control of the western spruce budworm (Lepidoptera:Tortricidae), *Can. Entomol.* **109**:1153.

Brooks, M. H., Stark, R. W., and Campbell, R. W., 1978, The Douglas-fir tussock moth: A synthesis, U.S. Department of Agriculture, Technical Bulletin 1858, 321 pp., Washington, D.C.

Brown, L. R., and Eads, C. O., 1975, Nantucket pine tip moth in Southern California: Identity and insecticidal control, *J. Econ. Entomol.* **68**:380.

Brown, L. R., Eads, C. O., Crisp, C. E., and Page, M., 1979, Control of a Jeffrey pine needleminer by spraying and trunk implantation and resultant acephate residues, *J. Econ. Entomol.* **72**:51.

Buckner, C. H., McLeod, B. B., and Lidstone, R. G., 1976, Environmental impact studies of spruce budworm (*Choristoneura fumiferana* Clemens) control programs in New Brunswick in 1976, *Chem. Control. Res. Inst. Ottawa Inf. Rep. CC-X* 135.

Burke, R. E., and Hulsey, C. T., 1979, Spruce budworm research in Maine: A user's guide, Maine Forest Service, Maine Department of Conservation, Augusta, Maine.

CANUSA, 1979, Request for research, development and application proposals. Western component. Canada/U.S. Spruce Budworms Program–West, U.S. Department of Agriculture Forest Service Miscellaneous Paper, Pacific Northwest Forest and Range Experiment Station, 30 pp., Portland, Oregon.

Carson, R., 1962, *Silent Spring*, Houghton Mifflin, Boston.

Ciesla, W. M., 1976, Historical and present approach to spruce budworm control in the United States, in: Proceedings of the Symposium on Spruce Budworm (W. H. Klein, Technical coordinator), pp. 51–56. U.S. Department of Agriculture Miscellaneous Publication 1327, Washington, D.C.

Ciesla, W. M., 1977, Douglas-fir tussock moth: Direct control with chemical and microbial insecticides, *Bull. Entomol. Soc. Am.* **23**:174.

Conney, A. H., and Burns, J. J., 1972, Metabolic interactions among environmental chemicals and drugs, *Science* **178**:576.

Crafts, A. S., and Crisp, C. E., 1971, *Phloem Transport in Plants*, Freeman, San Francisco.

Cramer, H. E., and Boyle, D. G., 1976, The micrometeorology and physics of spray particle behavior, in: *Pesticide Spray Application, Behavior, and Assessment: Workshop Proceedings* (R. B. Roberts, ed.), pp. 27–39, U.S. Department of Agriculture Forest Service General Technical Report PSW-15, Pacific Southwest Forest Range and Experiment Station, Berkeley, California.

Crisp, C. E., 1972, The molecular design of systemic insecticides and importance of certain organic functional groups in translocation, *Pestic. Chem.* **1**:211.

Crisp, C. E., and Look, M., 1979, Phloem loading and transport of weak acids, in: *Advances in Pesticide Science* (H. Geissbuhler, ed.), pp. 430–437, Pergamon Press, Oxford.

Crisp, C. E., Koerber, T. W., Richmond, C. E., and Roettgering, B. H., 1979, Acropetal translocation of acephate in terminal shoots of Jeffrey pine for chemical control of western pine shoot borer, in: *Symposium on Systemic Chemical Treatments in Tree Culture* (J. J. Kielbaso, ed.), pp. 307–324, Michigan State University Press, East Lansing, Mich.

Cunningham, P. A., 1976, Effects of Dimilin (TH-6040) on reproduction in the brine shrimp, *Artemia salina*, *Environ. Entomol.* **5**:701.

Deck, E., 1975, Federal and state pesticide regulation and legislation, *Annu. Rev. Entomol.* **20**:119.

Dewey, J. E., 1979, Registration, in *The Douglas-Fir Tussock Moth–A Synthesis* (M. H. Brooks, R. W. Stark, and R. W. Campbell, eds.), pp. 129–130, U.S. Department of Agriculture Technical Bulletin 1585, Washington, D.C.

Dewey, J. E., McGregor, M. D., Marsalis, R. L., Barry, J. W., Williams, C. B., and Ciesla, W. M., 1974, Mexacarbate and *Bacillus thuringiensis* for control of pine butterfly infestations, Report 74-10, Division State and Private Forestry, U.S. Department of Agriculture, Northern Region, Missoula, Montana.

Durham, W. F., and Williams, C. H., 1972, Mutagenic, teratogenic, and carcinogenic properties of pesticides, *Annu. Rev. Entomol.* **17**:123.

Ellis, H. C., 1978, Pine tip moth control, *Insecticide and Acaricide Tests* **3**:147.

Fellin, D. G., 1980, The western spruce budworm in the American Rocky Mountains, Canada–United States Spruce Budworms Program, *Newsletter* **8**:1.

Fettes, J. J., and Buckner, C. H., 1976, Historical sketch of the philosophy of spruce budworm control in Canada, in: *Proceedings of the Symposium on Spruce Budworm* (W. H. Klein, technical coordinator), pp. 57–60, U.S. Department of Agriculture Miscellaneous Publication 1327, Washington, D.C.

Gillette, N. L., Robertson, J. L., and Lyon, R. L., 1978, Bioassays of TH 6038 and diflubenzuron applied to western spruce budworm and Douglas-fir tussock moth, *J. Econ. Entomol.* **71**:310.

Graham, D. A., Mounts, J., and Dewey, A., 1975, Cooperative Douglas fir tussock moth control project, Oregon, Washington, Idaho, U.S. Department of Agriculture, Pacific Northwest Region.

Graham, F., Jr., 1975, The rise and fall of a safe pesticide, *Audubon* **77**(B):112.

Granett, J., 1978, Insect growth regulators for eastern spruce budworm control, Life Sciences and Agriculture Experiment Station, University of Maine (Orono), Miscellaneous Report 198.

Granett, J., and Dunbar, D. M., 1975, TH 6040: Laboratory and field trials for control of gypsy moths, *J. Econ. Entomol.* **68**:99.

Hallett, D. J., Weinberger, P., and Prasad, R., 1973, A preliminary study on the fate of fenitrothion in forest seeds. Determination of residues in eastern white pine (*Pinus strobus* L.) and their effects on amino acid metabolism, *Chem. Control Res. Inst. Ottawa Inf. Rep.* CC-X 50.

Hallett, D. J., Weinberger, P., Greenhalgh, R., and Prasad, R., 1974, Fate of fenitrothion in forest trees. V. The formation of metabolites in *Pinus strobus* L. and their detection by gas chromatography and mass spectroscopy, *Chem. Control Res. Inst. Ottawa Inf. Rep.* CC-X 78.

Hallett, D. J., Greenhalgh, R., Weinberger, P., and Prasad, R., 1975, The absorption of fenitrothion during germination of stratified and nonstratified white pine seeds and identification of metabolites formed, *Can. J. For. Res.* **5**:84.

Hard, J. S., 1979, Field experiments, in: *The Douglas-fir Tussock Moth—A Synthesis* (M. H. Brooks, R. W. Stark, and R. W. Campbell, eds.), pp. 117–118, U.S. Department of Agriculture Technical Bulletin 1585, Washington, D.C.

Hard, J. S., Ward, J. D., and Ilnytzky, S., 1977*a*, Douglas-fir tussock moth control on Douglas-fir, *Insecticide and Acaricide Tests* **2**:113.

Hard, J. S., Meso, S., and Haskett, M. J., 1977b, Larch casebearer control on western larch, *Insecticide and Acaricide Tests* 2:116.

Hard, J. S., Ward, J. D., and Ilnytzky, S., 1978, Control of Douglas-fir tussock moth by aerially applied Dimilin (TH 6040), U.S. Department of Agriculture Forest Service Research Paper PSW-130, Pacific Southwest Forest and Range Experiment Station, Berkeley, California.

Hastings, F. L., and Jones, A. S., 1976, Contact toxicity of 29 insecticides to southern pine beetle adults, U.S. Department of Agriculture Forest Service Research Note SE-245, Southeastern Forest Experiment Station, Asheville, North Carolina.

Himel, C. M., and Moore, A. D., 1967, Spruce budworm mortality as a function of aerial spray droplet size, *Science* 156:1250.

Hobart, J., 1977, Pesticides in forestry: An introduction, in: *Ecological Effects of Pesticides* (F. H. Pering and K. Mellanby, eds.), pp. 61–88, Academic Press, New York.

Holcomb, R. W., 1970, Insect control: Alternatives to the use of conventional pesticides, *Science* 168:456.

Honing, F. W., 1976, Objectives and philosophies of direct control of the spruce budworm, in: *Proceedings of the Symposium on Spruce Budworm* (W. H. Klein, technical coordinator), pp. 57–60, U.S. Department of Agriculture Miscellaneous Publication 1329, Washington, D.C.

Hopewell, W. W., 1977, Field evaluation of the pyrethroid NRDC-143, compared with fenitrothion, acephate and chlorpyrifos-methyl as simulated aerial spray deposit for control of the spruce budworm, *Choristoneura fumiferana*, *Chem. Control Res. Inst. Ottawa Inf. Rep. CC-X* 132.

Hopewell, W. W., and Nigam, P. C., 1974, Field evaluation of Orthene, phoxim, and fenitrothion against spruce budworm (*Choristoneura fumiferana*), applied as simulated aerial spray, *Chem. Control Res. Inst. Ottawa Inf. Rep. CC-X* 83.

Irving, C. W., Jr., 1970, Agricultural pest control and the environment, *Science* 168:1419.

Johnson, N. E., 1965, A test of 12 insecticides for the control of the Sitka-spruce weevil, *Pissodes sitchensis, J. Econ. Entomol.* 58:572.

Johnson, N. E., and Lawrence, W.H., 1977, Role of pesticides in the management of American forests, in: *Pesticides in the Environment*, Vol. 3, (R. White-Stevens, ed.), pp. 135–255, Marcel Dekker, New York.

Kenaga, E. E., 1972, Guidelines for environmental study of pesticides: Determination of bioconcentration potential, *Residue Rev.* 44:73.

Kingsbury, P. D., 1976, Studies of the impact of aerial applications of synthetic pyrethroid NRDC-143 on aquatic ecosystems, *Chem. Control Res. Inst. Ottawa Inf. Rep. CC-X* 127.

Krebs, C. F., 1976, The spruce budworm problem in North America: The current situation and outlook, in: *Proceeding of the Symposium on Spruce Budworm* (W. H. Klein, technical co-ordinator), pp. 9–13, U.S. Department of Agriculture Miscellaneous Publication 1329, Washington, D.C.

Kulman, H. M., 1971, Effects of insect defoliation on growth and mortality of trees, *Annu. Rev. Entomol,* 16:289.

Lang, J. M., 1970, Reduction in the fertility of female *Choristoneura occidentalis* by Lannate, *J. Econ. Entomol.* 63:1619.

Lang, J. M., and Miskus, R. P., 1967, Zectran fed orally to mice—cholinesterase levels in blood determined, U.S. Department of Agriculture Forest Service Research Note PSW-140, Pacific Southwest Forest and Range Experiment Station, Berkeley, California.

Lewis, R., Jr., and Filer, T. H., Jr., 1977, Screening of fungi and bacteria for control of the forest tent caterpillar, *Insecticide and Acaricide Tests* 2:115.

Linane, J. P., 1978, Ground tests with insecticides against the Douglas-fir tussock moth in New Mexico, *Insecticide and Acaricide Tests* 3:146.

Look, M., Crisp, C. E., and Richmond, C. E., 1976, Chemical alteration of translocation characteristics of insecticides—*O,O*-dimethylthiophosphoramide (Monitor or Tamaron), *Am. Chem. Soc. Proc.* **172**(Pest):51.

Luck, R. F., van den Bosch, and Barcia, R., 1977, Chemical insect control—A troubled pest management strategy, *BioScience* **27**:606.

Lyon, R. L., 1971, Contact toxicity of 17 insecticides applied topically to adult bark beetles, U.S. Department of Agriculture Forest Service Research Note PSW-249, Pacific Southwest Forest and Range Experiment Station, Berkeley, California.

Lyon, R. L., 1974, The status of chemicals for suppression of spruce budworm in the United States, in: *Proceedings of the Symposium on Spruce Budworm* (W. H. Klein, technical coordinator), pp. 91–116, U.S. Department of Agriculture Miscellaneous Publication 1329, Washington, D.C.

Lyon, R. C., 1976, Unconventional chemicals, in: *Proceedings of the Symposium on Spruce Budworm* (W. H. Klein, technical coordinator), pp. 127–129, U.S. Department of Agriculture Miscellaneous Publication 1329, Washington, D.C.

Lyon, R. L., and Brown, S. J., 1970, Contact toxicity of insecticides applied to fall cankerworm reared on artificial diet, *J. Econ. Entomol.* **63**:1970.

Lyon, R. L., and Brown, S. J., 1971, Contact toxicity of 14 insecticides tested on pine butterfly larvae, U.S. Department of Agriculture Forest Service Research Note PSW-257, Pacific Southwest Forest and Range Experiment Station, Berkeley, California.

Lyon, R. L., and Camp, H. W. 1972, The Forest Service's insecticide evaluation program, Western Forestry and Conservation Association, Permanent Assoc. Comm., Proc., December, pp. 48–50, Seattle, Washinton.

Lyon, R. L., and Flake, H. W., Jr., 1966, Rearing Douglas-fir tussock moth larvae on synthetic media, *J. Econ. Entomol.* **59**:696.

Lyon, R. L., Page, M., and Brown, S. J., 1968, Tolerance of spruce budworm to malathion, U.S. Department of Agriculture Forest Service Research Note PSW-173, Pacific Southwest Forest and Range Experiment Station, Berkeley, California.

Lyon, R. L., Flake, H. W., and Ball, L., 1970, Laboratory tests of 55 insecticides on Douglas-fir tussock moth larvae, *J. Econ. Entomol.* **63**:513.

Lyon, R. L., Brown, S. J., and Robertson, J. L., 1972a, Contact toxicity of 16 insecticides applied to forest tent caterpillars reared on artificial diet, *J. Econ. Entomol.* **65**:928.

Lyon, R. L., Richmond, C. E., Robertson, J. L., and Lucas, B. A., 1972b, Rearing diapause and diapause-free western spruce budworm *(Choristoneura occidentalis)* (Lepidoptera: Tortricidae) on an artifical diet, *Can. Entomol.* **104**:417.

Maksymiuk, B., and Orchard, R. D., 1974, Techniques for evaluating *Bacillus thruingiensis* and spray equipment for aerial application against forest defoliating insects, U.S. Department of Agriculture Forest Service Research Paper PNW 183, Pacific Northwest Forest and Range Experiment Station, Portland, Oregon.

Markin, G. P., 1977, Western spruce budworm control with three dosages of Orthene, *Insecticide and Acaricide Tests* **2**:115.

Markin, G. P., and Shea, P. J., 1978, Development and registration of the insecticide Orthene for control of western forest insect pests (speech), p. 12, U.S. Department of Agriculture Forest Service, Washington, D.C. [presented at the 25th National Meeting of the Entomological Society of America, November 26–30, 1978, Houston, Texas].

Markin, G. P., and Wilcox, H., III, 1977, Douglas-fir tussock moth spray tests, *Insecticide and Acaricide Tests* **2**:113.

Markin, G. P., Batzer, H. O., and Brewer, J. W., 1978, Effectiveness of three insecticides applied at two droplet sizes for control of the Douglas-fir tussock moth and western spruce budworm,

U.S. Department of Agriculture Forest Service Research Note PNW-321, Pacific Northwest Forest and Range Experiment Station, Portland, Oregon.

Mauck, W. L., Olson, L. E., and Marking, L. L., 1976, Toxicity of natural pyrethrins and five pyrethroids to fish, *Arch. Environ. Contam. Toxicol.* **4:**18.

McGuire, J. R., 1976, Forest environmental protection: Challenges in insect and disease management, in: *Proceedings of the Symposium on Spruce Budworm* (W. H. Klein, technical coordinator), pp. 3–8, U.S. Department of Agriculture Miscellaneous Publication 1329, Washington, D.C.

McKnight, M. E., 1976, Control methodologies available or planned for near future, in: *Proceedings of the Symposium on Spruce Budworm* (W. H. Klein, technical coordinator), pp. 73–76, U.S. Department of Agriculture Miscellaneous Publication 1329, Washington, D.C.

Merkel, E. P., 1970, Trunk-implanted systemic insecticides for slash pine cone insect control, *Fl. Entomol.* **53:**143.

Miskus, R. P., Look, M., Andrews, T. L., and Lyon, R. L., 1968, Biological activity as an effect of structural changes in aryl *N*-methylcarbamates, *J. Agric. Food Chem.* **16:**605.

Moody, R. P., Prasad, R., Greenhalgh, R. J., and Weinberger, P., 1976, Fate of fenitrothion in forest trees. VII. Persistence, translocation and metabolism of 14C-fenitrothion in conifers, *Chem. Control Res. Inst. Ottawa Inf. Rep. CC-X* 122.

Moody, R. P., Prasad, R., Greenhalgh, R., Weinberger, P., 1977*a*, Translocation of ring-labelled 14C-fenitrothion in Conifers, in: *Proceedings of the Symposium on Fenitrothion: Longterm Effects of Its Use in the Forest Ecosystems*, pp. 217–231, National Research Council of Canada, Environmental Secretariat Publication NRCC 16073, Ottawa.

Moody, R. P., Prasad, R., Greenhalgh, R., and Weinberger, P., 1977*b*, Fate of fenitrothion in forest trees. VI. Some factors affecting rate of dissipation from balsam fir and white spruce, in: *Pesticide Management and Insecticide Resistance* (D. L. Watson and A. W. Brown, eds.), pp. 583–598, Academic Press, New York.

Moore, A. D., 1969, Pesticides—New facts, old problems, new developments in forest insect problems, *Trans. North. Am. Wildl. Nat. Resour. Conf.* **39:**55.

Morris, O. N., 1977, Long term study of the effectiveness of aerial application of *Bacillus thuringiensis*-acephate combinations against the spruce budworm, *Choristoneura fumiferana* (Lepidoptera: Tortricidae), *Can. Entomol.* **109:**1239.

Morris, R. C., 1976, Cottonwood leaf beetle control, *Insecticide Acaricide Tests* **1:**139.

Morrison, T. A., and Dimond, J. B., 1978, Field trials for control of spruce budworm in Maine: A history and bibliography, Maine Bureau of Forestry, Entomology Division, Technical Report No. 6.

Mrak, E. M. (ed.), 1969, Report of the Secretary's Commission on Pesticides and Their Relationship to Environmental Health, Department of Health, Education and Welfare Publication, Food and Drug Administration, Washington, D.C.

National Academy of Sciences (USA), 1975*a*, Decision making for regulating chemicals in the environment, Washington.

National Academy of Sciences (USA), 1975*b*, Pest control: An assessment of present and alternative technologies. IV. Forest pest control, Washington.

National Academy of Sciences (USA), 1975*c*, Principles for evaluating chemicals in the environment, Washington.

National Academy of Sciences (USA), 1978, Pesticide decision making, Washington.

Neisess, J., Marking, G. P., and Schaefer, R., 1976, Field evaluations of acephate and dimilin against the Douglas-fir tussock moth, *J. Econ. Entomol.* **69:**783.

Nigam, P. C., 1977, A summary of the 1977 Forest Pest Management Institute (Ottawa) field and laboratory studies, Proceedings of the Canadian Forest Pest Control Forum, Forest Pest Management Institute, Canadian Forestry Service, Environment Canada, Sault Ste. Marie, Ontario.

Nigam, P. C., 1978, Summary of laboratory evaluation of insecticides against various species of forest insect pests during 1978, Rep. FP-10, Proceedings of the Canadian Forestry Pest Control Forum, Forest Pest Management Institute, Canadian Forestry Service, Environment Canada, Sault Ste. Marie, Ontario.

Ospenson, J. N., 1977, Development and registration requirements for agricultural chemicals, *Vortex* **38**:16.

Page, M., and Lyon, R. L., 1973, Insecticides applied to western tussock moth reared on artificial diet: Laboratory tests, *J. Econ. Entomol.* **66**:53.

Page, M., and Lyon, R. L., 1975, Contact toxicity of insecticides applied to cottonwood leaf beetle, *J. Econ. Entomol.* **69**:147.

Page, M., and Robertson, J. L., 1976, Western spruce budworm, bioactivity of mexacarbate during long-term storage, *Insecticide Acaricide Tests* **1**:104.

Page, M., Lyon, R. L., and Green, L. E., 1974, Contact toxicity of eleven insecticides applied to the spring cankerworm, *J. Econ. Entomol* **64**:460.

Peck, H. M., 1966, Evaluating the safety of drugs, *BioScience* **16**:696.

Pieper, G. R., and Miskus, R. P., 1967, Determination of Zectran residues in aerial forest spraying, *J. Agric. Food Chem.* **15**:915.

Pimentel, D., Krummel, J., Gallahan, D., Hough, J., Merrill, A., Schreiner, I., Vittum, P., Koziol, F., Back, E., Yen, D., and Fiance, S., 1978, Benefits and costs of pesticide use in U.S. food production, *BioScience* **28**:772.

Pomber, L., Weinberger, P., and Prasad, R., 1973, A preliminary study on the fate of fenitrothion in forest seeds. II. Some effects on the morphogenetic characteristics of germinating white pine (*Pinus strobus* L.) seeds in relation to forest regeneration, *Chem. Control Res. Inst. Ottawa Inf. Rep. CC-X* 51.

Pomber, L., Weinberger, P., and Prasad, R., 1974*a*, Some physiological and phytotoxic effects of fenitrothion on germination and seedling growth of *Pinus strobus* L, *Chem. Control Res. Inst. Ottawa Inf. Rep. CC-X* 0-80,

Pomber, L., Weinberger, P., and Prasad, R., 1974*b*, The phytotoxicity of fenitrothion as assessed by germination and early growth of *Betula alleghaniensis* Britt, *Chem. Control Res. Inst. Ottawa Inf. Rep. CC-X* 79.

Pomber, L. A., Weinberger, P., and Prasad, R., 1975*a*, Some physiological effects of fenitrothion on the germination and seedling growth of *Betula Alleghaniesis* Britt, and *Picea glauca* (Moench) Voss, *Chem. Control Res. Inst. Ottawa Inf. Rep. CC-X* 108.

Pomber, L., Weinberger, P., and Prasad, R., 1975*b*, Studies on phytotoxicity of fenitrothion to some forest seeds and seedlings under laboratory conditions, *Chem. Control Res. Inst. Ottawa Inf. Rep. CC-X* 106.

Pomber, L. A., Weinberger, P., and Prasad, R., 1976, Some responses of white spruce and yellow birch seeds to organophosphorous insecticides during germination, *Chem. Control Res. Inst. Ottawa, Inf. Rep. CC-X* 131.

Prasad, R., 1977, Persistence, translocation and fate of fenitrothion in *Pinus banksiana* Lamb, Proceedings of the 24th Meeting of the Canadian Pest Management Society, Guelph, Canada, August, pp. 46–54.

Prasad, R., and Moody, R. P., 1974, Fate of fenitrothion in forest trees. III. Development of a histoautoradiographic technique for investigating foliar penetration in balsam fir and white spruce, *Chem. Control Res. Inst. Ottawa Inf. Rep. CC-X* 70.

Prasad, R., and Moody, R. P., 1976, Fate of fenitrothion in forest trees. VIII. Persistence, translocation and metabolism of 14C-fenitrothion in jack pine (*Pinus banksiana* Lamb.) in relation to sawfly mortality, *Chem. Control Res. Inst. Ottawa Inf. Rep. CC-X* 126.

Pschorn-Walcher, H., 1977, Biological control of forest insects, *Ann. Rev. Entomol.* **22**:1.

Quistad, G. B., Staiger, L. E., and Schooley, D. A., 1975, Environmental degradation of the insect growth regulator methoprene (Isopropyl (2E,4E-11-Methoxy-3,7,11-tri-methyl-2,4-dodecadienoate). III. Photodecomposition, *J. Agric. Food Chem.* **23**:299.

Ragenovich, I. R., and Coster, J. E., 1974, Evaluation of some carbamate and phosphate insecticides against southern pine beetle and *Ips* bark beetles, *J. Econ. Entomol.* **67**:763.

Randall, A. P., 1976, Insecticides, formulations, and aerial application technology for spruce budworm control, in: *Proceedings of the Symposium on Spruce Budworm* (W. H. Klein, technical coordinator), pp. 77–90, U.S. Department of Agriculture Miscellaneous Publication 1329, Washington, D.C.

Randall, A. P., and Nigam, P. C., 1966, Toxicity of phosphorous carbamate insecticides to spruce budworm and two species of sawflies, *Bi-Mon. Res. Notes Can. For. Serv.* **22**:3.

Richmond, C. E., 1972, Juvenile hormone analogues tested on larvae of western spruce budworm, *J. Econ. Entomol.* **65**:950.

Richmond, C. E., Averill, R. D., and Crisp, C. E., 1978, Protection of Douglas-fir foliage from western spruce budworm (Lepidoptera: Tortricidae) damage by early applications of acephate (Orthene 75S), *Can. Entomol.* **110**:1127.

Richmond, C. E., Crisp, C. E., Larson, J. E., and Pieper, G. R., 1979, A simple method for extraction, clean-up and identification of acephate and methamidophos residues in plant tissues by GLC, *Bull. Environ. Contam. Toxicol.* **22**:512.

Roberts, R., 1978. Chemical analysis of spray deposits, in: *Methods for Sampling and Assessing Deposits of Insecticidal Sprays Released over Forests* (J. W. Barry, R. B. Ekblad, G. P. Markin, and G. C. Trostle, eds.), pp. 104–106, U.S. Department of Agriculture Technical Bulletin 1596. Washington, D.C.

Roberts, R. B. (ed.), 1976, *Pesticide Spray Application, Behavior, and Assessment: Workshop Proceedings*, U.S. Department of Agriculture Forest Service General Technical Report PSW-15, Pacific Southwest Forest and Range Experiment Station, Berkeley, California.

Roberts, R. B., Miskus, R. P., Duckles, C. K., and Sakai, T. T., 1969, *In vivo* fate of the insecticide Zectran in spruce budworm, tobacco budworm, and housefly larvae, *J. Agric. Food Chem.* **17**:107.

Roberts, R. B., Lyon, R. L., Duckles, C. K., and Look, M., 1972, Influence of selected synergists on the action of five insecticides on larval western spruce budworm: Absence of synergism and *in vitro* oxidation of Zectran, *J. Econ. Entomol.* **65**:1277.

Roberts, R. B., Fisher, D. A., and Schroen, C. K., 1976, Cuticle of the western spruce budworm (Lepidoptera:Tortricidae): Its morphology and role in insecticide poisoning, Anniversary Publication 9, pp. 61–69, Department of Entomology, University of Idaho, Moscow.

Roberts, R. B., Look, M., Haddon, W. F., and Dickerson, T. C., 1978, A new degradation product of the insecticide mexacarbate found in fresh water, *J. Agric. Food Chem.* **16**:55.

Robertson, J. L., 1972, Toxicity of Zectran aerosol to the California oakworm, a primary parasite, and a hyperparasite, *Environ. Entomol.* **1**:115.

Robertson, J. L., 1976, Western black-headed budworm laboratory spray tests, *Insecticide and Acaricide Tests* **1**:104.

Robertson, J. L., 1978*a*, Laboratory bioassays, in: *The Douglas-fir Tussock Moth—A Synthesis* (M. H. Brooks, R. W. Stark, and R. W. Campbell, eds.), pp. 112–115, U.S. Department of Agriculture Technical Bulletin 1585, Washington, D.C.

Robertson, J. L., 1978*b*, Feeding tests of insecticides, *Insecticide and Acaracide Tests* **3**:146.

Robertson, J. L., 1979, Rearing the western spruce budworm, U.S. Department of Agriculture, Canada United States Spruce Budworm Program [GPO-1979-699-944].

Robertson, J. L., and Boelter, L. M., 1979a, Toxicity of insecticides to Douglas-fir tussock moth *Orgyia pseudotsugata* (Lepidoptera: Lymantriidae). I. Contact and feeding toxicity, *Can. Entomol.* **111**:1145.

Robertson, J. L., and Boelter, L. M., 1979b, Toxicity of insecticides to Douglas-fir tussock moth, *Orgyia pseudotsugata* (Lepidoptera: Lymantriidae). II. Residual toxicity and rainfastness, *Can. Entomol.* **111**:1161.

Robertson, J. L., and Gillette, N. L., 1973, Western tent caterpillar: Contact toxicity of ten insecticides applied to the larvae, *J. Econ. Entomol.* **65**:629.

Robertson, J. L., and Gillette, N. L., 1978, Contact toxicity of insecticides to western pine beetle, *Insecticide and Acaricide Tests* **3**:148.

Robertson, J. L., and Kimball, R. A., 1979a, Effects of insect growth regulators on the western spruce budworm *(Choristoneura occidentalis)* (Lepidoptera: Tortricidae). I. Lethal effects of last instar treatments, *Can. Entomol.* **111**:1361.

Robertson, J. L., and Kimball, R. A., 1979b, Effects of insect growth regulators on the western spruce budworm *(Choristoneura occidentalis)* (Lepidoptera: Tortricidae). II. Fecundity and fertility reduction following last instar treatments, *Can. Entomol.* **111**:1369.

Robertson, J. L., and Lyon, R. L., 1973a, Elm spanworm: Contact toxicity of ten insecticides applied to the larvae, *J. Econ. Entomol.* **66**:627.

Robertson, J. L., and Lyon, R. L., 1973b, Western spruce budworm: Nonresistance to Zectran, *J. Econ. Entomol.* **66**:801.

Robertson, J. L., and Lyon, R. L., 1973c, Douglas-fir tussock moth: Contact toxicity of 20 insecticides applied to the larvae, *J. Econ. Entomol.* **66**:1255.

Robertson, J. L., and Rappaport, N. G., 1979, Direct, indirect, and residual toxicities of insecticide sprays to western spruce budworm, *Choristoneura occidentalis* (Lepidoptera: Tortricidae), *Can. Entomol.* **111**:1219.

Robertson, J. L., Lyon, R. L., Shon, F. L., and Page, M., 1973, Western blackheaded budworm: Toxicity of five insecticides to two populations, *J. Econ. Entomol.* **66**:274.

Robertson, J. L., Lyon, R. L., and Gillette, N. L., 1975, Contact toxicity of 38 insecticides to pales weevil adults, *J. Econ. Entomol.* **68**:124.

Robertson, J. L., Gillette, N. L., Look, M., Lucas, B. A., and Lyon, R. L., 1976, Toxicity of selected insecticides applied to western spruce budworm, *J. Econ. Entomol,* **69**:99.

Robertson, J. L., Boelter, L. M., and Gillette, N. L., 1977, Laboratory tests of insecticides on western spruce budworm, *Insecticide Acaricide Tests* **2**:110.

Robertson, J. L., Boelter, L. M., Russell, R. M., and Savin, N. E., 1978a, Variation in response to insecticides by Douglas-fir tussock moth, *Orgyia pseudotsugata* (Lepidoptera: Lymantriidae), populations, *Can. Entomol.* **110**:325.

Robertson, J. L., Gillette, N. L., Lucas, B. A., Russell, R. M., and Savin. N. E., 1978b, Comparative toxicity of insecticides to *Choristoneura* species (Lepidoptera: Tortricidae), *Can. Entomol.* **110**:399.

Robertson, J. L., Lyon, R. L., Andrews, T. L., Moellman, E. E., and Page, M., 1979, Moellman spray chamber: Versatile research tool for laboratory bioassays, U.S. Department of Agriculture Forest Service Research Note PSW-335, Pacific Southwest Forest and Range Experiment Station, Berkeley, California.

Robertson, J. L., Russell, R. M., and Savin, N. E., 1980, POLO: A user's guide to Probit or LOgit analysis, U.S. Department of Agriculture, General Technical Report PSW-38, Pacific Southwest Forest and Range Experiment Station, Berkeley, California.

Rose, A. H., 1958, The effect of defoliation on foliage production and radial growth of quaking aspen, *Forest Sci.* **4**:335.

Rumker, R., von., Guest, H. R., and Upholt, W. M., 1970, The search for safer, more selective, and less persistent pesticides. A questionnaire survey of pesticide manufacturers, *BioScience* **20**:1004.

Russell, R. M., and Robertson, J. L., 1979, Programming probit analysis, *Bull. Entomol. Soc. Am.* **25**:191.

Russell, R. M., Robertson, J. L., and Savin, N. E., 1977, POLO: A new computer program for probit analysis, *Bull Entomol. Soc. Am.* **23**:209.

Sanders, C. J., 1976, Pest management strategy of epicenter control, in: *Proceedings of the Symposium on Spruce Budworm* (W. H. Klein, technical coordinator), pp. 61–63, U.S. Department of Agriculture Miscellaneous Publication 1327, Washington, D.C.

Savin, N. E., Robertson, J. L., and Russell, R. M., 1977, A critical evaluation of bioassay in insecticide research: Likelihood ratio tests of dose-mortality regression, *Bull. Entomol. Soc. Am.* **23**:257.

Shea, P. J., 1977, Testing of chemical and microbial insecticides for safety . . . Some techniques, *Bull. Entomol. Soc. Am.* **23**:176.

Shea, P. J., 1979, Environmental safety, in: *The Douglas-Fir Tussock Moth—A synthesis* (M. H. Brooks, R. W. Stark, and R. W. Campbell, eds.), pp. 122–129, U.S. Department of Agriculture Technical Bulletin 1585, Washington D.C.

Shea, P. J., Cecil, H. C., Schaefer, C. H., Steelman, C. D., and Zinkle, J. G., 1978: Effects of diflubenzuron (Dimilin) on nontarget avian and aquatic organisms, and its fate in the environment, Pacific Southwest Forest and Range Experiment Station, Berkeley, California.

Singh, P., 1977, *Artificial Diets for Insects, Mites, and Spiders,* Plenum Press, New York.

Smith, R. F., 1971, Juveno-mimetic effects of lannate in sublethal doses on western spruce budworm *(Choristoneura occidentalis), J. Invert. Pathol.* **17**:132.

Solomon, J. D., and Oliveria, F. L., 1977, Aphid control on cottonwood with carbofuran, *Insecticide and Acaricide Tests* **2**:111.

Stock, M. W., and Robertson, J. L., 1979, Differential response of Douglas-fir tussock moth, *Orgyia pseudotsugata* (Lepidoptera: Lymantriidae), populations and sibling groups to acephate and carbaryl: Toxicological and genetic analyses, *Can. Entomol.* **111**:1231.

Sundaram, K. M. S., 1978, Studies on dispersal, persistence, cycling and accountability of aerially applied insecticides in the forest environment, Proceedings of the Canadian Forest Pest Control Forum, Forest Pest Management Institute Report FP-11-198, Canadian Forestry Service Environment Canada, Sault Ste. Marie, Ontario.

Sundaram, K. M. S., and Hopewell, W. W., 1976, Distribution, persistence and translocation of Orthene in spruce trees after simulated aerial spray application, *Chem. Control Res. Inst. Ottawa Inf. Rep. CC-X* 121.

Sundaram, K. M. S., and Hopewell, W. W., 1977, Fate and persistence of aminocarb in conifer foliage and forest soil after simulated aerial application. *Can. Dept. Fish Environ. Inf. Rep. FPM-X* 6.

Sundaram, K. M. S., Hopewell, W. W., and LaFrance, G., 1977, Uptake, translocation and metabolism of C-14 acephate in spruce trees, *Chem. Control Res. Inst. Ottawa Inf. Rep. CC-X* 139.

United States Department of Agriculture, 1976*a*, Forest Service Pesticide Use Reports: 1976., Washington, D.C.

United States Department of Agriculture, 1976*b*, Supplement to the principal laws relating to Forest Service activities, U.S. Department of Agriculture Handbook 453.

United States Department of Agriculture, 1977*a*, Pesticide use reports: 1977, Washington, D.C.

United States Department of Agriculture, 1977*b*, United States Department of Agriculture-Department of Environment Canada. Charter: Research, development and applications program, Canada-U.S. Spruce Budworms Program, Memorandum of Understanding, Washington, D.C.

United States Department of Agriculture, 1978*a*, Forest Service Pesticide Use Reports: 1978, Washington, D.C.
United States Department of Agriculture, 1978*b*, Douglas-fir tussock moth program accomplishments report. U.S. Department of Agriculture *Information* Bulletin 417.
Valovage, W. D., and Kulman, H. M., 1977, *Pristiphora erichsonii* control with Dimilin on larch, *Insecticide Acaricide Tests* 2:116.
Washburn, R. K., Livingston, R. L., and Markin, G. P., 1977, An aerial test of Orthene against the larch casebearer, U.S. Department of Agriculture Forest Service Research Note INT-226, Intermountain Forest and Range Experiment Station, Ogden, Utah.
Weinberger, P., Pomber, L., and Prasad, R. 1978*a*, The response of white spruce and yellow birch to some selected organophosphorus insecticides and the adjuvants Atlox and Arotex, *J. Exp. Bot.* 29:479.
Weinberger, P., Pomber, L., and Prasad, R., 1978*b*, Phytotoxicity of fenitrothion to white pine seeds and seedlings, *Can. J. For. Res.* 8:155.
Weinberger, P., Pomber, L., and Prasad, R., 1978*c*, Some toxic effects of fenitrothion on seed germination and early seedling growth of jack pine, spruce and birches, *Can. J. For. Res.* 8:243.
Wernz, J., and Markin, G. P., 1977, Flow rates and characteristics of Dimilin, Dylox 1.5, Orthene 75S, and Sevin 4-Oil, U.S. Department of Agriculture Forest Service Research Note PNW-300, Pacific Northwest Forest and Range Experiment Station, Portland, Oregon.
Williams, C. B., Jr., 1973, Field tests of four insecticides against the Douglas-fir tussock moth in Oregon, Western Forestry and Conservation Association, Permanent Assoc. Comm. Proc., Portland, Oregon, December, pp. 77–83.
Williams, C. B., Jr., and Walton, G., 1968, Effects of naled and Zectran on the budworm *Choristoneura occidentalis* and associated insects in Montana, *J. Econ. Entomol.* 61:784.
Williams, C. B., Walton, G. S., and Tiernan, C. F., 1969, Zectran and naled affect incidence of parasitism of the budworm *Choristoneura occidentalis* in Montana, *J. Econ. Entomol.* 62:310.
Williams, C. B., Jr., Markin, G. P., and Shea, P. J., 1978*a*, Effects of carbaryl, trichlorfon, and DDT on collapsing Douglas-fir tussock moth populations in Oregon, U.S. Department of Agriculture Forest Service Research Note PSW-334, Pacific Southwest Forest and Range Experiment Station, Berkeley, California.
Williams, C. B., Jr., Shea, P. J., Maksymiuk, B., Neiess, J. A., and McComb, D., 1978*b*, Aerial application of mexacarbate and stabilized pyrethrins on Douglas-fir tussock moth populations, U.S. Department of Agriculture Forest Service Research Note PSW-332, Pacific Southwest Forest and Range Experiment Station, Berkeley, California.
Williams, C. B., Jr., Shea, P. J., and McGregor, M. D., 1979, Effects of aerially applied mexacarbate on western spruce budworm larvae and their parasites in Montana, U.S. Department of Agriculture Forest Service Research Paper PSW-144, Pacific Southwest Forest and Range Experiment Station, Berkeley, California.
Wood, D. L., 1977, Manipulation of forest pests, in: *Chemical Control of Insect Behavior* (H. H. Shorey and J. R. McKelvey, eds.), pp. 369–384, John Wiley, New York.

8

The Use of Biodegradable Pesticides in Public Health Entomology

Gene R. DeFoliart

8.1. INTRODUCTION

In his presidential address to the American Society of Tropical Medicine and Hygiene, W. C. Reeves (1972) asked: "Can the war to contain infectious diseases be lost?" That remains a good question today. One must realize how fragile our ability is to control arthropod-borne disease. After malaria was reduced in India from 750 million cases and 750,000 deaths per year prior to 1953 (Wattal, 1971) to only 100,000 cases per year during the mid-1960s, we have witnessed a resurgence to 5 million cases in 1976 and to 10 million cases during the first 9 months of 1977 (Akhtar and Learmonth, 1977). In India, 122 million people live at risk of filariasis (Wattal, 1971). Outbreaks of dengue and chikungunya viruses occur repeatedly, and less than a year ago an epidemic of Japanese encephalitis resulted in 5359 confirmed and clinically suspected cases and 1869 deaths (U.S. Department of Health, Education and Welfare, 1978).

In the United States, a temperate zone country, vector-borne problems pale in comparison to those of India. Nevertheless, we have more than 1000 cases of Rocky Mountain spotted fever annually, and the number is increasing. Only 4 years ago we experienced the greatest epidemic of mosquito-borne human encephalitis in the U.S. since the 1930s, with more than 2000 cases of St. Louis encephalitis (U.S. Department of Health, Education and Welfare, 1976). Near

Gene R. DeFoliart • Department of Entomology, University of Wisconsin, Madison, Wisconsin 53706

disaster struck in 1971 when epidemic Venezuelan equine encephalitis (VEE) surged into Texas, resulting in more than 1500 equine deaths and 110 human cases (Sudia *et al.*, 1975). More than 3 million horses were vaccinated and more than 8 million acres were sprayed with insecticide before this invasion was brought under control.

The preceding are only some of the more notable examples. Tick-borne Kyasanur Forest Disease virus and mosquito-borne West Nile virus occur in India, and there are several important mosquito-borne encephalitis viruses in the United States. Leishmaniasis, both visceral and cutaneous, is endemic to India, and large-scale epidemics numbering up to 20,000 cases were not infrequent prior to 1953. Some Indian workers predict a comeback for leishmaniasis if for any reason intradomiciliary spraying for malaria control should cease (Shanmugham *et al.*, 1977; Sharma *et al.*, 1973a,b). Bubonic plague, which harassed India until the mid-twentieth century with 12.5 million deaths between 1896 and 1948, and an outbreak of 600 cases as recently as 1962 in Mysore State (Wattal, 1971), still lurks in sylvatic foci in both countries. Although human cases are sporadic, continued vigilance will be essential.

8.2. THE NATURE AND DIVERSITY OF ARTHROPOD-BORNE DISEASE

The majority of arthropod-borne disease agents are, in Pavlovsky's terminology, *zooanthroponoses*, i.e., disease agents perpetuated in wild vertebrate–arthropod cycles that infect man only incidentally. Man becomes infected by entering the orbit of the wild cycles or occasionally they spill over in epidemic proportions into human populations. The enzootic foci of most of these zooanthroponoses are so widely dispersed that there is little or no hope for their elimination in the foreseeable future. The main line of defense against these agents is good surveillance and the ability to quickly mobilize vector control technology when an epidemic threatens.

Anthroponoses, i.e., disease agents transmissible directly from human to human via an arthropod vector (no extrahuman reservoir) seem generally more amenable to elimination or containment by vector control and/or other means. Even these agents present extremely complex challenges, however, as demonstrated by the resurgence of malaria in many areas, and by the recurring epidemics of dengue in both Eastern and Western Hemispheres.

One cannot help but marvel at the uneven state of the art in medical entomology. On the one hand we embarked on the global eradication of malaria; on the other hand, after 100 years, we do not know how to make an imbedded tick detach voluntarily from one of our own appendages. Undoubtedly this is due in part to simply the sheer number of different arthropod-borne vertebrate-pathogenic entities and the variety of habitats and life styles of their vectors. The number of known arboviruses, for example, is nearing 400 (Berge, 1975); most are transmitted by mosquitoes, but some are transmitted by ticks, *Phlebotomus* sp. or *Culicoides* sp. Fortunately, many appear not to be associated with human disease, but more than 100 have been so associated.

The World Health Organization (WHO) and the United Nations Development Programme (UNDP) recently launched the Special Program for Research and Training in Tropical Diseases, which is in part an effort to focus top-flight research attention on six diseases that afflict more than 600 million people worldwide, especially in tropical regions. Four of the six diseases are arthropod-borne: malaria, filariasis, leishmaniasis, and trypanosomiasis. On the surface, four diseases sounds like a manageable number. The trouble is that this "Tropical Big Four" is composed of more than a dozen different parasites and literally scores of different epidemiological entities.

There are four species of human malaria plasmodia and more than 60 species of *Anopheles* are efficient vectors. Filariasis includes not only mosquito-borne *Wuchereria* and *Brugia* but also blackfly-transmitted onchocerciasis. Leishmaniasis involves an as yet unsettled number of *Leishmania* species, and epidemiological and clinical types. All are transmitted by phlebotomine sandflies, but some are anthroponoses and some are zooanthroponoses. Trypanosomiasis includes *Trypanosoma cruzi*, the etiologic agent of Chagas disease in the Western Hemisphere, transmitted by several species of triatomine bugs, and two species of human-infecting tsetse-transmitted trypanosomes in Africa. The two African diseases are of very different epidemiological patterns. In addition, several species of *Trypanosoma* that devastate livestock will have to be dealt with if the people of Africa are to be freed of the yoke of the tsetses.

8.3. INSECTICIDES: THE RECENT PAST

Some insight as to where we are today in public health entomology, and how we got there, may be gained by examining the situation that currently confronts organized mosquito control units in the United States and workers in the global malaria program.

8.3.1. Mosquito Control in the United States

Florida and California have been two of the areas of most intense mosquito control activity in the U.S., and a National Academy of Sciences study (NAS, 1976) draws an interesting comparison between the history of organized control and the current status of insecticide resistance in the two states. Historically, there have been some parallels in control strategies and also some differences, the latter being in part dictated by the differing nature of the mosquito problem in the two states.

In coastal Florida, the salt marsh breeders, *Aedes taeniorhynchus* and *Ae. sollicitans* have posed a serious threat to tourism and retirement. In the interior, the glades mosquito, *Psorophora confinnis,* breeds in vast areas of poorly drained flatwoods as well as in irrigated pastures and citrus groves. In California, the main problem stems from freshwater mosquitoes *Ae. nigromaculis* and *Ae. dorsalis* in irrigated pastures and other irrigated agricultural lands, abetted by *Culex tarsalis* and *Anopheles freeborni,* mainly in rice fields.

Both states have utilized source reduction, but Florida has fewer options in this respect. Its mosquitoes come from wildlands, and despite Provost's belief (1977) that salt marshes can be altered without ecological damage, salt marsh alterations have met with increasing opposition from environmentalists. In the case of *Psorophora,* the sheer dispersion and vastness of the breeding grounds preclude much effort at source reduction. For the same reasons that source reduction options are limited in Florida, larvicides would have limited utility. By contrast, California's mosquito problems are mostly man-made, thus more amenable to correction through prevention or, lacking prevention, the use of larvicides.

Chemical names of insecticides are listed in Table 8.1. Table 8.2 compares the use of mosquito insecticides in Florida and California, 1970–1972. Despite early exhortations by Herms (1949) and others for restraint in the use of larvicides and for continued emphasis on prevention, by 1954 resistance to all chlorinated hydrocarbons was widespread in California, and by 1970 mosquito control was in a state of crisis with *Ae. nigromaculis* and *C. tarsalis* widely resistant to all registered organophosphorous (OP) compounds. Note in Table 8.2 the decline in OP larvicides from 227,000 lb to only 98,000 lb in the 2-year period from 1970 to 1972. This decrease was made up for by an increase in the use of larvicidal oils. The resistance situation in California rendered it extremely vulnerable if the VEE invasion of Texas in 1972 had spread to that state. Fortunately, the virus was stopped in Texas.

In Florida, because of the nature of the mosquito production grounds, and in a conscious effort to delay the appearance of resistance, the State Board of Health advised mosquito control districts to use organic insecticides only against adults, not against larvae, the rationale being that a thorough-going larvicide program selects for tolerance against the entire population while adulticiding exerts pressure only against the segment of the mosquito population that finds its way to urban areas. Note (Table 8.2) that Florida used 848,000 lb of adulticides in 1972 compared to 8000 lb by California and that, except for larvicidal oils

Table 8.1.   Chemical Names of Insecticides Mentioned in Text

Insecticide	Chemical name
Bioresmethrin	5-Benzyl-3-furylmethyl (+) *trans* chrysanthemate
Chlorpyrifos (Dursban®)	O,O-Diethyl-O-(3,5,6-trichloro-2-pyridyl) phosphorothioate
DDT	1,1,1-Trichloro-2,2-bis(*p*-chlorophenyl) ethane
Decamethrin	(−)-(Cyano)-3-phenoxybenzyl-(+) *cis*-3-(2,2-Dibromovinyl)-2,2-dimethylcyclopropane-1-carboxylate
Dieldrin	Not less than 85% of 1,2,3,4,10-10-hexachloro-6-7-epoxy-1,4,4a,5,6,7,8,8a-*endo-exo*-5-8-dimethanonaphthalene
Diflubenzuron (Dimilin®)	1-(4-Chlorophenyl)-3-(2,6-diflurobenzoyl) urea
Fenitrothion	O-O-Dimethyl-O-(4-nitro-*m*-tolyl) phosphorothioate
Fenthion (Baytex®)	O-O-Dimethyl O-[3-methyl-4-(methylthio)phenyl] phosphorothioate
Flit MLO	Petroleum distillate of undisclosed nature
HCH	1,2,3,4,5,6-Hexachlorocyclohexane, mixed isomers
Malathion	Diethyl mercaptosuccinate S-ester with O,O-Dimethyl phosphorodithioate
Methoprene (Altosid®)	Isopropyl (2E, 4E)-11-methoxy-3,7,11-trimethyl-2,4-dodecadienoate
Methyl parathion	O,O-Dimethyl O-*p*-nitrophenyl phosphorothioate
Naled (Dibrom®)	1,2-Dibromo-2,2-dichloroethyl dimethylphosphate
Parathion	O,O-Diethyl O-*p*-nitrophenyl phosphorothioate
Paris green	Copper acetoarsenite $(CH_3COO)_2Cu \cdot 3Cu(AsO_2)_2$
Permethrin (Pounce®)	3-Phenoxybenzyl (±) *cis-trans*-3-(2,2-dichlorovinyl)-2,2-dimethylcyclopropane carboxylate
Propoxur (Baygon®)	O-Isopropoxyphenyl methylcarbamate
R-U 22974 (Decis®)	S-[Cyano(3-phenoxyphenyl)methyl] cis-(+)-3-(2,2-dibromoethenyl-2-2-dimethylcyclopropanecarboxylate
SD-43775 (Pydrin®)	α-Cyano-3-phenoxybenzyl 4-chloro-α-(1-methylethyl) phenylacetate
Temephos (Abate®)	O,O,O',O'-Tetramethyl O,O'-thiodi-*p*-phenylene phosphorothioate

Florida's use of larvicides, especially OP larvicides, was negligible. OP resistance remains a minor problem in the control of Florida mosquitoes (Boike and Rathburn, 1972, 1975; Boike *et al.*, 1978).

NAS (1976)* summarized the California–Florida comparison as follows:

> For quite different reasons, mosquito control in California and Florida must henceforth be much more sophisticated than it was when insecticides ruled. Both states are in trouble. California's big problem is mosquito resistance to insecticides. The state is taking the only rational options left to it: enforcement of laws against producing

---

*Reproduced from NAS (1976), with the permission of the National Academy of Sciences, Washington, D.C.

Table 8.2. Insecticide Use in Florida and
California, 1970–1972[a]

Insecticide	Pounds used	
	1970	1972
California		
Adulticides		
Propoxur	5,779	8,693
Larvicides		
Fenthion	109,912	51,332
Parathion, ethyl	72,603	18,691
Parathion, methyl	28,327	11,709
Malathion	10,478	11,267
Chlorpyrifos	5,128	4,793
Totals	227,140	98,507
Larvicidal oils (gal)	339,216	528,800
Florida		
Adulticides		
Malathion	420,001	605,835
Naled	233,407	223,282
Fenthion	12,311	19,323
Totals	665,719	848,440
Larvicides		
Paris green	51,800	14,885
Temephos	1,215	16,320
Totals	53,015	31,175
Larvicidal oils (gal)	1,222,910	1,476,618

[a] Source: NAS (1976).

mosquitoes and source reduction through cooperation with agriculturists. It can easily manage the current legitimate concern over environmental quality because so little of its mosquito-producing terrain is natural environment. In Florida, the situation is nearly the reverse. There is no severe problem with insecticide resistance, but everywhere there is conflict with protectors of the environment. . . . Mosquito control can no longer be a unilateral operation. Collaboration is now essential with landowners, agricultural scientists, conservationists, engineers of several sorts, a great variety of public agencies, and, most assuredly, land-use planners. Mosquito control is now an integral part of land and water management in the public interest.

8.3.2. Malaria Control

The strategy for attempted global eradication of malaria, a goal now revised (WHO, 1978), was based on the premise that plasmodial infection in the human population will die out within 2–3 years in a given area if mosquito transmission can be interrupted for that length of time. Although the transmission dynamics of malaria varies from one locality to another, depending upon climate, species of parasites and species of vectors present, and customs of the people (Macdonald, 1957, and others), most malaria transmission takes place inside houses at night. The main method of attack therefore has been application of residual insecticides to the inside walls of domiciles.

For various reasons, the attack phase with insecticides lasted longer than expected in many areas and, as is well known, the greatest deterrent to success in the program has been development of resistance by many of the major vector species to a succession of insecticides used as intradomiciliary sprays. DDT resistance has developed in populations of 15 anopheline vector species and dieldrin resistance in populations of 37 species (Brown *et al.*, 1976). In India, four of the nine vector anophelines are resistant to DDT—*An. culicifacies, An. stephensi, An. fluviatilis,* and *An. philippinensis,* with the first two also resistant to BHC and dieldrin (Brown *et al.*, 1976; Sharma, 1972) and with *An. culicifacies* now starting to show resistance to malathion (Rajagopal, 1977). In southern Turkey, *An. sacharovi* is not only DDT- and dieldrin-resistant but has gone the route through malathion and propoxur resistance. In El Salvador and Nicaragua, the same is true of *An. albimanus. An. albimanus* is one of a number of examples of the importance of agricultural insecticides in bringing selection pressure to bear on important vectors. The malathion and propoxur resistance of *An. albimanus* in El Salvador has been mainly induced by the use of malathion, methyl parathion, and carbaryl on cotton fields (Georghiou, 1972). As resistance appears, substitutions become expensive, malathion costing 5 times and propoxur 20 times more than DDT when substituted for it in the late 1960s and early 1970s (Brown *et al.*, 1976). In tests in India against *An. culicifacies,* Bhatnagar *et al.* (1974) found that three rounds of fenitrothion would be required to cover one malaria transmission season, compared to two rounds for DDT, and the substitution of fenitrothion for DDT would result in a 10.66-fold cost increase.

A number of other factors have contributed to the currently complicated situation: the appearance of parasite resistance to chloroquine and related 4-aminoquinolines in many areas of southeast Asia and South America (Peters, 1974); exophily of vectors, in which the vector bites outdoors and thus does not contact the wall deposits, for example, *An. balabacensis* in southeast Asia (Scanlon and Sandhinand, 1965); the excito-repellent effect of DDT deposits, causing some species to exit from houses soon after biting; absorption of insecticide applied to mud walls, thereby reducing its availability to vectors; DDT resistance in bedbugs and other household pests, thus making spraymen less welcome (Rafatjah, 1971); nomadism of the people in some geographic areas; operational problems caused by reduced finanacial support from international sources; inflation; and shortages of insecticides (Brown *et al.*, 1976). Despite the systematic screening of more than 1400 compounds by WHO in its search for suitable DDT substitutes (Wright, 1971), only a few promising compounds have surfaced.

8.4. INTEGRATED PEST AND VECTOR MANAGEMENT

The DDT and immediate post-DDT era pinpointed problems that result from a unifactor approach to insect control using nondegradable, broad-spectrum insecticides:

1. Incorporation and concentration in food chains, hence the current insistence that new insecticides be biodegradable. An important exception is the use of DDT as an intradomiciliary spray for malaria control, as this presents no environmental hazard.
2. Destruction of beneficial parasites and predators by broad-spectrum insecticides, hence the desire for insecticides or other biocides of relatively narrow target specificity. This is the aim of much current research, but we know practically nothing about the impact of introducing an additional biocide into specific environments. Laird (1977) described how it required 9 years to secure simply a taxonomic inventory (incomplete) on more than 200 species of plants and animals that inhabited a small Canadian snow-melt pool only 2 m in diameter. A counterforce here is that insecticides of narrow specificity have smaller markets and therefore attract less interest from manufacturers. Reduced markets have jeopardized continued supplies of such well-established insecticides as DDT and Paris green (NAS, 1976).
3. Development of genetic resistance, hence the need to minimize the use of any one biocidal agent by developing approaches that integrate a variety of methods against a target species. It can be expected that any chemical approach will be vulnerable to the selection of resistant strains, as were the organochlorines (OC). OC- and OP-resistant house flies, *Musca domestica,* have exhibited cross-resistance to juvenoids (synthetic analogues of juvenile hormone) (Cerf and Georghiou, 1972, 1974; Plapp and Vinson, 1973) and direct selection by methoprene resulted in resistance levels of 80 to 400-fold in *Culex* (T. M. Brown and A. W. A. Brown, 1974; Georghiou *et al.,* 1974) and of greater than 1000-fold in *M. domestica* (Georghiou *et al.,* 1978). Cross-resistance to pyrethroids has been reported for OC- and OP-resistant house flies (Farnham, 1973; Farnham and Sawicki, 1976) and mosquitoes (Chadwick *et al.,* 1977), and a strain of *Culex p. quinquefasciatus* selected by *d-trans* permethrin developed >4000-fold resistance to this isomer by generation F_{18} along with cross-resistance to the *d-cis* isomer and to various other pyrethroids (Priester and Georghiou, 1978).

Brown (1977) described the progression of resistance in *Ae. nigromaculis* in California as follows: to organochlorines by 1951, to parathion by 1960, to fenthion by 1965, and to chlorpyrifos by 1970. He also stated that in Denmark, between 1951 and 1967, each OP compound was effective against *M. domestica* for about 2 years. One of the main goals in devising integrated control programs is to increase the number of years that an insecticide can be used before it loses its effectiveness. Applied entomologists should become familiar with the genetics of resistance. Georghiou and Taylor (1977*a,b*) and Taylor and Georghiou (1979) have shown that, depending on the initial frequency and dominance of alleles which confer resistance, the rate of evolution of resistance can be slowed by several partly controllable operational factors such as the initial population size, rate of inward migration of unselected individuals, presence of untreated refugia within a treated area, and dose and timing of insecticide application.

For mosquito control, currently available resources for integration include source reduction, conservation of natural predators and parasites, several mass-producible biocontrol agents, and a number of insecticides and methods of applying them. One of the main problems in devising integrated control programs is how to integrate methods in such a way that the effects are additive rather than disruptive. The additive effects of components integrated by workers in California (Dr. J. R. Anderson and co-workers) and North Carolina (Dr. R. C. Axtell and co-workers) for control of flies that develop in manure under caged poultry are readily apparent. The program as it eventually evolved in North Carolina (Axtell, 1970*a,b*) is aimed at control of the house fly, *M. domestica*, and the lesser house fly, *Fannia canicularis*, and is based on the preservation of two species of manure-inhabiting predatory mites, *Machrocheles muscae-domesticae* and *Fuscuropoda vegetans*, plus judicious use of fly adulticides. Fly control, as often practiced in caged poultry houses, consisted of periodic removal of manure plus weekly application of larvicides, this amounting in North Carolina to 16–18 applications per season. A search for suitable selective larvicides, i.e., not deleterious to the mites, was not successful (Axtell, 1966, 1968). Since the mites repopulate more slowly than the flies after manure removal, various schemes of partial removal have been suggested (Anderson, 1965; Axtell, 1970*a*; Legner and Brydon, 1966; Peck and Anderson, 1970). Willis and Axtell (1968) found that the two mite species complemented each other in several ways. The density of *M. muscaedomesticae* became maximum after 2–3 weeks of manure accumulation, then slowly declined, while *F. vegetans* increased more slowly, becoming the dominant species after 5–6 weeks of manure accumulation. Also, *M. muscaedomesticae*, which prefer fly eggs, were found mainly in the outermost layer of manure and near the peak of the manure cone, while *F. vegetans*, which prey only on first-instar fly larvae, were found in aggregations 2–4 cm within the manure. Finally, it was determined that adulticides applied to the upper parts of the sheds had no deleterious effects on the mites and that five to six such applications at 2- to 5-week intervals during the season provided control equivalent to that obtained by larviciding (Axtell, 1970a). It was estimated that larviciding requires about five times as much insecticide and two and one-half times as many man-hours as required for the integrated program (Axtell, 1970b).

It would be nice to end the story there, as an example of a complete success for integrated control. However, in the attempted management of wild populations solutions seldom prove to be simple or final. Axtell and Edwards (1970) and others have reported the failure of house flies to develop in the presence of the soldier fly, *Hermetia illucens,* because the latter make manure physically unsuitable for housefly development. However, the soldier flies themselves may become a nuisance, and since they are not satisfactorily reduced by the integrated method, a decision is sometimes necessary as to whether a larvicide should be applied for their control. Such a decision must be made with care as the larvicide application decimates the mite populations and commits the producer to a single course of action—continued larviciding for the remainder of the season to control house flies.

In contrast to the North Carolina program, the work of Hoy and colleagues on rice field mosquito control in California is instructive as to how the introduction of a new component can disrupt effective natural control. Hoy *et al.* (1971) concluded that in rice fields, of which there are more than 400,000 acres in California, reasonable control of *C. tarsalis* and *An. freeborni* could be achieved by early-season stocking of *Gambusia affinis* at the rate of 300 mature females per acre. In a later test (Hoy *et al.,* 1972), however, they compared two fish-stocking rates (0.2 and 0.6 lb/acre) and chlorpyrifos (0.0125 lb*/acre) and found that the fields stocked at the higher rate of fish did not produce significantly fewer mosquitoes than the untreated fields. The authors attributed the poor results to disruption of notonectids and other invertebrate predators. The mosquito population in the fields sprayed with chlorpyrifos surged to several times greater than that found in the undisturbed control fields. The relatively low numbers of larvae in the control fields also suggested the presence of an effective invertebrate predator population.

As these results illustrate, we still do not know, in most cases, what degree of control is contributed by indigenous natural control agents. While waiting for the development of new more selective insecticides and other biocides usable as inundation techniques, much more research is needed on the ecology and behavior of native fishes, predatory Hemiptera, Coleoptera, and other invertebrates and pathogens that share the habitats of vector and pest targets.

The preceding example also suggests that, as more integrated programs

---

* Throughout this chapter, insecticide application rates are stated as amounts of actual ingredient applied.

reach the operational stage, an increased investment in surveillance will become necessary. In a recent survey of U.S. organized mosquito abatement districts, surveillance, including mapping, inspection, and processing of mosquito collections, accounted for 13–58% of the mosquito control effort and averaged 35% (NAS, 1976). To this it will be necessary to add surveillance of other components of the invertebrate fauna in order to avoid disruption of natural systems that provide a significant degree of control.

8.5. SOURCE REDUCTION

Source reduction is probably the area in which existing knowledge and technology is most underutilized. The initial cost of source reduction and other cultural control methods is often cited as a deterrent to their use. Following a survey of several mosquito control districts in Florida, however, Provost (1977) reported that the cost of ditching or impounding salt marsh was recovered, on an average, in 2 or 3 years of savings on larvicide alone. Sarhan *et al.* (1979), using an empirical model of mosquito control practices in a California abatement district, concluded that physical source reduction methods were more efficient in both the short and long run.

Source reduction alone is usually not adequate, but source reduction has been a basic component of some of the most successful integrated control programs. Source reduction is not a viable option in some situations because of environmental considerations. It is particularly inviting in situations where human activity has already damaged or destroyed the natural ecology, such as by sprawling urbanization or poor agricultural practice. With regard to uncontrolled urbanization, *Culex pipiens,* a polluted water breeder and the vector of filariasis in India and of arboviruses in the United States, immediately comes to mind. Das (1971) states that this species could best be controlled in India by building more modern sewerage systems than now exist in urban areas and by the use of such techniques as canalization, interception of seepage, insect proofing of septic tank ventilation pipes, and installation of manhole covers.

Sharma (1974) reviewed some of the culturally based methods used for mosquito control in India prior to the DDT era. Deweeding of slow-moving water channels for *An. fluviatilis* control, streamlining water flow in irrigation channels for control of *An. culicifacies,* sealing of wells for control of *An. stephensi,* and the institution of "dry days" in which all domestic and peridomestic water containers were emptied at least once per week for *Ae. aegypti* and *An. stephensi* control were among the methods that were used effectively, in some cases in conjunction with *Gambusia* or limited application of insecticides.

8.5.1. Salt Marsh Mosquitoes

Ae. sollicitans and *Ae. taeniorhynchus* are the salt marsh mosquitoes of the Atlantic and Gulf coasts. Control efforts have traditionally depended on source reduction—diking, ditching, dredging, and filling of marshlands—supplemented by the use of adulticides. There is increasing opposition to most types of salt marsh minipulation, however, despite excellent and painstaking studies showing that source reduction can be practiced on salt marshes without damage to the delicate ecology of tidelands and estuaries.

Salt marsh *Aedes* inhabit the high marsh, while the biota to be protected utilize the low marsh and the estuaries. Larvicides cannot be applied to the high marsh because they may be washed into the estuaries by tides and rain. Provost (1977) advocates that the open-marsh management system developed in New Jersey (Ferrigno, 1970; Ferrigno and Jobbins, 1968; Ferrigno *et al.*, 1969) is applicable with slight modification to salt marshes everywhere. Ditches are dug only to connect mosquito-breeding depressions to tidewater or to ponds. This insures that temporary water does not stand long enough for mosquitoes to develop and permits access of minnows to all parts of the marsh. Permanent ponds and pools that serve as shrimp nurseries are not connected to the ditching system. If done properly, ditching increases marsh and estuarine productivity by expediting the flushing of detritus into the lower marsh and estuary (Provost, 1974).

Impoundments can also be ecologically safe if they are constructed to permit exchange of impoundment and estuarine waters, permitting movement of aquatic life, preservation of the natural vegetation, and release of nutrients to the estuary. The Gumbo Island (Florida) impoundment described by Provost (1974) has proven completely effective in preventing mosquito development, while not damaging the normal functioning of the marsh (Provost, 1977).

8.5.2. Aedes vexans

Ae. vexans, the major pest species in the north-central U.S., breeds in temporarily flooded woods, fields, and river floodplains, from whence it invades populated areas. Since much of the breeding is on wildlands, source reduction opportunities are limited. However, the work of Dixon and Brust (1972) is a good example of how careful surveillance can constitute "source reduction" as far as reducing the need for insecticides is concerned. They conducted intensive larval surveys in a perimeter around Winnipeg, Manitoba, and found that only 20–25% of the pools sampled produced mosquitoes. The mosquito-producing pools totaled only 5 acres out of 5120 acres surveyed, and the area requiring larval-control measures was only 3% of the uncultivated land area. If treated indiscriminately by air, 97% of the insecticide would be applied to land where none was required.

8.5.3. Aedes aegypti

Within the context of source reduction, *Ae. aegypti* is an enigma. It is the sole vector of dengue viruses in the Western Hemisphere and in much of the Eastern Hemisphere, yet dengue epidemics continue to surge and resurge in both hemispheres. In most places, *Ae. aegypti* is a domestic or peridomestic species, with its breeding restricted to small containers of water. If there is an important vector mosquito that should be amenable to control by simplistic measures, it is *Ae. aegypti*. It cannot breed if such water containers as old tires and tins are eliminated and essential water storage containers made mosquito-proof (Reuben and Panicker, 1975, and many others). Yet, as stated by Reeves (1972), "we seem to be in the unenviable position that we have a wealth of research knowledge that continues to build while we have little or no immediate hope of preventing dengue epidemics."

Wattal (1971) states that there is no concerted effort to control *Ae. aegypti* in India, although the species could be controlled by mosquito-proof storage of water and elimination of the breeding foci. In the U.S. apparently only one organized mosquito abatement district, Dade County, Florida, regularly attempts *Ae. aegypti* control. This district conducted 59,900 premise inspections in 1972 (NAS, 1976). There was an eradication effort in the United States during the decade of the sixties, but *Ae. aegypti* persists in cities in the southern part of the country, and the U.S. remains vulnerable, therefore, to the reappearance of dengue.

8.5.4. Aedes triseriatus

The vector species that I work on, *Ae. triseriatus,* may be second only to *Ae. aegypti* as a species amenable to simplistic measures of control. *Ae. triseriatus* is the vector of La Crosse (LAC) virus, one of the California encephalitis group. A hundred cases, more or less, are reported annually from the eastern two-thirds of the United States. The virus is transmitted transovarially (Watts *et al.*, 1973) and overwinters in the diapausing eggs of the mosquito (Watts *et al.*, 1974). Chipmunks and tree squirrels are the vertebrate hosts involved in summer amplification of the virus (Moulton and Thompson, 1971).

In the last few years it has become our goal to model the transmission dynamics of the LAC system in order, hopefully, to predict the conditions under which transmission would be interrupted. As is usually the case, the deeper a problem is probed, the more complicated it gets. So far, about 40 parameters have been identified that affect the survival of the virus in nature (DeFoliart, 1978), and undoubtedly others have not yet been detected. Suitable quantification of those parameters could require several lifetimes of research.

In the meantime, *Ae. triseriatus* is an enticing target for control by source reduction. The natural breeding sites are treeholes that contain water, and in western Wisconsin, where LAC virus is endemic, large gallery forests are the main centers of production and dispersion. Control or elimination of the vector from these large forests is not feasible with current technology. However, *Ae. triseriatus* also breeds readily in discarded tires and other man-made containers that collect water. Quantitative documentation is lacking, but the available evidence suggests that a high proportion of La Crosse encephalitis cases in Wisconsin could be prevented through simple sanitation—the removal of old tires and other man-made containers from the vicinity of human habitations. Such containers around farm and suburban hillside homes and in shaded residential neighborhoods are readily colonized by female mosquitoes emigrating from their woodland haunts, and with transovarial transmission of virus to progeny, they serve as long-term foci of infection that are in intimate contact with humans.

Source reduction may also be warranted in some cases for reducing *Ae. triseriatus* populations in small woodland areas within or adjacent to areas of high human population density. Admittedly, treehole detection and closure is a labor-intensive method, but treehole-filling materials are now known that last 3 years or longer (Scholl and DeFoliart, 1979), so that an area once worked would not need to be reworked for several years. A previous attempt to reduce *Ae. triseriatus* by basal treehole closure was considered only moderately successful (Garry and DeFoliart, 1975). Measured by oviposition, the mean reduction in four test plots ranging in size from 8 to 20 acres was 67%. Deterrents to higher reductions in that study were considered to be open barrier zones of insufficient width to prevent infiltration from adjacent wooded areas, failure to remove old tires, and the possible presence of arboreal treeholes. In retrospect, it also would probably have been better to tabulate results on the basis of biting counts, as there is reason to suspect that there is a significant amount of mortality between oviposition and the ensuing bloodmeal.

Two questions must be answered, however, in order to place source reduction efforts on a sound footing. Scholl *et al.* (1979) found a biting rate of 28 per hour at ground level in a hyperendemic locality, but the level of biting activity at which virus transmission to humans is interrupted or significantly reduced remains unknown. Secondly, the proportion of an *Ae. triseriatus* population produced by arboreal treeholes, i.e., those not readily detectable by ground level inspection, is unknown. The ratio of arboreal to basal treeholes is probably small, but undoubtedly varies somewhat depending on age, type, and history of a given woodlot. A relevant factor is the presence of a competitor species, *Ae. hendersoni;* although closely related to *Ae. triseriatus, Ae. hen-*

dersoni cannot transmit LAC virus (Watts *et al.* 1975). These two species differ in their vertical stratification when studied with ovitraps, 60–76% of oviposition by *Ae. triseriatus* being in basal (ground level) traps, and 74–96% of oviposition by *Ae. hendersoni* being in arboreal traps (Loor and DeFoliart, 1970; Scholl and DeFoliart, 1977; Sinsko and Grimstad, 1977). Closure of basal treeholes would reduce the available ground-level habitat and force *Ae. triseriatus* to compete with *Ae. hendersoni* on the latter's "home grounds." The probable outcome of this competition is not known, but regardless of the outcome, *Ae. triseriatus* populations could probably be further reduced, if necessary, by the supplementary use of ovitraps containing slow-release formulations of insecticides.

8.6. MASS-PRODUCED BIOCONTROL AGENTS

Except for larvivorous fish, the current armamentarium is quite slender, but a number of promising pathogens are under development. The status of various candidate biological control agents in WHO's five-stage scheme for screening and evaluating their efficacy, safety, and environmental impact is shown in Table 8.3. Only first-priority organisms are included. In this protocol, stages I and II are confined to the laboratory and include identification and characterization, assessment against selected vectors, preliminary attempts at mass-rearing, mammalian safety tests, and preliminary assessment against nontarget species. Stage III involves preliminary field trials; stage IV, additional testing for safety to mammals and nontarget organisms; and stage V, large-scale field tests.

The compilation of literature by Jenkins (1964) on pathogens, parasites, and predators has recently been updated for pathogens and parasites by Roberts and Strand (1977).

Table 8.3. WHO First-Priority-Candidate Biocontrol Agents; Stages Completed and Planned Date of Stage V Testing[a]

Class of organism	Name (and number of species or strains)	Stage completed (year)	Stage V (planned)
Bacteria	*Bacillus sphaericus* (3)	II (1976)	1978–1979
	Bacillus thuringiensis (1)	I (1970–1976)	1978–1979
Fungi	*Coelomomyces* spp. (8)	I (1974–1978)	1980
	Lagenidium giganteum	III (1976)	1980
	Metarrhizium anisopliae	III (1975)	1979
Protozoa	*Nosema algerae*	II (1976)	1978
Nematodes	*Romanomermis culicivorax*	III (1974–1977)	1978–1980
	Romanomermis muspratti		

[a] Source: WHO (1977).

8.6.1. Larvivorous Fish

Many successful instances of the use of *Gambusia* and other larvivorous fish can be cited. Green and Imber (1977) recently reported excellent control of *C. pipiens* for a distance of 3 miles from stocking sites in two urban polluted stream systems in New Jersey. In India, for control of the urban malaria vector, *An. stephensi,* breeding in wells, Sitaraman *et al.* (1975) found *G. affinis* as effective as either pure petrol or Paris green, and use of fish resulted in a considerable cost reduction. Menon and Rajagopalan (1977) studied the mosquito control potential of 13 species of indigenous fishes and found 2 of them to have advantages in certain situations over *G. affinis* against *An. stephensi* in wells. *Oryzias melastigma* and *Aplocheilus blochii* demonstrated higher tolerances for temperature, salinity and pollution than did *Gambusia.*

The introduction of exotic fish can have a heavy impact on an aquatic ecosystem and, as the longest-used antimosquito biocontrol agent, *Gambusia* is illustrative of the types of considerations that come into play, both as to effectiveness and environmental impact, in the choice of a living organism for insect control. The following advantages and disadvantages are summarized from NAS (1976) and Legner *et al.* (1974): A surface feeder (1) is generally less effective against culicines than against *Anopheles*; (2) lives easily in the confined water of artificial containers, making it effective against such species as *Ae. aegypti*; (3) grazes selectively on zooplankton in small habitats, thereby causing phytoplanktonic blooms, which in turn may cause other undesirable side effects such as odor; (4) has high reproductive capacity and the capability of existing at high population densities; (5) has fair pollution tolerance, but not as good as that of the common guppy, *Poecilia reticulata*; (6) tolerates a fairly wide temperature range but has insufficient cold tolerance for year-round survival in northern temperate zones; (7) has good shoaling behavior—into shallow water after larvae—but is less able to penetrate algal mats and some aquatic weed growths than are some other fish, such as *Heterandria formosa*, a very small live-bearer that penetrates these readily; (8) has been known to eliminate native fish species; and (9) has caused significant reductions in native invertebrate predators such as notonectids, dytiscids, and hydrophilids by predation upon them.

Studies have shown that *Gambusia* is fairly tolerant to insecticides used as larvicides and is therefore compatible with larvicides in an integrated mosquito control program. Malathion is toxic to *Gambusia* at larvicidal levels (70% mortality 48 hr posttreatment at 0.5 lb/acre) (Mulla and Isaak, 1961), but temephos, fenthion, and chlorpyrifos (Darwazeh and Mulla, 1974; Ferguson *et al.,* 1966) have appeared safe (Table 8.4). Chlorpyrifos, however, was shown to produce some fish toxicity at only two to four times larvicidal rates, so caution would be necessary to avoid overdosing with this insecticide in areas where fish are present (Darwazeh and Mulla, 1974).

Table 8.4. Toxicity of Mosquito Larvicides to *Gambusia affinis*[a]

Chemical and formulation	Concentration	Average percent mortality (48 hr)
In 20-gal tubs		
Temephos EC[b]	1.0 ppm	0
	5.0 ppm	0
Chlorpyrifos (tech.)	0.1 ppm	0
	0.5 ppm	0
Chlorpyrifos EC	1.0 ppm	92
	5.0 ppm	100[c]
Fenthion EC	1.0 ppm	0
	5.0 ppm	40
In ponds		
Chlorpyrifos EC[d]	0.05 lb/acre	0
	0.10 lb/acre	40
	0.50 lb/acre	100

[a] Source: Darwazeh and Mulla (1974).
[b] Emulsifiable concentrate.
[c] At 24 hr posttreatment.
[d] Larvicidal rate: 0.025–0.05 lb/acre.

Even the compounds more toxic to fish can be used if applied several days prior to fish stocking. When *Gambusia* were added to water 48 hr posttreatment with chlorpyrifos at 0.5 lb/acre, cumulative toxicity reached a maximum of 56% on day 2 (Darwazeh and Mulla, 1974). Similarly, with malathion, mortality was not more than 10% in fish added 48 hr after insecticide treatment (Mulla and Isaak, 1961). Since weed control is practiced in rice fields and also by mosquito abatement districts in some other aquatic environments, Darwazeh and Mulla (1974) tested six soil-sterilant-type herbicides for toxicity to *Gambusia*. No acute mortality was observed.

8.6.2. Insectan Predators

The insectan predator *Toxorhynchites brevipalpis* has been mass-produced on living *Ae. aegypti* larvae (Trpis and Gerberg, 1973) and field tested (Gerberg and Visser, 1978) but appears to have limited potential for either inundation or effective recycling (Trpis, 1973).

8.6.3. Bacterial Pathogens

Bacillus sphaericus is readily cultured *in vitro* (Singer *et al.*, 1966) and is considered to have high promise against mosquito larvae. The toxic material appears to be associated with the bacterial cell at the outset of sporulation; treatment that kills the cells but not the spores reduces toxicity (Davidson and Singer, 1973). Singer (1975a) reported that strain SS11-1, isolated from larvae collected in Delhi, India, was 1000 times more active than previously examined strains. It was more toxic to *Culex* spp. than to *Ae. aegypti* and *Anopheles* sp. (Singer, 1975b). Strains 1593-4 from Indonesia and 1404-9 from the Philippines were toxic to *Culex* and more toxic to *Anopheles* than had been demonstrated by SS11-1 in the earlier investigation (Singer and Murphy, 1976). *Psorophora columbiae* and *Culex nigripalpus* have been shown susceptible to all three strains (Ramoska *et al.*, 1977).

In a field test against *C. nigripalpus* larvae, in which a mixture of the three strains was applied, the 48 hr posttreatment reduction was 89%, with fourth instars exhibiting lower susceptibility than earlier instars (Ramoska *et al.*, 1978). In two tests against *P. columbiae* in which the broods are more synchronous, strain 1593 produced 100% mortality within 30 and 48 hr posttreatment.

8.6.4. Fungi

In *Coelomomyces* spp. host specificity is high (Federici *et al.*, 1975, and others) so several species have been chosen for development in the WHO testing program. High temporary infection rates, from 59% to more than 95%, have been observed in natural populations: *Co. indicus* in *Anopheles gambiae* 95% + (Muspratt, 1962); *Co. punctatus* in *An. quadrimaculatus* up to 81% (Umphlett, 1968); up to 80% + in Louisiana (Chapman *et al.*, 1967); *Co. punctatus* and *Co. dodgei* up to 67% and 59%, respectively, in *An. crucians* (Chapman and Glenn 1972); *Coelomomyces* sp. in *An. gambiae* up to 77% (Service, 1973), and infection may prolong the larval stage thus increasing susceptibility to other mortality factors (Umphlett; 1970). The sporangium survives in dry mud, enabling recycling year after year in the mosquito environment (Roberts, 1967); 5 years after introduction of *Co. stegomyiae* on the Tokelau Islands, 37% of *Ae. polynesiensis* and *Ae. vexans nocturnus* larvae sampled were parasitized (Laird, 1967).

The greatest obstacle to the eventual commercial development of *Coelomomyces* is that it is an obligate parasite requiring an alternation of hosts. Mass production can be achieved in the laboratory (Couch, 1972) but only by duplicating the cycle that involves both a mosquito and the intermediate host, usually a copepod (Federici and Roberts, 1976; Whisler *et al.*, 1974, 1975). As to mammalian safety of using *Coelomomyces*, no systematic tests have yet been conducted (WHO, 1977).

Metarrhizium anisopliae can be mass propagated by industrial fermentation and infects mosquito larvae when the asexual conidia are introduced into the larval habitat. *In vitro*, the fungus mycelium produces destruxins A and B, which are also toxic to mosquito larvae (Roberts, 1967). Applied to the water surface *Metarrhizium* is effective against *Anopheles:* some strains are highly virulent to culicines in fresh, brackish, or organically polluted waters (WHO, 1977). *M. anisopliae* has shown survival but not replication in mammals (WHO, 1977). According to Laird (1977), *M. anisopliae* has been mass-produced and used in the field in the USSR without any reported adverse health or environmental effects. However, its wide host range compared to that of most entomopathogens—more than 200 species being susceptible in a variety of insect orders—would appear to be a factor limiting its use in some integrated-control programs. As the fungus is not normally associated with mosquitoes, repeated applications would be necessary (Roberts, 1970).

Lagenidium giganteum (= *L. culicidum)* (Umphlett, 1973) is a promising mosquito control agent. A saprophyte, it should be propagatable by fermentation techniques similar to those for bacteria. *Anopheles* are susceptible (Couch and Romney, 1973) as well as virtually all freshwater culicines (McCray, 1973, and others). Larval death is usually simultaneous with sporangial formation and occurs about 60 hr after ingestion of motile zoospores (McCray, 1973). Young larvae are more susceptible than older ones, but more than 80% of larvae of all stages are killed at high dosages (Umphlett and Huang, 1972). By modifications of its life cycle, the fungus recycles in both permanent water and intermittently flooded areas, and field tests by McCray *et al.* (1973) in both types of situations resulted in dramatically reduced mosquito populations. No infections were found in 1400 nontarget organisms (small crustaceans and insects) sampled from the treated sites. WHO has assigned high priority to studies on *L. giganteum* with emphasis on *in vitro* propagation and finding methods for storage and transportation of the zoospores (WHO, 1977).

8.6.5. Protozoa

The main impact of *Nosema algerae* (= *N. stegomyiae)* is on the longevity and reproductive capacity of adult mosquitoes [*An. albimanus* (Anthony *et al.,* 1972, 1978); *An. stephensi* (Undeen and Alger, 1975); *C. fatigans* (Reynolds, 1971)]. High larval mortality sometimes occurs in anophelines (Savage and Lowe, 1970). Anthony *et al.* (1978) found that first and second instars were only slightly more susceptible to infection (100%) than were third and fourth instars (88% and 92%, respectively) when exposed to 5×10^4 spores/ml of water. From their data on the number of viable eggs produced, they estimated that *N. algerae* introduced into populations consisting of mixed larval instars could reduce the F_1 progeny of infected females by 54%. Anthony *et al.* (1972) proposed a population model showing that an infection of *N. algerae* that reduced the female LT-90 by 50% (as shown by laboratory data) would reduce malaria transmission by 85–97%.

There are indications that, despite the planned stage V testing in 1978 (Table 8.3), this species may be slow in progressing to commercial production. Spores of good viability are produced in huge numbers in corn earworms (Undeen and Maddox, 1973; Undeen and Alger, 1975), but this *in vivo* method of production is expensive. Improved formulations are needed, and there are unsettled questions as to mammalian safety.

Two field tests have been encouraging. One, in Pakistan, resulted in infection of 50% of *An. stephensi* larvae. In field tests against *An. albimanus* in Panama, infection rates were dose dependent, ranging from 16% in an area given a single dose, to 86% in an area given four treatments.

8.6.6. Nematodes

Romanomermis culicivorax (= *Reeseimermis nielseni*) is the first mosquito pathogen to be registered and marketed in the United States (Fairfax's Skeeter Doom). Numerous field surveys and laboratory studies have demonstrated its wide host range among mosquitoes (Chapman *et al.*, 1969, 1970; Petersen, 1975; Petersen and Willis, 1971; Petersen *et al.*, 1968, 1969), and its safety to nontarget organisms (Ignoffo *et al.*, 1973, and others). As yet, mass production is only by *in vivo* methods developed at the USDA's Gulf Coast Mosquito Research Laboratory at Lake Charles, Louisiana (Petersen, 1973a–c, 1978; Petersen and Willis, 1970, 1972a).

Field releases have given varied results depending on the mosquito species and aquatic conditions pertaining (Brown *et al.*, 1977; Hoy and Petersen, 1973; Mitchell *et al.*, 1972; Petersen and Willis, 1972b, 1974; Petersen *et al.*, 1972, 1973). The largest and most recent test was conducted against *An. albimanus* and *An. pseudopunctipennis* at Lake Apastepeque in El Salvador (Petersen *et al.*, 1978a,b). The lake is about 2.5 km in circumference and the breeding habitat is a 2- to 5-m band of marginal floating and surface vegetation extending around nearly the entire margin. Eleven applications over a 7-week period reduced the larval population by 94% by the end of the release period, although the average parasitism during the release period was only 58%. In order to carry out the planned treatment of 144,000 m^2 at a dosage rate of about 4800 preparasites per square millimeter of surface area, a total of 14.1 lb of postparasitic nematodes and 425 cultures (15 g) were produced. Five weeks after cessation of treatment, larval populations had increased by more than three times.

Although the nematodes can sometimes establish and recycle (Petersen and Willis, 1972b, 1975, and others), the incidence of infection is usually too low for adequate control, so repeated applications are necessary. Also, as infected larvae die before pupation (Petersen *et al.*, 1969, and others), there is little natural dispersion of the organisms.

Romanomermis muspratti, which unlike *R. culicivorax* is active in polluted waters, holds special promise for use against *C. fatigans* (Muspratt, 1963, 1965).

Data by Winner and Steelman (1978) indicate that insecticide application would have to be carefully monitored in integrated programs involving *R. culicivorax*. Dosage mortality data showed that infective stage nematodes could not survive concentrations equivalent to that in a 1-square-acre body of water 0.15 m in depth treated at the maximum rate on the insecticide label for naled and chlorpyrifos. Under these conditions, however, fenthion, malathion, temephos, propoxur, diflubenzuron, and methoprene would have no adverse effect on the motility of the preparasites, nor would there be any adverse effect on the egg or postparasitic stages. Although viable postparasites were recovered from infected larvae that had received a lethal concentration of insecticide, insect growth regulators (IGRs) such as methoprene and diflubenzuron have an advantage in this respect in that they tend to increase duration of the larval period, thus allowing more postparasitic stage nematodes to emerge.

8.7. INSECTICIDES FOR MOSQUITO CONTROL

Table 8.2 includes most of the EPA-registered insecticides for mosquito control in the United States. These insecticides are also, with the exception of some used as interior wall sprays, the major insecticides available for use elsewhere.

8.7.1. Conventional Larvicides

As larvicides, temephos (Abate) and chlorpyrifos (Dursban) have been tested widely and have proven effective under a variety of conditions (Table 8.5), with chlorpyrifos being especially effective in waters of high organic pollution. Temephos, on the other hand, has increasingly become the insecticide of choice in aquatic environments where nontarget organisms are of concern, because of its relative safety to these organisms (Cooney and Pickard, 1974; Frank and Sjogren, 1978; see former for additional references) as well as to humans, domestic animals, and fish. Glancey *et al.* (1968) observed more than 34 weeks of complete control of *Ae. aegypti* with both emulsifiable concentrate (EC) and granular formulations of temephos at 1 ppm in concrete water jars in Thailand. Chlorpyrifos EC at 1 ppm provided only 4–5 weeks of control in these tests. In India, temephos at 1 ppm in water containers (drinking water containers were not treated) gave control for 8–12 weeks in an isolated test area and for 4–6 weeks in an area subject to infiltration (Geevarghese *et al.*, 1977). Against floodwater *Aedes,* Cooney and Pickard (1974) obtained from more than 11 days

Table 8.5. Efficacy of Several Mosquito Larvicides

Reference	Insecticide and formulation[a]	Dosage: actual insecticide	Species	Residual duration
Glancey et al. (1968)	Temephos EC	1.0 ppm	*Ae. aegypti*	>34 weeks
	Temephos gf	1.0 ppm		>34 weeks
	Chlorpyrifos EC	1.0 ppm		4–5 weeks
Geevarghese et al. (1977)	Temephos	1.0 ppm	*Ae. aegypti*	8–12 weeks
	Temephos	1.0 ppm	*Ae. aegypti*	4–6 weeks
Cooney and Pickard (1974)	Chlorpyrifos gf	0.10 lb/acre	Floodwater mosquitoes	>11–>25 days
	Temephos gf	0.10 lb/acre		4 days
	Chlorpyrifos gf, pr	0.10 lb/acre		>30 days
	Chlorpyrifos EC, pr	0.10 lb/acre		>14 days
	Temephos gf, pr	0.10 lb/acre		<14 days
Fontaine and Rosen (1973)	Temephos gf	1.0 ppm	*An. gambiae*	27 days
	Temephos EC	1.0 ppm		24 days
McNeill et al. (1968)	Chlorpyrifos gf	0.5 lb/acre	*C. quinquefasciatus*	72 days
	Chlorpyrifos EC	0.5 lb/acre		108 days
Steelman et al. (1967)	Chlorpyrifos EC	1.0 ppm	*C. quinquefasciatus*	144 days
	Temephos EC	1.0 ppm		20 days
	Propoxur EC	1.0 ppm		20 days
	Naled EC	1.0 ppm		19 days
	Fenthion EC	1.0 ppm		18 days
	Malathion EC	1.0 ppm		2 days
Lewis et al. (1966)	Chlorpyrifos EC	1.0 ppm	*C.p. pipiens*	23 days
	Fenthion EC	1.0 ppm		14 days
Mulla et al. (1970)	Chlorpyrifos EC	0.3 lb/acre	*Culex* spp.	77 days
	Temephos EC	0.3 lb/acre		>28 days
	Fenthion EC	0.4 lb/acre		7–21 days

[a] EC, emulsifiable concentrate; gf, granular formulation; pr, preflood application.

to more than 25 days of control with granular chlorpyrifos applied as a posthatch treatment at the rate of 0.1 lb/acre, and more than 30 days at the same rate applied as a preflood treatment. Temephos at a similar dosage was comparatively ineffective.

Chlorpyrifos has exhibited especially long-lasting residual activity in organically polluted waters. McNeill *et al.* (1968) observed an average of 72 and 108 days of complete control of *C. quinquefasciatus* larvae in septic ditches in Texas when chlorpyrifos granular and EC, respectively, were applied at the rate of 0.5 lb/acre. They attributed the residual activity to absorption of the insecticide on organic matter in the ditches. In waste disposal lagoons in Louisiana, chlorpyrifos at 1 ppm (EC) provided 144 days of complete control of *C. quinquefasciatus* compared to only 18–20 days for temephos and several other insecticides, and only 2 days for malathion (Steelman *et al.*, 1967). In Oregon log ponds, chlorpyrifos at 0.1 lb/acre gave 23 days of control of *C. p. pipiens* compared to 14 days for fenthion (Lewis *et al.*, 1966). Against four species of *Culex* in sewage oxidation ponds in California, chlorpyrifos EC at 0.3–0.4 lb/acre gave complete control for 77 days compared with 28 + days for temephos and 7–21 days for fenthion (Mulla *et al.*, 1970).

A consequence of the increasing dearth of effective residuals that are economically practical for wall spraying in malaria control has forced a move toward greater consideration of larvicides. Fontaine and Rosen (1973) found that temephos, in floating granule formulations, was effective for about 27 days at 1 ppm against *An. gambiae* in northern Nigeria during the dry- to wet-season transition period. During the wet season, temephos 1% sand granules and emulsion formulations at 1 ppm prevented larvae from developing beyond the first instar for a 24-day period, suggesting a sorption–release mechanism as described above for chlorpyrifos.

Larvicidal oils, including some newly developed ones, are receiving increased usage, especially where resistance to organic insecticides is high, such as in California. Flit MLO is effective against larvae and pupae of *Anopheles* and *Culex* at only 1 gal/acre compared to 10–40 gal/acre for older formulations. Resistance to Flit MLO was not induced in *C. fatigans* in 20 generations of selection pressure (Micks *et al.*, 1968).

The NAS Public Health Study Team (NAS, 1976) made a plea for the resurrection of Paris green as a larvicide more readily available for mosquito control. They detailed the excellent safety record of the insecticide when it was used in large quantities worldwide for malaria control (Bishopp, 1940, 1949); its rapid disappearance when added to soil or water (Rathburn, 1966); the development of formulations that made it effective against culicines (Rogers and Rathburn, 1958, 1960*a,b*) as well as against anophelines; and the failure of mosquitoes to develop any significant tolerance to it (Rathburn and Boike, 1973). The study team suggested that Paris green might well be the method of last resort for control of resistant larvae if petroleum derivatives should be declared environmentally unacceptable. Also, its use as a larvicide could prolong the life of residual organic insecticides by delaying the development of resistance.

8.7.1.1. Controlled-Release Formulations

The terms *controlled release* and *slow release* have been used rather indiscriminately for various methods of prolonging toxicant release, from adsorption or absorption on clays, silicas, or charcoal, to incorporation or encapsulation in elastomeric or plastic matrices. Cardarelli (1976) restricted the term *controlled release* to formulations that deliver the proper dosage at a constant rate over a long period of time, in contrast to *slow release* of toxicant at variable rates over a long period.

Controlled-release technology has not only added greatly to the potential of juvenoids and other IGRs, for which timing of application is critical, but has been used to increase the residual of OP compounds such as temephos and chlorpyrifos. In one of the earliest semifield evaluations, chlorpyrifos in various plastic-based formulations demonstrated effective control for 21 to more than 24 weeks in outdoor artificial pools (Miller *et al.*, 1973; L. W. Roberts *et al.*, 1973). At dosages effective for larval control, nontarget populations of gerrids, chaoborids, and chironomids were reduced but not eliminated (D. R. Roberts *et al.*, 1973). More recently, Nelson *et al.* (1976) tested a 10.6% controlled-release formulation of chlorpyrifos against *P. confinnis* in Arkansas rice plots. In plots treated at 0.25, 0.5, 1.0, and 2.0 ppm based on a theoretical total release of all active ingredients, average mortalities over an 11-week period were 22, 58, 79, and 99% respectively. Chlorpyrifos residues recovered from test water averaged 0.0004, 0.0006, 0.0009, and 0.0014 ppm, respectively.

Keenan (1978) reported excellent control of larvae, including several species, in southern Maryland with a controlled-release formulation of chlorpyrifos (Dursban® 10 CR). Control lasted throughout the entire 12–18 weeks of observation when pools and ditches were treated to yield a dosage rate of 1.5 ppm. Except on one overdosed sewage basin, where notonectids were killed and did not reappear for 4 weeks, no adverse effects were noted on nontarget organisms.

Against adult mosquitoes, long-term control (2–4 months) has been obtained by dichlorvos formulated in wax, polyvinyl chloride resins, and permeable plastic in storm sewer catch basins (Brooks *et al.*, 1963, 1965) and in huts (Schoof *et al.*, 1963).

One disadvantage of controlled-release and slow-release formulations is that a considerable amount of sublethal dosing is probably unavoidable. A result is an increased potentiality for development of resistance among target species.

8.7.1.2. Ultra-Low-Volume Application

The unique feature of ultra-low-volume (ULV) application methodology in public health entomology is that it provides an efficient "last-resort" tool for aborting impending epidemics. The common mosquito adulticides are usually applied at rates of 3 fl oz/acre or less (compared to 32–192 fl oz/acre formerly in aerial sprays), and this permits the treatment of large areas in a short period of time. The reduced volumes also result in greatly reduced costs because of increased payloads.

The practicality of ULV for disease control was first demonstrated during an outbreak of St. Louis encephalitis in Dallas, Texas, in 1966. Malathion, at 3 fl oz/acre, was applied by aircraft to 475,000 acres during an 8-day period, with a consequent reduction of 90–95% in the density of the vector, *C. quinquefasciatus* (Kilpatrick and Adams, 1967). An even more spectacular demonstration of the efficacy of ULV in an emergency situation was, as referred to earlier, the application of malathion to more than 8 million acres during the 1971 outbreak of VEE in Texas.

Lofgren (1970) reviewed the use of ULV-applied insecticides against mosquito adults and larvae and discussed technical and operational considerations related to droplet size, application equipment and conditions of application. Since then there have been many reports of improved techniques of application; operational, technical, meteorological, and environmental conditions that influence the results obtained; evaluations of newer insecticides; nontarget effects; and additional tests of the old standards, malathion, naled, and fenthion. A few representative examples will suffice to indicate results that can be expected and the variability encountered in field tests.

The results of Mount *et al.* (1972) (Table 8.6) against rice field mosquitoes in Arkansas are typical of what can be expected from ULV applications against mosquito species that disperse readily and, therefore, can rapidly infiltrate a treated area. They tested malathion, naled, and chlorpyrifos against the rice field mosquito, *P. confinnis* at Lonoke, Arkansas. All three compounds gave good control at 1–2 hr posttreatment (86–100%) applied as ground aerosols but at 24 hr posttreatment, applications every other night and every night, averaged only 66% and 87% control, respectively. The authors concluded that nightly applications would be necessary for satisfactory control.

The salt marsh mosquitoes, *Ae. taeniorhynchus* and *Ae. sollicitans,* also disperse rapidly. Mount and Lofgren (1967) compared conventional sprays of naled, fenthion, and malathion with ULV against these species in citrus groves located near salt marshes in Florida. Naled gave about the same control with both methods, and neither method gave residual control. A dosage rate of 0.2 lb/acre was required to obtain more than 90% control 6 hr after application.

Table 8.6.   Applications of Ground and Aerial ULV Adulticides

Investigator(s), locality, target species	Insecticide	Dose: actual insecticide/ acre[a]	Percent reduction (posttreatment interval in parentheses)	
Mount *et al.* (1972),	Malathion	0.03–0.04 lb (G)	94 (1–2 hr)	17 (24 hr)
Arkansas	Naled	0.0175–0.021	97 (1–2 hr)	68 (24 hr)
Ps. confinnis	Chlorpyrifos	0.0114–0.015	86 (1–2 hr)	88 (24 hr)
Mount and Lofgren (1967),	Naled	0.05 lb (A)	65 (6 hr)	17 (24 hr)
Florida		0.1	88 (6 hr)	36 (24 hr)
Ae. taeniorhynchus		0.2	94 (6 hr)	78 (24 hr)
Ae. sollicitans	Fenthion	0.05 lb (A)	79 (6 hr)	60 (24 hr)
		0.1	72 (6 hr)	84 (48 hr)
		0.2	75 (6 hr)	77 (48 hr)
Mount and Pierce (1974), Florida *Ae. taeniorhynchus*	Naled	0.02 lb (G)?	81–94 (30–45 min)	
Mount *et al.* (1978),	Propoxur	0.020 lb (G)	56 (45 min)	
Florida		0.038	72 (45 min)	
Ae. taeniorhynchus	Naled	0.033	85 (45 min)	
Brooke *et al.* (1974),	Bioresmethrin	3.0 g (G)	92 (24 hr)	
Grand Cayman		1.5	89 (24 hr)	
Ae. taeniorhynchus				

[a] A, aerial application; G, ground application.

Fenthion as a conventional spray gave excellent control at 0.5 to 0.2 lb/acre for 6 hr and good residual control for 48 hr at the highest rate, 0.2 lb/acre; the ULV treatment gave only fair control at 6 hr but good residual at 24 and 48 hr (Table 8.6). Poor results with malathion were attributed to resistance. In later tests with naled ULV in residential sections of Sugarloaf Key, Florida, Mount and Pierce (1974) obtained 81–94% reductions (average 86%) 30–45 min after applications at the rate of 0.02 lb/acre (Table 8.6). Posttreatment counts at 12 or 24 hr, depending on time of application, revealed a rapid reinfestation, thus necessitating repeated applications for satisfactory control.

Sutherland *et al.* (1978) obtained, at best, only fair results from aerial applications of naled and malathion against *Ae. sollicitans* in New Jersey. The treated area consisted of mixed forest and fields with sparse shrub and ground cover. With naled at 1 oz/acre, they obtained a reduction greater than 60% one day after application only 52% of the time and noted an increase 22% of the time. Comparable data from malathion at 3 oz/acre were 40% and 20%, respectively.

Propoxur, not currently registered for ULV aerosol use, was compared with naled by Mount *et al.* (1978) against *Ae. taeniorhynchus* at Crescent Beach,

Florida. Poor coverage at some stations where mosquito landing rates were taken was attributed to dense vegetation and/or shifts in wind direction during application. Although this resulted in a low mean percent reduction (Table 8.6), the authors stated that naled and the higher rate of propoxur (0.038 lb/acre) gave complete control at many of the landing stations.

Bioresmethrin, a synthetic pyrethroid, proved effective against *Ae. taeniorhynchus* when applied by ground equipment as a ULV cold aerosol to dense mangrove swamp on Grand Cayman (Brooke *et al.*, 1974) (Table 8.6).

Against a sedentary mosquito such as *Ae aegypti*, successful control has been obtained with applications made at wider intervals. Eliason *et al.* (1970) found that oviposition by *Ae. aegypti* was almost totally interrupted by aerial applications of malathion at 3 fl oz/acre twice per week. The premises index was 20.1% prior to treatment but only 1.3% at the end of 25 treatments. The posttreatment index in the control area was 17.9%.

Based mainly on experience with malathion, ULV sprays appear generally safe to nontarget aquatic organisms (Tagatz *et al.*, 1974; see exceptions cited by these authors) and to nontarget terrestrial organisms (Hill *et al.*, 1971). The latter, however, observed significant reductions of Homoptera and Hymenoptera associated with spraying and substantial apiary losses occurred when hives were not covered. Caron (1979) reported that daytime applications of malathion and naled were more harmful to bees than was pyrethrins, while none of the insecticides had a discernible effect on bees when applied at night.

8.7.2. Synthetic Pyrethroids

The photostabilization of pyrethroids has opened new horizons for their use as agricultural and public health insecticides. High cost and lack of persistence limited their use in the past despite their high insecticidal activity, low mammalian toxicity, and rapid biodegradability. Based on published acute LD_{50} values (mg/kg) for rats and four species of insects (topical application), Elliott (1977) calculated a general ratio of insect-to-mammal toxicity of 4500 for pyrethroids compared with 91 for OC compounds, 33 for OP compounds, and 16 for carbamates.

A main feature of pyrethroids is that they are flexible molecules, and as knowledge of structure–activity relationships has increased, it has been possible to devise insecticides of greatly increased insect toxicity and stability without sacrificing low mammalian toxicity (Elliott *et al.*, 1973; Miyamoto, 1976; Verschoyle and Barnes, 1972) or environmental biodegradability (Barlow *et al.*, 1977; Kaufman *et al.*, 1977). For example, decamethrin, a compound stable enough for field use, shows an LD_{50} of 0.0003 µg per female house fly compared with 0.33 µg for pyrethrin I, a 1000-fold increase in potency (Elliott, 1977). Decamethrin is 600 times as active as DDT to *An. stephensi* (Barlow *et al.*,

1977; Hadaway *et al.*, 1977) and hundreds of times more toxic than dieldrin to tsetse flies as a residual application on leaf surfaces.

Pyrethroids have some disadvantages. In aquatic situations, in addition to mayfly nymphs, they are somewhat toxic to fish (Mauck *et al.*, 1976; NAS, 1976). Although there have been no cases as yet of resistance developed to pyrethroids by natural populations, OP- and OC-resistant strains are somewhat cross-tolerant to them and resistance can be expected as they come into regular use. Finally, Holmstead *et al.* (1977) have raised a question as to whether further stabilization may increase the risk of unfavorable environmental persistence.

In field tests with several synthetic pyrethroids as larvicides, Mulla *et al.* (1978) observed good control for up to 2 weeks or longer in experimental ponds containing a mixture of *C. tarsalis, Culiseta inornata,* and *An. franciscanus* (Table 8.7). Decamethrin (FMC-45498) was the most effective material, giving 80% control of larvae and pupae 2 weeks after treatment at the rate of 0.001 lb/acre. SD-43775 gave good control for longer than 2 weeks at the rate of 0.025 lb/acre, compared with only 1 week for permethrin applied at the same rate. Against multiresistant *Ae. nigromaculis* decamethrin was again the most effective material, producing almost complete mortality of larvae 6 hr posttreatment at rates of 0.001–0.005 lb/acre. Against this species the authors estimated that the effective range of permethrin and SD-43775 will be approximately 0.01–0.02 and 0.01–0.05 lb/acre, respectively. Ephemeroptera naiads were adversely affected by all of the pyrethroids at larvicidal rates with SD-43775 being the most toxic. Dragonfly naiads and diving beetle larvae were only slightly affected by the treatments except, again, by SD-43775.

Lewis and Tucker (1977) tested the pyrethroid Roussel-Uclaf 22974 (Decis®) in 1-m^2 sod-lined ponds containing a mixture of *C. tarsalis, C. peus,* and *C. quinquefasciatus,* and they state, without accompanying data, that a minimum

Table 8.7. Evaluation of Synthetic Pyrethroids against Mosquito Larvae in California Experimental Ponds[a,b]

Insecticide[c]	Application rate (actual insecticide lb/acre)	Percent reduction (days)	
		7	14
FMC-33297 (permethrin)	0.025	100	0
SD-43775 (Pydrin®)	0.025	95	81
	0.050	100	97
FMC-45498 (decamethrin)	0.0005	90	44
	0.0010	100	80

[a] Source: Mulla *et al.* (1978).
[b] Species present: all aquatic stages of *C. tarsalis* (40%), *Culiseta inornata* (50%), and *An. franciscanus* (10%).
[c] All formulations were emulsifiable concentrates.

residual effectiveness of 15 days was obtained at an application rate of 0.01 lb/ acre. The LC_{50} against fourth instar *C. quinquefasciatus* in the laboratory was 0.15 ppb, indicating a toxicity between that of permethrin (FMC-33297) and decamethrin (FMC-45498), since Mulla *et al.* (1978) found an LC_{50} of 1.40 and 0.02 ppb, respectively, for the latter two pyrethroids against *C. quinquefasciatus*.

Thompson and Meisch (1978) tested the residual effectiveness of permethrin against adult ricefield mosquitoes on plywood panels hung indoors in the laboratory and outdoors on the back walls of open sheds. The latter are favorite resting sites for adult mosquitoes in the Mississippi delta region of Arkansas. At application rates considered by the authors to be minimum for long-term residual efficacy, high mortalities were observed throughout the 10- to 11-week test period (Table 8.8). These are among accumulating results indicating that pyrethroids may have promise as residual wall sprays for malaria control.

8.7.3. Insect Growth Regulators

Chamberlain (1975) reviewed research on IGRs for use against insects of medical and veterinary importance. The results of Schaefer and Wilder (1973) with methoprene are typical of the early work on mosquitoes which showed the influence of stage, species, and formulation on results obtained. In small pool tests, in which only fourth instar *Ae. nigromaculus* were treated, dosages as low as 0.0125 lb/acre produced a final field population mortality of 100%, while against third instars a dosage of 0.1 lb/acre produced only 90% mortality. A slow-release formulation (SR 10; 10% flowable liquid, microencapsulated, water base) applied by aircraft to pastures at rates of 0.025–0.05 lb/acre produced 100% mortality of all instars except the first. Similar results were obtained with

Table 8.8. Mortality of Arkansas Rice Field Mosquitoes Exposed for 1 hr to Permethrin-Treated Plywood Panels[a]

Species	Application rate (g/m^2)	Percent mortality at posttreatment weeks[b]	
		8–9	10–11
Indoors			
Ps. columbiae	0.125	96.2	97.0
An. quadrimaculatus	0.125	98.1	88.1
Outdoors			
Ps. columbiae	0.50	91.4	87.0
An. quadrimaculatus	0.250	100.0	86.6

[a] Source: Thompson and Meisch (1978).
[b] Eight and 10 weeks for *An. quadrimaculatus* and 9 and 11 weeks for *Ps. columbiae*, respectively. Mortality was determined 24 hr postexposure.

SR 10 against *Ae. melanimon,* but against *C. tarsalis* dosages as high as 0.2 lb/ acre gave unsatisfactory control of all instars including the fourth.

Slow-release formulations have greatly increased the potential efficacy of juvenoids and other IGRs. Dunn and Strong (1973) reported that polyurethane wafers of 3% methoprene content (by weight) gave a high degree of control of *C. pipiens* in catch basins for more than 53 days following application of a wafer. Against *C. pipiens* in sewage water, Hoppe *et al.* (1974) found that 1 ppm methoprene gave 93% inhibition of adult emergence when applied as a granular formulation at 3-week intervals. By contrast, only 55% inhibition of emergence was obtained when methoprene was applied as an emulsifiable concentrate. Rathburn and Boike (1977) found that methoprene briquets were almost completely effective against *Ae. taeniorhynchus* for 31 days after initial application, while a black sand granular formulation applied at 0.01 lb/acre had no residual activity 7 days after application. When exposed 21 days as a preflood application, the briquets displayed complete residual effectiveness for at least 7 days after flooding (later tests were not made).

Case and Washino (1978) tested two formulations of methoprene, the standard microencapsulated form, and a 10F charcoal formulation against *C. tarsalis* in California rice fields. The insecticide was applied aerially at the rate of 0.1 lb/acre. By the 7th day posttreatment, emergence rates in treated fields were not significantly different from those before treatment began. Failure to achieve better control was attributed to water flow through the test plots and the asynchronous age structure of *C. tarsalis* populations.

Self *et al.* (1978) compared diflubenzuron (TH-6040) (= Dimilin®) [25% wettable powder (WP)] and methoprene (= Altosid® 10F briquette formulation) against *C. quinquefasciatus* in Jakarta, Indonesia. At a dosage of 1 ppm, the compounds were highly effective in preventing adult emergence for 2 and 5 weeks, respectively, after one application.

Early work with diflubenzuron, a urea-type compound that inhibits chitin formation, has yielded impressive results. Mulla *et al.* (1974) tested EC and WP formulations against asynchronous field populations of *C. tarsalis* and found them equally effective, producing high to complete inhibition of adult emergence for 5–15 days posttreatment. In subsequent tests in which the material was applied at 0.025 and 0.05 lb/acre against *C. tarsalis* in ponds, adult emergence from treated larvae held in floating units was almost completely inhibited for at least 11 days posttreatment (Mulla *et al.,* 1975). Against third instar *Ps. columbiae* in rice plots, Steelman *et al.,* (1975) found that diflubenzuron provided 100% control 24 hr posttreatment at the lowest dosage tested, 0.001 lb/acre. Methoprene, by comparison, provided 100% control at dosages as low as 0.05 lb/acre but only 40% at 0.001 lb/acre. Finally, Mulla and Darwazeh (1976) reported complete control of the synchronous floodwater mosquito, *Ps. confinnis,* in irrigated alfalfa hay fields and complete inhibition of emergence for more than

27 days of *C. tarsalis* and *An. franciscanus* from ponds treated at 0.0025 lb/ acre.

The general pattern of activity of IGRs against nontarget organisms has been that a few nontarget populations show temporary reductions but soon recover after treatment ceases. A number of investigators have studied the acute effects of methoprene on nontarget aquatic organisms, with, in some cases, contradictory conclusions (Breaud *et al.*, 1977; Dunn *et al.*, 1974; Miura and Takahashi, 1973; Norland and Mulla, 1975; Schaefer *et al.*, 1974; Steelman *et al.*, 1975; Takahashi and Miura, 1975). This is due in part to differences in species, water conditions, formulation, and dosage rate, but Steelman *et al.* (1975) have pointed to the importance of long-term evaluations of toxicity because of the long life cycles of some nontarget organisms and the nature of the mechanisms of action of IGRs. In evaluations of methoprene and three other IGRs made 80 days post-treatment in rice fields, they found significant reductions ($P < 0.01$) in *Tropisternus* ssp. adults (Coleoptera) and dragonfly immatures, a finding contrary to previous reports by other investigators. *Tropisternus* larvae were in the fields at the time of treatment and mortality probably occurred at a larval molt. They found no significant reductions ($P > 0.05$) in *Notonecta* adults at application rates as high as 0.25 lb/acre.

Breaud *et al.* (1977) observed that six applications of methoprene applied at 11.3 g/acre to a Louisiana coastal marsh during an 18-month period had no effect on 28 species of aquatic organisms but significantly reduced populations of 14 others (Table 8.9). None of the adversely affected species were eliminated, however, and repopulation from adjacent untreated marsh occurred following a drought. Populations of five species were observed to increase, which the authors attributed to control of predator species by the methoprene applications.

Table 8.9. Aquatic Organisms Reduced but Not Eliminated by Six Aerial Applications of Methoprene[a,b]

Scud, *Hyalella azteca*, adults and young
Opossum shrimp, *Taphromysis louisianae*, adults and young
Freshwater prawns, *Palaemonetes paladosus*, adults and young
Mayflies, *Callibaetis* sp., naiads
Dance flies, *Notophila* sp., larvae
Midges, Chironomidae, larvae
Freshwater snail, *Physa* sp., adults and young
Damselflies and dragonflies, *Enallagma, Anax*, and *Belonia* spp., naiads
Burrowing water beetles, *Suphisellus* sp., adults, and *Hydrocanthus* sp., adults
Water scavenger beetles, *Suphisellus* sp., adults, and *Hydrocanthus* sp., adults
Water scavenger beetles, *Berosus infuscatus*, adults, and *Berosus* spp., larvae

[a] Source: Breaud *et al.* (1977).
[b] Applied at the rate of 11.3 g actual insecticide per acre over a period of 18 months.

With diflubenzuron, cladocerans (*Daphnia* spp.) and mayfly nymphs appear particularly susceptible. Mulla *et al.* (1975) found that populations of both, plus copepods and chironomid larvae, were temporarily depressed, while ostracods, diving beetle larvae and adults, and odonate naiads were not affected. Miura and Takahashi (1975) found that water fleas, in addition to mayfly nymphs and cladocerans, suffered temporary reductions, but monthly treatments during a 4-month period did not eliminate any of the populations. Adult aquatic beetles were tolerant, and *Pardosa* and *Lycosa* spiders were not affected. Julin and Sanders (1978) concluded that at rates effective against mosquito larvae (0.02–0.04 lb/acre) diflubenzuron would have no effect on fish but that populations of daphnids (*Daphnia magna*) and scuds (*Gammarus pseudolimnaeus*) would be reduced.

8.8. THE NEED TO APPLY EXISTING KNOWLEDGE

Because of the initial successes with DDT, part of our problem today may be that we have become so fascinated by the search for new "magic bullets" that we have lost sight of the real goal—the delivery of health to people. There is no doubt that new technology is needed and that we need more, not less, basic research, but I think that there is a widening feeling among working scientists within the biomedical sciences that we are not doing a very good job in applying the technology that we have. In a recent editorial in *Tropical Medicine and Hygiene News*, Gibson (1977) stated, in part:

> On the one hand we can continue in the course of elite professionalism which has marked most of our actions in the past. We can keep on running our immunoelectrophoresis experiments, studying our electronmicrographs, reporting at annual meetings, and publishing the results in prestigious journals. We can, in other words, continue to be a Society which is almost completely research-oriented, with little or no attempt to insure that our efforts help someone have better health. This is the main highway, clearly marked out, well traveled, and relatively free of risks, except the risk of complacency.
>
> On the other hand, we can elect to travel from time to time on the poorly-marked and less populated byway which branches off from the highway, now and again touching the isolated villages and city slums of the Third World where live so many millions of the world's undernourished, overdiseased, unproductive people. In other words, we can become a Society concerned not only with new knowledge, but also with the *use* of knowledge to improve the world's health, especially in the tropics. This will be the more difficult path to follow, and we run the risk of finding ourselves in the strange company of sociologists, agronomists, sanitarians, economists, and perhaps even politicians!

In response to the preceding, Thurber (1978) stated:

> We can learn all there is to know about enzyme systems, fine structure, DNA metabolism, immune mechanisms, etc., and still make no inroads against tropical dis-

eases. Some place along the line, some one must study the implementation of disease prevention/control programs. Somehow populations must be educated as to the why and how, then be motivated to use sanitary and hygienic methods to diminish the incidence of disease.

As the 1972 Charles Franklin Craig Lecturer of the American Society of Tropical Medicine and Hygiene, Dr. Carlos Sanmartín (1973) of Colombia spoke in a similar vein:

> In general, I should say that a revision of public health training and research policies is mandatory in our countries. . . . We should concentrate on the most urgent needs. We should not be ashamed of teaching and insisting that the careful examination of a thick film for malaria, the opportune and correct diagnosis of meningitis, the responsible identification of the different stages of *Entamoeba histolytica*, the search for coliform organisms in drinking water, proper knowledge of the poisonous snakes and the adequate treatment of their victims, the ability to recognize the presence of *Aedes aegypti* in a locality and so forth are legitimate, useful and even respectable activities. . . . So many things, in a word, that are attainable without resorting to complicated methods.

In an earlier paragraph I stated that good surveillance is our first line of defense against zoonoses, but Sanmartín cites how a huge dengue epidemic swept through Barranquilla and other Caribbean urban centers of Colombia for 6 months, producing at least one-half million cases, without any national or international public health agency having any suspicion. He cites, in addition, an equine outbreak of VEE, in close proximity to the Cali international airport, that went 3 weeks before detection. These occurrences were in 1972 and 1967, respectively.

Narrowing from this broader scope to a consideration of public health entomology, I believe that there is a need to develop and support more researchers who are target-species-oriented rather than technology-oriented, researchers who will devote themselves to studying a target species long enough to define the problem that it poses, to understand the ecological interrelationships in the target habitat, and to search for points at which, and methods by which, the system may be most safely and efficiently manipulated. In perusing the applied literature, it becomes apparent that, in reporting the results of technology testing, we seldom define the specific health or nuisance problem posed, seldom interpret the results in relation to the biology of the target species, and seldom discuss what the results mean in relation to alleviating the problem.

Economic thresholds have received a great deal of attention in agricultrual entomology. It is difficult to place a value on human health or on increased comfort resulting from reduced exposure to anthropophilic and synanthropic insects. Nevertheless, an equivalent term, which might be called the "tolerance limit," is needed in medical entomology. For example, a ULV application of insecticide may reduce the adult mosquito density in an area by 85%, 6 hr posttreatment. But does an 85% reduction bring the landing rate down to 1/min or 0.1/min? Is either of these rates acceptable in the situation pertaining? For what period of time does the target species ordinarily occur at densities above the tolerance limit, thereby dictating the number of applications necessary and the seasonal cost of the procedure per unit of area?

Similarly with larvicides, if a larvicide at a range of dosage rates produces high mortality for 7, 14, and 21 days, respectively, what does this mean relative to its possible utilization against specific targets having, for example, synchronous or asynchronous broods? Again, depending on the biology of the target species, how many applications will be needed per season, so that comparative costs of treatments can be estimated? A high proportion of our published technology testing is largely a comparison of mortalities achieved at a range of dosage rates with little attempt to describe how the results might be useful in relation to a real problem that exists.

The tolerance limit in the case of vectors is more difficult to define. But the critical initial question is not whether a vector population can be reduced by 80–90% using a particular control method, but to what level must the population be reduced in order to interrupt transmission in endemic foci, or lacking that, to prevent or reduce transmission to human populations at risk. More, and more precise, epidemiological models are needed from which critical vector population levels can be predicted and, therefore, the degree of control that must be exerted.

Disease Control through Public Education.   A recently launched program in South Carolina (Burgdorfer *et al.*, 1975) is a good example of an effort to apply existing knowledge, imperfect as it may be, to reduce the incidence of human cases of a zoonotic disease. Rocky Mountain spotted fever *(Rickettsia rickettsii)*, the major tick-borne disease in the United States, is a disease that is benefiting from new technology, but in addition requires management beyond scientific endeavor. Like most arthropod-borne diseases of importance in the United States, it is a zooanthroponosis and there is no chance that it can be eradicated. The rickettsia is maintained in nature in cycles involving several tick vectors and their host mammals (Burgdorfer, 1975).

In the eastern United States increased suburbanization and recreation have brought people into closer contact with the zoonotic foci with the result that the annual number of reported cases increased from fewer than 200 in 1959 to 1118 in 1977. Despite the fact that cases recover when treated properly with broad-spectrum antibiotics, the yearly case fatality rates have varied between 3% and 10% since 1948 (Hattwick, *et al.*, 1973). Deaths result because people fail to seek proper medical care and because physicians are not familiar with the disease and do not recognize it, particularly in its early stages, thereby delaying specific treatment.

Research advances hold promise in the future for development of effective vaccines. In the meantime, the hemolymph test, in conjunction with direct fluorescent antibody staining, permits fairly rapid detection of *R. rickettsii* in ticks and prediction of the possible occurrence of a spotted fever case. As pointed out by Burgdorfer (1975), however, "such techniques are of little help where the public and physicians are unaware of the disease and the potential danger of ticks." An educational program initiated in South Carolina in 1973 received an overwhelming response from the public and the medical profession (Burgdorfer *et al.*, 1975). Information was distributed via pamphlets, newspaper releases, and educational television and radio programs. In addition, the general public and the medical profession were invited to submit for examination live ticks collected from vegetation, animals, and humans. The distributed card containing shipping instructions also contained information on early clinical signs suggestive of spotted fever. As a result of this program, a total of 1186 ticks were submitted during 1973 and 1974. A more comprehensive educational program was initiated in 1974 by the South Carolina Department of Health and Environmental Control (Loving *et al.*, 1978). The volume of ticks submitted soon made it necessary to restrict examination to ticks removed only from people. As a result of the South Carolina programs, Burgdorfer *et al.* (1975) state that education is by far the best means of preventing spotted fever.

REFERENCES

Akhtar, R., and Learmonth, A., 1977, The resurgence of malaria in India 1965–76, *Geojournal* **1**:69. (Additional information in *Abst. Rev. Appl. Entomol. Ser. B* **66**:371, 1978.)

Anderson, J. R., 1965, A preliminary study of integrated fly control on northern California poultry ranches, *Proc. Calif. Mosq. Control Assoc.* **33**:42.

Anthony, D. W., Savage, K. E., and Weidhaas, D. E., 1972, Nosematosis: Its effect on *Anopheles albimanus* Weidemann and a population model of its relation to malaria transmission, *Proc. Helminthol. Soc. Wash.* **39**:428.

Anthony, D. W., Lotzhar, M. D., and Avery, S. W., 1978, Fecundity and longevity of *Anopheles albimanus* exposed at each larval instar to spores of *Nosema algerae*, *Mosq. News* **38**:116.

Axtell, R. C., 1966, Comparative toxicities of insecticides to house fly larvae and *Macrocheles muscaedomesticae*, a mite predator of the house fly, *J. Econ. Entomol.* **59**:1128.

Axtell, R. C., 1968, Integrated house fly control: Populations of fly larvae and predaceous mites, *Macrocheles muscaedomesticae* in poultry manure after larvicide treatment, *J. Econ. Entomol.* **61**:245.

Axtell, R. C., 1970a, Integrated fly-control program for caged-poultry houses, *J. Econ. Entomol.* **63**:400.

Axtell, R. C., 1970b, Fly control in caged-poultry houses: Comparison of larviciding and integrated control programs, *J. Econ. Entomol.* **63**:1734.

Axtell, R. C., and Edwards, T. D., 1970, *Hermetia illucens* control in poultry manure by larviciding, *J. Econ. Entomol.* **63**:1786.

Barlow, F., Hadaway, A. B., Flower, L. S., Grose, J. E. H., and Turner, C. R., 1977, Some laboratory investigations relevant to the possible use of new pyrethroids in control of mosquitoes and tsetse flies, *Pestic. Sci.* **8**:291.

Berge, T. O. (ed.), 1975, *International Catalogue of Arboviruses*, U.S. Department of Health, Education and Welfare Publication No. (CDC) 75-8301.

Bhatnagar, V. N., Wattal, B. L., Sharma, K. L., Joshi, G. C., and Mathur, P. S., 1974, Field trials with fenitrothion [O,O-dimethyl O-(4-nitro-*m*-tolyl), phosphorothioate] against DDT resistant *Anopheles culicifacies* in Siliser Area, District Alwar, Rajasthan, *J. Commun. Dis.* **6**:241.

Bishopp, F. C., 1940, Cooperative investigations of the relation between mosquito control and wildlife conservation, *Science* **92**:201.

Bishopp, F. C., 1949, Larvicides, in: *Malariology* (M. F. Boyd, ed.), pp. 1339–1359, W.B. Saunders, Philadelphia.

Boike, A. H., Jr., and Rathburn, C. B., Jr., 1972, The susceptibility of mosquito larvae to insecticides in Florida, 1969–71, *Mosq. News* **32**:328.

Boike, A.H., Jr., and Rathburn, C. B., Jr., 1975, Laboratory susceptibility tests of some Florida strains of *Aedes taeniorhynchus* (Wied.) and *Culex nigripalpus* Theob. to malathion and naled, 1972–1974, *Mosq. News* **35**:137.

Boike, A. H., Jr., Rathburn, C. B., Jr., Hallmon, C. F., and Cotterman, S. G., 1978, Insecticide susceptibility tests of *Aedes taeniorhynchus* and *Culex nigripalpus* in Florida, 1974–1976, *Mosq. News* **38**:210.

Breaud, T. P., Farlow, J. E., Steelman, C. D., and Schilling, P. E., 1977, Effects of the insect growth regulator methoprene on natural populations of aquatic organisms in Louisiana intermediate marsh habitats, *Mosq. News* **37**:704.

Brooke, J. P., Giglioli, M. E. C., and Invest, J., 1974, Control of *Aedes taeniorhynchus* Wied. on Grand Cayman, with ULV bioresmethrin, *Mosq. News* **34**:104.

Brooks, G. D., Elmore, C. M., Schoof, J. F., and Carmichael, G. R., 1963, Field evaluations of three types of DDVP dispensers for the control of *Culex pipiens quinquefasciatus* Say in catch basins, in: Proceedings of the 50th Annual Meeting of the New Jersey Mosquito Extermination Association and the 19th Annual Meeting of the American Mosquito Control Association, p. 355.

Brooks, G. D., Carmichael, G. T., and Schoof, J. F., 1965, Evaluation of large-scale treatment with dichlorvos for the control of *Culex pipiens quinquefasciatus* Say, *Mosq. News* **25**:427.

Brown, A. W. A., 1977, The progression of resistance mechanisms developed against insecticides, in: *Pesticide Chemistry in the 20th Century* (J. R. Plimmer, ed.), pp. 21–34, ACS Symposium Series 37, American Chemical Society, Washington, D.C.

Brown, A. W. A., Haworth, J., and Zahar, A. R., 1976, Malaria eradication and control from a global standpoint, *J. Med. Entomol.* **13**:1.

Brown, B. J., Platzer, E. G., and Hughes, D. S., 1977, Field trials with the mermithid nematode, *Romanomermis culicivorax*, in California, *Mosq. News* **37**:603.

Brown, T. M., and Brown, A. W. A., 1974, Experimental induction of resistance to a juvenile hormone mimic, *J. Econ. Entomol.* **67**:799.

Burgdorfer, W., 1975, A review of Rocky Mountain spotted fever (tick-borne typhus), its agent, and its tick vectors in the United States, *J. Med. Entomol.* **12**:269.

Burgdorfer, W., Adkins, T. R., Jr., and Priester, L. E., 1975, Rocky Mountain spotted fever (tick-borne typhus) in South Carolina: An educational program and tick-rickettsial survey in 1973 and 1974, *Am. J. Trop. Med. Hyg.* **24**:866.

Cardarelli, N., 1976, *Controlled Release Pesticides Formulations*, CRC Press, Cleveland, Ohio.

Caron, D. M., 1979, Effects of some ULV mosquito abatement insecticides on honey bees, *J. Econ. Entomol.* **72**:148.

Case, T. J., and Washino, R. K., 1978, Effects of the growth regulator methoprene on *Culex tarsalis* and non-target organisms in California rice fields, *Mosq. News* **38**:191.

Cerf, D. C., and Georghiou, G. P., 1972, Evidence of cross-resistance to a juvenile hormone analogue in some insecticide-resistant house flies, *Nature (London)* **239**:401.

Cerf, D. C., and Georghiou, G. P., 1974, Cross-resistance to juvenile hormone analogues in insecticide-resistant strains of *Musca domestica* L., *Pestic. Sci.* **5**:759.

Chadwick, P. R., Invest, J. F., and Bowron, M. J., 1977, An example of cross-resistance to pyrethroids in DDT-resistant *Aedes aegypti*, *Pestic. Sci.* **8**:618.

Chamberlain, W. F., 1975, Insect growth regulating agents for control of arthropods of medical and veterinary importance, *J. Med. Entomol.* **12**:395.

Chapman, H. C., and Glenn, F. E., Jr., 1972, Incidence of the fungus *Coelomomyces punctatus* and *C. dodgei* in larval populations of the mosquito *Anopheles crucians* in two Louisiana ponds, *J. Invertebr. Pathol.* **19**:256.

Chapman, H. C., Woodard, D. B., and Petersen, J. J., 1967, Pathogens and parasites in Louisiana Culicidae and Chaoboridae, *Proc. N.J. Mosq. Exterm. Assoc.* **54**:54.

Chapman, H. C., Clark, T. B., Petersen, J. J., and Woodard, D. B., 1969, A two-year survey of pathogens and parasites of Culicidae, Chaoboridae, and Ceratopogonidae in Louisiana, *Proc. N.J. Mosq. Exterm. Assoc.* **56**:203.

Chapman, H. C., Clark, T. B., and Petersen, J. J., 1970, Protozoans, nematodes, and viruses of anophelines, *Misc. Publ. Entomol. Soc. Am.* **7**:134.

Cooney, J. C., and Pickard, E., 1974, Field tests with Abate and Dursban insecticides for control of floodwater mosquitoes in the Tennessee Valley Region, *Mosq. News* **34**:12.

Couch, J. N., 1972, Mass production of *Coelomomyces*, a fungus that kills mosquitoes, *Proc. Natl. Acad. Sci.* **69**:2043.

Couch, J. N., and Romney, S. V., 1973, Sexual reproduction in *Lagenidium giganteum*, *Mycologia* **65**:250.

Darwazeh, H. A., and Mulla, M. S., 1974, Toxicity of herbicides and mosquito larvicides to the mosquito fish *Gambusia affinis*, *Mosq. News* **34**:214.

Das, M., 1971, Prospect of management of *Culex pipiens fatigans* through integrated actions, *J. Commun. Dis.* **3**:83.

Davidson, E. W., and Singer, S., 1973, Pathogenesis of *Bacillus sphaericus* infections in mosquito larvae, Abstract of Paper Presented at the 5th International Colloquium on Insect Pathology and Microbial Control, Oxford, p. 5.

DeFoliart, G. R., 1978, Transovarial transmission of LaCrosse virus: Implications for viral persistence in *Aedes triseriatus* populations, Symposium on the Transovarial Transmission of Arboviruses by Mosquitoes, Annual Meeting of the American Society of Tropical Medicine and Hygiene, Chicago, November.

Dixon, R. D., and Brust, R. A., 1972, Mosquitoes of Manitoba. III. Ecology of larvae in the Winnipeg area, *Can. Entomol.* **104**:961.

Dunn, R. L., and Strong, F. E., 1973, Control of catch-basin mosquitoes using Zoecon ZR515 formulated in a slow release polymer—A preliminary report, *Mosq. News* **33**:110.

Dunn, R. L., Case, T. J., and Washino, R. K., 1974, Mosquito control studies in northern California with juvenile hormone analogues: A progress report, *Proc. Calif. Mosq. Control Assoc.* **42**:153.

Eliason, D. A., Kilpatrick, J. W., and Babbitt, M. F., 1970, Evaluation of the effectiveness of the ultra low volume aerial application of insecticides against *Aedes aegypti* (L.) in Florida, *Mosq. News* **30**:430.

Elliott, M., 1977, Synthetic pyrethroids, in: *Synthetic Pyrethroids* (M. Elliott, ed.), pp. 1–28, ACS Symposium Series, American Chemical Society, Washington, D.C.

Elliott, M., Farnham, A. W., Janes, N. F., Needham, P. H., Pulman, D. A., and Stevenson, J. H., 1973, A photostable pyrethroid, *Nature (London)* **246**:169.

Farnham, A. W., 1973, *Introduction to Quantitative Genetics*, Ronald Press, New York.

Farnham, A. W., and Sawicki, R. M., 1976, Development of resistance to pyrethroids in insects resistant to other insecticides, *Pestic. Sci.* **7**:278.

Federici, B. A., and Roberts, D. W., 1976, Experimental laboratory infection of mosquito larvae with fungi of the genus *Coelomomyces*. II. Experiments with *Coelomomyces punctatus* in *Anopheles quadrimaculatus, J. Invertebr. Pathol.* **27**:333.

Federici, B. A., Smedley, G., and Van Leuken, W., 1975, Mosquito host range tests with *Coelomomyces punctatus, Ann. Entomol. Soc. Am.* **68**:669.

Ferguson, D. E., Gardner, D. T., and Lindley, A. L., 1966, Toxicity of Dursban to three species of fish, *Mosq. News* **26**:80.

Ferrigno, F., 1970, Preliminary effects of open marsh water management on the vegetation and organisms of the salt marsh, *Proc. N.J. Mosq. Exterm. Assoc.* **57**:79.

Ferrigno, F., and Jobbins, D. M., 1968, Open marsh water management, *Proc. N.J. Mosq. Exterm. Assoc.* **55**:104.

Ferrigno, F., MacNamara, L. G., and Jobbins, D. M., 1969, Ecological approach for improved management of coastal wetlands, *Proc. N.J. Mosq. Exterm. Assoc.* **56**:188.

Fontaine, R. E., and Rosen, P., 1973, Evaluation of Abate insecticide formulations as larvicides against *Anopheles gambiae* in northern Nigeria, *Mosq. News* **33**:428.

Frank, A. M., and Sjogren, R. D., 1978, The effect of temephos and chlorpyrifos on Crustacea, *Mosq. News* **38**:138.

Garry, C. E., and DeFoliart, G. R., 1975, The effect of basal treehole closure on suppression of *Aedes triseriatus* (Diptera: Culicidae), *Mosq. News* **35**:289.

Geevarghese, G., Dhanda, V., Ranga Rao, P. N., and Deobhankar, R. B., 1977, Field trials for the control of *Aedes aegypti* with Abate in Poona city and suburbs, *Indian J. Med. Res.* **65**:466.

Georghiou, G. P., 1972, Studies on resistance to carbamate and organophosphorus insecticides in *Anopheles albimanus, Am. J. Trop. Med. Hyg.* **21**:797.

Georghiou, G. P., and Taylor, C. E., 1977*a*, Genetic and biological influences in the evolution of insecticide resistance, *J. Econ. Entomol.* **70**:319.

Georghiou, G. P., and Taylor, C. E., 1977*b*, Operational influences in the evolution of insecticide resistance, *J. Econ. Entomol.* **70**:653.

Georghiou, G. P., Lin, C. S., and Pasternak, M. E., 1974, Potentiality of *Culex tarsalis* for development of resistance to carbamate insecticides and insect growth regulators, *Proc. Calif. Mosq. Control Assoc.* **42**:117.

Georghiou, G. P., Lee, S., and De Vries, D. H., 1978, Development of resistance to the juvenoid methoprene in the house fly, *J. Econ. Entomol.* **71**:544.

Gerberg, E. J., and Visser, W. M., 1978, Preliminary field trial for the biological control of *Aedes aegypti* by means of *Toxorhynchites brevipalpis*, a predatory mosquito larva, *Mosq. News* **38**:197.

Gibson, C. L., 1977, Oh well—what's the difference?, *Trop. Med. Hyg. News* **26**(5):3.

Glancey, B. M., Moussa, M. A., Scanlon, J. E., and Lofgren, C. S., 1968, Abate® and Dursban® against *Aedes aegypti* (L.) breeding in concrete water jars in Bangkok, Thailand, *Mosq. News* **28**:205.

Green, M. F., and Imber, C. F., 1977, Applicability of *Gambusia affinis* to urban mosquito problems in Burlington County, New Jersey, *Mosq. News* **37**:383.

Hadaway, A. B., Barlow, F., Turner, C. R., and Flower, L. S., 1977, The search for new insecticides for tsetse fly control, *Pestic. Sci.* **8**:172.

Hattwick, M. A. W., Peters, A. H., Gregg, M. B., and Hanson, B., 1973, Surveillance of Rocky Mountain spotted fever, *J. Am. Med. Assoc.* **225**:1338.

Herms, W. B., 1949, Looking back half a century for guidance in planning and conducting mosquito control operations, *Proc. Calif. Mosq. Control Assoc.* **17**:89.

Hill, E. F., Eliason, D. A., and Kilpatrick, J. W., 1971, Effects of ultra low volume applications of malathion in Hale County, Texas. III. Effect on non-target animals, *J. Med. Entomol.* **8:**173.

Holmstead, R. L., Casida, J. E., and Ruzo, L. O., 1977, Photochemical reactions of pyrethroid insecticides, in: *Synthetic Pyrethroids* (M. Elliott, ed.), pp. 137–146, ACS Symposium Series, American Chemical Society, Washington, D.C.

Hoppe, T., Isler, H., and Vogel, W., 1974, Biological activity of juvenile hormone analogues against larvae of *Culex pipiens pipiens* tested in small-scale field trials, *Mosq. News* **34:**293.

Hoy, J. B., and Petersen, J. J., 1973, Fish and nematodes—Current status of mosquito control techniques, *Proc. Calif. Mosq. Control Assoc.* **41:**49.

Hoy, J. B., O'Berg, A. G., and Kauffman, E. E., 1971, The mosquitofish as a biological control agent against *Culex tarsalis* and *Anopheles freeborni* in Sacramento Valley rice fields, *Mosq. News* **31:**146.

Hoy, J. B., Kauffman, E. E., and O'Berg, A. G., 1972, A large-scale field test of *Gambusia affinis* and chlorpyrifos for mosquito control, *Mosq. News* **32:**161.

Ignoffo, C. M., Biever, K. D., Johnson, W. W., Sanders, H. O., Chapman, H. C., Peterson, J. J., and Woodard, D. B., 1973, Susceptibility of aquatic vertebrates and invertebrates to the infective stage of the mosquito nematode *Reesimermis nielseni, Mosq. News* **33:**599.

Jenkins, D. W., 1964, Pathogens, parasites, and predators of medically important arthropods, *Bull. WHO Suppl.* **30.**

Julin, A. M., and Sanders, H. O., 1978, Toxicity of the IGR, diflubenzuron, to freshwater invertebrates and fishes, *Mosq. News* **38:**256.

Kaufman, D. D., Haynes, S. C., Gordan, E. G., and Kayser, A. J., 1977, Permethrin degradation in soil and microbial cultures, in: *Synthetic Pyrethroids* (M. Elliott, ed.), pp. 147–161, ACS Symposium Series, American Chemical Society, Washington, D.C.

Keenan, C. M., 1978, Use of a controlled release larvicide in southern Maryland, *Mosq. News* **38:**203.

Kilpatrick, J. W., and Adams, C. T., 1967, Emergency measures employed in the control of St. Louis encephalitis epidemics in Dallas and Corpus Christi, Texas, *Proc. Calif. Mosq. Control Assoc.* **35:**53.

Laird, M., 1967, A coral island experiment: A new approach to mosquito control, *WHO Chron.* **21:**18.

Laird, M., 1977, Enemies and diseases of mosquitoes; their natural population regulatory significance in relation to pesticide use, and their future as marketable components of integrated control, *Mosq. News* **37:**331.

Legner, E. F., and Brydon, H. W., 1966, Suppression of dung-inhabiting fly populations by pupal parasites, *Ann. Entomol. Soc. Am.* **59:**638.

Legner, E. F., Sjogren, R. D., and Hall, I. M., 1974, The biological control of medically important arthropods, *Crit. Rev. Environ. Control* **4:**85.

Lewis, L. F., and Tucker, T. W., 1977, Toxicity of the pyrethroid Roussel-Uclaf 22974 to mosquito larvae in laboratory and semifield tests, *Mosq. News* **37:**718.

Lewis, L. F., Christenson, D. M., and Eddy, G. W., 1966, Results of tests with Dursban and fenthion for the control of mosquito larvae in log ponds of western Oregon, *Mosq. News* **26:**579.

Lofgren, C. S., 1970, Ultralow volume applications of concentrated insecticides in medical and veterinary entomology, *Annu. Rev. Entomol.* **15:**321.

Loor, K. A., and DeFoliart, G. R., 1970, Field observations on the biology of *Aedes triseriatus, Mosq. News* **30:**60.

Loving, S. M., Smith, A. B., DiSalvo, A. F., and Burgdorfer, W., 1978, Distribution and prevalence of spotted fever group rickettsiae in ticks from South Carolina, with an epidemiological survey of persons bitten by infected ticks, *Am. J. Trop. Med. Hyg.* **27:**1255.

Macdonald, G., 1957, *The Epidemiology and Control of Malaria*, Oxford University Press, London.

Mauck, W. L., Olson, L. E., and Marking, L. L., 1976, Toxicity of natural pyrethrins and five pyrethroids to fish, *Arch. Environ. Contam. Toxicol.* **4**:18.

McCray, E. M., Jr., 1973, Laboratory studies on a new fungal pathogen of mosquitoes, *Mosq. News* **33**:54.

McCray, E. M., Jr., Womeldorf, D. J., Husbands, R. C., and Eliason, D. A., 1973, Laboratory observations and field tests with *Lagenidium* against California mosquitoes, *Proc. Calif. Mosq. Control Assoc.* **41**:123.

McNeill, J. C., IV, Miller, W. O., and Wleczyk, C. M., 1968, Evaluation of Dursban as a larvicide in septic ditches, *Mosq. News* **28**:160.

Menon, P. K. B., and Rajagopalan, P. K., 1977, Mosquito control potential of some species of indigenous fishes in Pondicherry, *Indian J. Med. Res.* **66**:765.

Micks, D. W., Chambers, G. V., Jennings, J., and Barnes, K., 1968, Laboratory evaluation of a new petroleum derivative, Flit MLO, *J. Econ. Entomol.* **61**:647.

Miller, T., Nelson, L. L., Young, W. W., Roberts, L. W., Roberts, D. R., and Wilkinson, R. N., 1973, Polymer formulations of mosquito larvicides. I. Effectiveness of polyethylene and polyvinyl chloride formulations of chlorpyrifos applied to artificial field pools, *Mosq. News* **33**:148.

Mitchell, C. J., Chen, P. S., and Chapman, H. C., 1972, Exploratory trials utilizing a mermithid nematode as a control agent for *Culex* mosquitoes in Taiwan (China), *Formosan Med. Assoc. J.* **73**:241.

Miura, T., and Takahashi, R. M., 1973, Insect developmental inhibitors. 3. Effects on non-target aquatic organisms, *J. Econ. Entomol.* **66**:917.

Miura, T., and Takahashi, R. M., 1975, Effect of the IGR TH-6040 on nontarget organisms when utilized as a mosquito control agent, *Mosq. News* **35**:154.

Miyamoto, J., 1976, Degradation metabolism and toxicity of synthetic pyrethroids, *Environ. Health Perspect.* **14**:15.

Moulton, D. W., and Thompson, W. H., 1971, California group virus infections in small forest-dwelling mammals of Wisconsin. Some ecological considerations, *Am. J. Trop. Med. Hyg.* **20**:474.

Mount, G. A., and Lofgren, C. S., 1967, Ultra-low volume and conventional aerial sprays for control of adult salt-marsh mosquitoes, *Aedes sollicitans* (Walker) and *Aedes taeniorhynchus* (Weidemann), in Florida, *Mosq. News* **27**:473.

Mount, G. A., and Pierce, N. W., 1974, Ultralow volume ground aerosols of naled for control of *Aedes taeniorhynchus* (Wiedemann) in the Florida Keys, *Mosq. News* **34**:268.

Mount, G. A., Meisch, M. V., Lee, J. T., Pierce, N. W., and Baldwin, K. F., 1972, Ultralow volume ground aerosols of insecticides for control of rice field mosquitoes in Arkansas, *Mosq. News* **32**:444.

Mount, G. A., Pierce, N. W., Baldwin, K. F., and Washington, F., 1978, Control of *Aedes taeniorhynchus* at Crescent Beach, Florida, with aerosols of propoxur (Baygon MOS) and naled (Dibrom 14), *Mosq. News* **38**:54.

Mulla, M. S., and Darwazeh, H. A., 1976, The IGR Dimilin and its formulations against mosquitoes, *J. Econ. Entomol.* **69**:309.

Mulla, M. S., and Isaak, L. W., 1961, Field studies on the toxicity of insecticides to the mosquito fish, *Gambusia affinis*, *J. Econ. Entomol.* **54**:1237.

Mulla, M. S., Darwazeh, H. A., and Peters, D. R., 1970, Mosquito control in sewage oxidation ponds with drip and pour-in larvicides, *Mosq. News* **30**:456.

Mulla, M. S., Darwazeh, H. A., and Norland, R. L., 1974, Insect growth regulators: Evaluation procedures and activity against mosquitoes, *J. Econ. Entomol.* **67**:329.

Mulla, M. S., Majori, G., and Darwazeh, H. A., 1975, Effects of the insect growth regulator Dimilin or TH-6040 on mosquitoes and some non-target organisms, *Mosq. News* **35**:211.

Mulla, M. S., Navvab-Gojrati, H. A., and Darwazeh, H. A., 1978, Biological activity and longevity of new synthetic pyrethroids against mosquitoes and some non-target insects, *Mosq. News* **38**:90.

Muspratt, J., 1962, Destruction of the larvae of *Anopheles gambiae* by a *Coelomomyces* fungus, WHO/EBL/2, WHO/Vector Control/2.

Muspratt, J., 1963, Progress report (May 1963) on investigations concerning three mosquito pathogens at Livingstone, Northern Rhodesia, WHO/EBL/12.

Muspratt, J., 1965, Technique for infecting larvae of the *Culex pipiens* complex with a mermithid nematode and for culturing the latter in the laboratory, *Bull. WHO* **33**:140.

National Academy of Sciences, 1976, *Pest Control: An Assessment of Present and Alternative Technologies,* Vol. V, *Pest Control and Public Health,* Washington, D.C.

Nelson, G. H., Evans, E. S., Jr., Pennington, N. E., and Meisch, M. V., 1976, Larval control of *Psorophora confinnis* (Lynch-Arribalzaga) with a controlled-release formulation of chlorpyrifos, *Mosq. News* **36**:47.

Norland, R. L., and Mulla, M. S., 1975, Impact of Altosid on related members of an aquatic ecosystem, *Environ. Entomol.* **4**:145.

Peck, J. H., and Anderson, J. R., 1970, Influence of poultry-manure removal schedules on various Diptera larvae and selected arthropod predators, *J. Econ. Entomol.* **63**:82.

Peters, W., 1974, Recent advances in antimalarial chemotherapy and drug resistance, *Adv. Parasitol.* **12**:69.

Petersen, J. J., 1973*a*, Factors affecting mass production of *Reesimermis nielseni* a nematode parasite of mosquitoes, *J. Med. Entomol.* **10**:75.

Petersen, J. J., 1973*b*, Relationship of density, location of hosts, and water volume to parasitism of larvae of the southern house mosquito by a mermithid nematode, *Mosq. News* **33**:516.

Petersen, J. J., 1973*c*, Role of mermithid nematodes in biological control of mosquitoes, *Exp. Parasitol.* **33**:239.

Petersen, J. J., 1975, Penetration and development of the mermithid nematode *Reesimermis nielseni* in eighteen species of mosquitoes, *J. Nematol.* **7**:207.

Petersen, J. J., 1978, Observations on the mass production of *Romanomermis culicivorax,* a nematode parasite of mosquitoes, *Mosq. News* **38**:83.

Petersen, J. J., and Willis, O. R., 1970, Some factors affecting parasitism by mermithid nematodes in southern house mosquito larvae, *J. Econ. Entomol.* **63**:175.

Petersen, J. J., and Willis, O. R., 1971, A two-year survey to determine the incidence of a mermithid nematode in mosquitoes in Louisiana, *Mosq. News* **31**:558.

Petersen, J. J., and Willis, O. R., 1972*a*, Procedures for the mass rearing of a mermithid parasite of mosquitoes, *Mosq. News* **32**:226.

Petersen, J. J., and Willis, O. R., 1972*b*, Results of preliminary field applications of *Reesimermis nielseni* (Mermithidae: Nematoda) to control mosquito larvae, *Mosq. News* **32**:312.

Petersen, J. J., and Willis, O. R., 1974, Experimental release of a mermithid nematode to control *Anopheles* mosquitoes in Louisiana, *Mosq. News* **34**:316.

Petersen, J. J., and Willis, O. R., 1975, Establishment and recycling of a mermithid nematode for the control of larval mosquitoes, *Mosq. News* **35**:526.

Petersen, J. J., Chapman, H. C., and Woodard, D. B., 1968, The bionomics of a mermithid nematode of larval mosquitoes in southwestern Louisiana, *Mosq. News* **28**:346.

Petersen, J. J., Chapman, H. C., and Willis, O. R., 1969, Fifteen species of mosquitoes as potential hosts of a mermithid nematode *Romanomermis* sp., *Mosq. News* **29**:198.

Petersen, J. J., Hoy, J. B., and O'Berg, A. G., 1972, Preliminary field tests with *Reesimermis nielseni* (Mermithidae: Nematoda) against mosquito larvae in California rice fields, *Calif. Vector Views* **19**:47.

Petersen, J. J., Steelman, C. D., and Willis, O. R., 1973, Field parasitism of two species of Louisiana rice field mosquitoes by a mermithid nematode, *Mosq. News* **33**:573.

Petersen, J. J., Willis, O. R., and Chapman, H. C., 1978*a*, Release of *Romanomermis culicivorax* for the control of *Anopheles albimanus* in El Salvador. I. Mass production of the nematode, *Am. J. Trop. Med. Hyg.* **27**:1265.

Petersen, J. J., Chapman, H. C., Willis, O. R., and Fukuda, R., 1978*b*, Release of *Romanomermis culicivorax* for the control of *Anopheles albimanus* in El Salvador. II. Application of the nematode, *Am. J. Trop. Med. Hyg.* **27**:1268.

Plapp, F. W., Jr., and Vinson, S. B., 1973, Juvenile hormone analogs: Toxicity and cross-resistance in the house fly, *Pestic. Biochem. Physiol.* **7**:261.

Priester, T. M., and Georghiou, G. P., 1978, Induction of high resistance to permethrin in *Culex pipiens quinquefasciatus*, *J. Econ. Entomol.* **71**:197.

Provost, M. W., 1974, Salt marsh management in Florida, *Proc. Tall Timbers Conf. Ecol. Anim. Control Manage.* **1973**:5.

Provost, M. W., 1977, Source reduction in salt-marsh mosquito control: Past and future, *Mosq. News* **37**:689.

Rafatjah, H. A., 1971, The problem of resurgent bed-bug infestation in malaria eradication programmes, *J. Trop. Med. Hyg.* **74**:53.

Rajagopal, R., 1977, Malathion resistance in *Anopheles culicifacies* in Gujarat, *Indian J. Med. Res.* **66**:27.

Ramoska, W. A., Singer, S., and Levy, R., 1977, Bioassay of three strains of *Bacillus sphaericus* in field collected mosquito larvae, *J. Invertebr. Pathol.* **30**:151.

Ramoska, W. A., Burgess, J., and Singer, S., 1978, Field application of a bacterial insecticide, *Mosq. News* **38**:57.

Rathburn, C. B., Jr., 1966, The arsenic content in soil following repeated applications of granular Paris green, *Mosq. News* **26**:537.

Rathburn, C. B., Jr., and Boike, A. H., Jr., 1973, Laboratory selection of *Culex nigripalpus* Theob. for resistance to Paris green, *Mosq. News* **33**:512.

Rathburn, C. B., Jr., and Boike, A. H., Jr., 1977, The efficacy of preflood and residual applications of two formulations of methoprene, *Mosq. News* **37**:620.

Reeves, W. C., 1972, Can the war to contain infectious diseases be lost?, *Am. J. Trop. Med. Hyg.* **21**:251.

Reuben, R., and Panicker, K. N., 1975, *Aedes* survey in five districts of Rajasthan, India, *J. Commun. Dis.* **7**:1.

Reynolds, D. G., 1971, Parasitism of *Culex fatigans* by *Nosema stegomyiae*, *J. Invertebr. Pathol.* **18**:429.

Roberts, D. R., Roberts, L. W., Miller, T. A., Nelson, L. L., and Young, W. W., 1973, Polymer formulations of mosquito larvicides. III. Effects of a polyethylene formulation of chlorpyrifos on non-target populations naturally infesting artificial field pools, *Mosq. News* **33**:165.

Roberts, D. W., 1967, Some effects of *Metarrhizium anisopliae* and its toxins on mosquito larvae, in: *Insect Pathology and Microbiological Control* (P. A. van der Laan, ed.), pp. 243–246, North-Holland, Amsterdam.

Roberts, D. W., 1970, *Coelomomyces, Entomophthora, Beauveria* and *Metarrhizium* as parasites of mosquitoes, *Misc. Publ. Entomol. Soc. Am.* **7**:140.

Roberts, D. W., and Strand, M. A. (ed.), 1977, Pathogens of medically important arthropods, *Bull. WHO Suppl.* **55**(1).

Roberts, L. W., Roberts, D. R., Miller, T. A., Nelson, L. L. and Young, W. W., 1973, Polymer formulations of mosquito larvicides. II. Effects of a polyethylene formulation of chlorpyrifos on *Culex* populations naturally infecting artificial field pools, *Mosq. News* **33**:155.

Rogers, A. J., and Rathburn, C. B., Jr., 1958, Tests with a new granular Paris green formulation against *Aedes, Anopheles* and *Psorophora* larvae, *Mosq. News* **18**:89.

Rogers, A. J., and Rathburn, C. B., Jr., 1960*a*, Improved methods of formulating granular Paris green larvicide, *Mosq. News* **20**:11.

Rogers, A. J., and Rathburn, C. B., Jr., 1960*b*, Airplane application of granular Paris green mosquito larvicide, *Mosq. News* **20**:105.

Sanmartín, C., 1973, Epidemiological experiences in over-developed subcountries, *Am. J. Trop. Med. Hyg.* **22**:291.

Sarhan, M. E., Howitt, R. E., and Moore, C. V., 1979, Pesticide resistance externalities and optimal mosquito management, *J. Environ. Econ. Manage.* **6**:69.

Savage, K. E., and Lowe, R. E., 1970, Studies of *Anopheles quadrimiaculatus* infected with a *Nosema* sp., *Proc. Int. Colloq. Insect Pathol.* **IV**:272.

Scanlon, J. E., and Sandhinand, U., 1965, The distribution and biology of *Anopheles balabacensis* in Thailand (Diptera: Culicidae), *J. Med. Entomol.* **2**:61.

Schaefer, C. H., and Wilder, W. H., 1973, Insect developmental inhibitors. 2. Effects on target mosquito species, *J. Econ. Entomol.* **66**:913.

Schaefer, C. H., Miura, T., Mulligan, F. S., III, and Dupras, E. F., Jr., 1974, Insect development inhibitors: Formulation research on Altosid, *Proc. Calif. Mosq. Control Assoc.* **42**:140.

Scholl, P. J., and DeFoliart, G. R., 1977, *Aedes triseriatus* and *Aedes hendersoni:* Vertical and temporal distribution as measured by oviposition, *Environ. Entomol.* **6**:355.

Scholl, P. J., and DeFoliart, G. R., 1979, Pipe insulating cement for closing treehole breeding sites of *Aedes triseriatus, Mosq. News* **39**:149.

Scholl, P. J., DeFoliart, G. R., and Nemenyi, P. B., 1979, Vertical distribution of biting activity by *Aedes triseriatus, Ann. Entomol. Soc. Am.* **72**:537.

Schoof, H. F., Pearce, G. W., and Willis, M., 1963, Dichlorvos as a residual fumigant in mud, plywood and bamboo huts, *Bull. WHO* **29**:227.

Self, L. S., Nelson, M. J., Pant, C. P., and Usman, S., 1978, Field trials with two insect growth regulators against *Culex quinquefasciatus, Mosq. News* **38**:74.

Service, M. W., 1973, Mortalities of the larvae of the *Anopheles gambiae* complex and detection of predators by the precipitin test, *Bull. Entomol. Res.* **62**:359.

Shanmugham, C. A. K., Roy, R. G., and Ganesan, A. V., 1977, Kala-azar in Tamil Nadu State during 1974–1975—A restrospective and prospective study, *Indian J. Med. Res.* **65**:796.

Sharma, M. I. D., 1972, Residual insecticides for the control of arthropod-borne diseases—The scope and limitations of their use with particular reference to India, *J. Commun. Dis.* **4**:208.

Sharma, M. I. D., 1974, Integrated control of mosquitoes with particular reference to India, *J. Commun. Dis.* **6**:136.

Sharma, M. I. D., Suri, J. C., and Kalra, N. L., 1973*a*, Studies on cutaneous leishmaniasis in India. I. A note on the current status of cutaneous leishmaniasis in north-western India as determined during 1973, *J. Commun. Dis.* **5**:73.

Sharma, M. I. D., Suri, J. C., Kalra, N. L., and Mohan, K., 1973*b*, Studies on cutaneous leishmaniasis in India. III. Detection of a zoonotic focus of cutaneous leishmaniasis in Rajasthan, *J. Commun. Dis.* **5**:149.

Singer, S., 1975*a*, Use of bacteria for control of aquatic insect pests, in: *Impact of the use of Microorganisms on the Aquatic Environment* (A. W. Bourquin, D. G. Ahearn, and S. P. Meyers, eds.), pp. 5–22, Environmental Protection Agency Ecology Research Service 660-375-001, Corvallis, Oregon.

Singer, S., 1975*b*, Isolation and development of bacterial pathogens of vectors, in: *Proceedings of the National Institutes of Health Workshops* (Mimeographed).

Singer, S., and Murphy, L. J., 1976, New insecticidal strains of *Bacillus sphaericus* useful against *Anopheles albimanus* larvae, *Proceedings of the Annual Meeting of the American Society for Microbiology*, Abstracts, p. 183.

Singer, S., Goodman, N. S., and Rogoff, M. H., 1966, Defined media for the study of bacilli pathogenic to insects, *Ann. N.Y. Acad. Sci.* **139**:16.

Sinsko, M. J., and Grimstad, P. R., 1977, Habitat separation by differential vertical oviposition of two treehole *Aedes* in Indiana, *Environ. Entomol.* **6**:485.

Sitaraman, N. L., Karim, M. A., and Reddy, G. V., 1975, Observations on the use of *Gambusia affinis holbrooki* to control *A. stephensi* breeding in wells. Results of two years study in Great Hyderabad City, India, *Indian J. Med. Res.* **63**:1509.

Steelman, C. D., Gassie, J. M., and Craven, B. R., 1967, Laboratory and field studies on mosquito control in waste disposal lagoons in Louisiana, *Mosq. News* **27**:57.

Steelman, C. D., Farlow, J. E., Breaud, T. P., and Schilling, P. E., 1975, Effects of growth regulators on *Psorophora columbiae* (Dyar & Knab) and non-target aquatic insect species in rice fields, *Mosq. News* **35**:67.

Sudia, W. D., Newhouse, V. F., Beadle, L. D., Miller, D. L., Johnston, J. G., Jr., Young, R., Calisher, C. H., and Maness, K., 1975, Epidemic Venezuelan equine encephalitis in North America in 1971: Vector studies, *Am. J. Epidemiol.* **101**:17.

Sutherland, K. J., Kent, R., and Downing, J., 1978, The effect of aerial ULV adulticiding with malathion and naled on field populations of *Aedes sollicitans, Mosq. News* **38**:488.

Tagatz, M. E., Borthwick, P. W., Cook, G. H., and Coppage, D. L., 1974, Effects of ground applications of malathion on salt-marsh environments in northwestern Florida, *Mosq. News* **34**:309.

Takahashi, R. M., and Miura, T., 1975, Insect developmental inhibitors: Multiple applications of Dimilin and Altosid to *Gambusia affinis* (Baird and Girard), *Proc. Calif. Mosq. Control. Assoc.* **43**:85.

Taylor, C. E., and Georghiou, G. P., 1979, Suppression of insecticide resistance by alteration of gene dominance and migration, *J. Econ. Entomol.* **72**:105.

Thompson, G. D., and Meisch, M. V., 1978, Residual efficacy of permethrin against adult ricefield mosquitoes contained on treated panels, *Mosq. News* **38**:275.

Thurber, G. A., 1978, Letters to the editor, *Trop. Med. Hyg. News* **27**(2):11.

Trpis, M., 1973, Interaction between the predator *Toxorhynchites brevipalpis* and its prey *Aedes aegypti, Bull. WHO* **49**:359.

Trpis, M., and Gerberg, E. J., 1973, Laboratory colonization of *Toxorhynchites brevipalpis, Bull. WHO* **48**:637.

Umphlett, D. J., 1968, Ecology of *Coelomomyces* infections of mosquito larvae, *J. Elisha Mitchell Sci. Soc.* **84**:108.

Umphlett, C. J., 1970, Infection levels of *Coelomomyces punctatus*, an aquatic fungus parasite, in a natural population of the common malaria mosquito, *Anopheles quadrimaculatus, J. Invertebr. Pathol.* **15**:299.

Umphlett, C. J., 1973, A note to identify a certain isolate of *Lagenidium* which kills mosquito larvae, *Mycologia* **65**:970.

Umphlett, C. J., and Huang, C. S., 1972, Experimental infection of mosquito larvae by a species of the aquatic fungus *Lagenidium, J. Invertebr. Pathol.* **20**:326.

Undeen, A. H., and Alger, N. E., 1975, The effect of the microsporidian *Nosema algerae* on *Anopheles stephensi, J. Invertebr. Pathol.* **25**:19.

Undeen, A. H., and Maddox, J. V., 1973, The infection of nonmosquito hosts by injection with spores of the microsporidian *Nosema algerae, J. Invertebr. Pathol.* **22**:258.

U.S. Department of Health, Education and Welfare, 1976, Vector topics No. 1: Control of St. Louis encephalitis.

U.S. Department of Health, Education and Welfare, 1978, *Morbidity Mortality Weekly Rep.* **27**:464.

Verschoyle, R. D., and Barnes, J. M., 1972, Toxicity of natural and synthetic pyrethrins to rats, *Pestic. Biochem. Physiol.* **2**:308.

Wattal, B. L., 1971, Vector-borne diseases in India, *J. Commun. Dis.* **3**:15.

Watts, D. M., Pantuwatana, S., DeFoliart, G. R., Yuill, T. M., and Thompson, W. H., 1973, Transoverial transmission of LaCrosse virus (California encephalitis group) in the mosquito, *Aedes triseriatus, Science* **182**:1140.

Watts, D. M., Thompson, W. H., Yuill, T. M., DeFoliart, G. R., and Hanson, R. P., 1974, Overwintering of LaCrosse virus in *Aedes triseriatus, Am. J. Trop. Med. Hyg.* **34**:697.

Watts, D. M., Grimstad, P. R., DeFoliart, G. R., and Yuill, T. M., 1975, *Aedes hendersoni:* Failure of laboratory-infected mosquitoes to transmit LaCrosse virus (California encephalitis group), *J. Med. Entomol.* **12**:451.

Whisler, H. C., Zebold, S. L., and Shemanchuk, J. A., 1974, Alternate host for mosquito parasite *Coelomomyces, Nature (London)* **251**:715.

Whisler, H. C., Zebold, S. L., and Shemanchuk, J. A., 1975, Life history of *Coelomomyces psorophorae, Proc. Natl. Acad. Sci. USA* **72**:693.

WHO, 1977, First scientific working group on biological control of insect vectors of disease, WHO TDR/BCV-SWG (1)/77.3.

WHO, 1978, Malaria control—A reoriented strategy, *WHO Chron.* **32**:226.

Willis, R. R., and Axtell, R.L., 1968, Mite predators of the house fly: A comparison of *Fuscuropoda vegetans* and *Machrocheles muscaedomesticae, J. Econ. Entomol.* **61**:1669.

Winner, R. A., and Steelman, C. D., 1978, Effects of selected insecticides on *Romanomermis culicivorax,* a mermithid nematode parasite of mosquito larvae, *Mosq. News* **38**:546.

Wright, J. W., 1971, The WHO programme for evaluation and testing of new insecticides, *Bull. WHO* **44**:11.

9

Pesticides for Stored Products

J. R. Plimmer

9.1. INTRODUCTION

If commodities are to be stored, transported, or processed, they must be protected from deterioration and loss caused by pests. Such losses place a heavy economic burden on the consumer, and their consequences may be disastrous in times of food shortage. Statistics indicate the magnitude of the problem. For example, in a 1947 FAO Survey it was reported that insects destroy at least 5% of the world production of cereal grains. In 29 countries the loss of cereals was 23,355,000 tons, of which 50% was attributed to insects (Cotton and Ashby, 1952).

This situation can be ameliorated somewhat by improvements in storage facilities and handling techniques, but some form of chemical treatment will continue to be essential. Chemical treatment to control stored-product pests and to prevent introduction of pests into quarantined areas presents special difficulties, and such applications differ considerably from those used for protection of crops or public health.

When chemicals are used for control of pests of any type, only a small fraction of the applied material is ingested or absorbed by the target organism. A considerably larger fraction is altered or dissipated in the environment. When

J. R. Plimmer ● Organic Chemical Synthesis Laboratory, Agricultural Research Service, U.S. Department of Agriculture, Beltsville, Maryland 20705.

pesticides such as the organophosphate insecticides are applied to an agricultural crop, they may be transformed biologically by the action of plant enzymes or soil microorganisms or they may be transformed chemically by the action of light, hydrolysis, oxidation, or reaction with soil or biological substrates. In addition, such physical means as volatilization, adsorption, leaching, and runoff may dissipate applied pesticides. The relative importance of each process will be governed by the physical and chemical properties of the pesticide and its interaction with environmental components.

For a long time, it was assumed that physical, chemical, and biological reactions occurring in the environment would readily transform residual pesticides into innocuous substances. The past two decades have taught us that this assumption must be examined very critically, and we now have sufficient experience to realize that the use of pesticides that are resistant to environmental transformation must be reduced or avoided. As a result, the development of alternative methods of pest control and the search for biologically active molecules that present fewer residue problems are now recognized as research priorities. Such innovations are accompanied by problems of technology transfer because a shift in emphasis away from conventional pesticide application techniques, or even the incorporation of new developments into integrated pest management programs, requires continued acquisition of data and experience and the development of new pest management skills.

In the case of chemical control of pests that affect stored products, there are additional special problems. Stored products must be protected from attack by insects, rodents, and microbial agents; therefore, chemicals used for control must have a broad spectrum of biocidal activity unless control is to be directed toward a limited number of species. The chemicals used for this purpose are usually applied in enclosed situations that afford continued protection against pests, such as bins, granaries, grain elevators, and holds; thus, the stored product itself becomes the major recipient of the chemical application, and any chemical in excess of that used to destroy the target organism is distributed throughout this commodity. Because the commodity is often intended for human or animal consumption, it is desirable that as little residual material as possible be retained and that any such residues be innocuous.

Microbial breakdown, which represents a major pathway for reduction of pesticide residues in most agricultural applications, is not an available route for chemicals used for insect control in stored products. Those residual chemicals that are not volatilized must be degraded by chemical reaction with the substrate, by hydrolysis, by oxidation, or by photodecomposition (to a limited extent).

Chemicals used for treatment of stored products fall into two major classes: *protectants* and *fumigants*. The former exert residual activity after application to the substrate or the container; the latter exert their activity in the vapor phase.

9.2. FUMIGANTS

Few chemicals are suitable for use as fumigants because of the stringent criteria that must be met. Fumigants must be biologically active and control pest species without phytotoxicity or damage to the substrate. They should be sufficiently volatile to diffuse rapidly into the substrate. They should not be adsorbed, and they should be rapidly removed by aeration. They should not be flammable. They should not react with metals. They should leave no residues that are hazardous to man or animals consuming the substrate. They should not adversely affect the nutritional quality, flavor, or processing characteristics of the substrate. It can easily be seen that no chemical behaves adequately with respect to each of the categories of desirable properties. The principal fumigants now in use are indicated in Table 9.1; however, current research findings on health-related aspects suggest that continued use of some of these fumigants may be undesirable.

Investigation of the toxicology of several fumigants in recent years, together with information attained as a result of improved analytical methodology, points to the widespread occurrence of undesirable residues. Fishbein (1976) gives a summary of some potential hazards of fumigant residues: ethylene dibromide is mutagenic and carcinogenic; ethylene oxide in wheat and flour gives ethylene bromohydrin, a mutagen; chronic exposure of workers to ethylene dibromide or dibromochloropropane may have adverse effect on human male reproduction; carbon tetrachloride produces liver tumors in mice, hamsters, and rats; methyl bromide and many other fumigants are alkylating agents and may possess mutagenic properties; several fumigants (ethylene dibromide, carbon tetrachloride,

Table 9.1. Commodity Fumigants

Compound	Formula	Boiling point (°C)
Acrylonitrile	$CH_2\!\!=\!\!CHCN$	77°
Carbon disulfide	CS_2	46.3°
Carbon tetrachloride	CCl_4	76.8°
Chloropicrin	$CCl_3\,NO_2$	112°
1,2-Dichloropropene	$CHCl\!\!=\!\!CCl\!\!-\!\!CH_3$	77°
Ethylene dibromide	CH_2BrCH_2Br	131.6°
Ethylene dichloride	CH_2ClCH_2Cl	83.5°
Ethylene oxide	$(CH_2)_2O$	10.7°
Hydrogen cyanide	HCN	26.1°
Methyl bromide	CH_3Br	3.6°
Phosphine	PH_3	$-87°$

1,3-dibromochloropropane, chloroform, trichloroethylene, and chloroethylene) are carcinogenic and/or heptatotoxic.

Conventional Fumigants. One of the most important fumigants in the U.S. is methyl bromide, which is widely used in the stored food and beverage industry. In 1974, 13.8 million kg were produced in the U.S. (Fowler and Mahan, 1976). Of 11 million kg produced in 1972, 1 million kg were exported, 4 million kg were used for soil fumigation, and 6 million kg were used commercially, mainly for treatment of stored grains and feeds (von Rumker *et al.*, 1974).

Methyl bromide is low boiling (b.p. 3.6°C) and is rapidly dissipated by desorption or reaction. The most common residue that results from its use is inorganic bromide. However, methyl bromide is a reactive methylating agent, and in a classic series of studies with ^{14}C-labeled methyl bromide, Winteringham, Bridges, and their co-workers at Slough (Winteringham *et al.*, 1955) were able to show that it reacted with certain components of flour; if too much methyl bromide was used, the reaction products gave off-flavors to baked goods. Levels of bromide ion have been determined in many commodities after fumigation with methyl bromide, but the presence of unknown background levels of bromide ion of natural origin has cast some doubt on the significance of these figures.

The effect of ^{14}C-labeled methyl bromide on wheat flour provided an indication of the fate of the compound in commodities. Free mercapto groups such as those present in wheat germ as reduced glutathione were methylated rapidly. The gluten or protein fraction of wheat accounted for 80% of the decomposition of methyl bromide. Methylation occurred, and *N*-methyl derivatives (50%), dimethyl sulfonium derivatives (30%), and methoxy and methylthio derivatives (20%) were formed.

Hydrolysis of the protein fraction from methyl-bromide-treated flour showed that most basic sites were methylated. The histidine residue was the principal site of reaction (Bridges, 1955), and 1-methylhistidine, 3-methylhistidine, and 1,3-dimethylhistidine were present in the hydrolysate. The nutritional and toxicological implications of these findings are probably not significant. Winteringham (1955) considered the possibility of human exposure to very small quantities of methanol, methyl glucose, *S*-methyl cysteine, methyl methionine sulfonium salts, and *N*-methyl derivatives of histidine. He concluded from feeding studies that there was little potential for risk to human health from these residues. There was little evidence of nutritional loss, and the major problem was that of "sulfide taint," the unpleasant odor that arises when dimethyl sulfonium derivatives, which are formed in flour treated with unduly high levels of methyl bromide, decompose and release sulfide compounds when the flour is baked.

Ethylene dibromide is another important fumigant. It has a boiling point of 131.6°C; this relatively high boiling point makes it useful for fumigation in tropical climates. It has been used in the U.S. for fumigation of citrus and other fruits, but it does not penetrate wheat well, and high residues remain in the surface layers. Ethylene dibromide is not very reactive, but some ethylene glycol is formed in wheat on heating. It is highly sorbed, and the low rate of desorption on airing may result in unchanged residual fumigant. When grain treated with ethylene dibromide was fed to hens, their egg-laying capacity was affected (Bierer and Vickers, 1959), and degeneration of spermatazoa occurred in bulls fed with ethylene-dibromide-treated corn (Amir and Volcani, 1965). Treated feeds do not produce symptoms of chronic toxicity in rats (Alumot *et al.*, 1974), but β-hydroxyethyl derivatives of glutathione were isolated from the rats' livers (Nachtomi, 1970). It has been recognized that spermatogenesis in humans is affected by ethylene bromide. It is a mutagen, and 0.15–0.8 ml/animal per day fed to rats or mice by chronic oral intubation caused a high incidence of carcinomas of the stomach after 10 weeks (Olson *et al.*, 1973). The related compound dibromochloropropane (a soil fumigant) also caused carcinomas in rats.

Phosphine, another major fumigant in the stored food and beverage industry, boils at -87°C. Although it is flammable and toxic, its use as a fumigant is increasing because it can be conveniently generated from tablets containing aluminum phosphide and ammonium carbamate (Phostoxin®), and it appears to present little long-term hazard. Residues are quite low, and the phosphorus-containing residue is mainly phosphite and hypophosphite.

Ethylene oxide and propylene oxide are toxic to microorganisms as well as to insects. They are quite reactive; ethylene oxide may react by nucleophilic ring fission to give low-molecular-weight derivatives or addition products such as ethylene chlorohydrin, ethylene bromohydrin, or ethylene glycol. It also may react with functional groups in constituents of food or commodities to give the corresponding hydroxyethylated compounds of, for example, sugars and amino acids.

Most conventional fumigants contain reactive halogen atoms and are capable of alkylation reactions; ethylene oxide is also a reactive nucleophilic molecule. Nevertheless, in the quantities recommended for fumigation, these compounds are expected to produce little change in the flavor, processing qualities, or nutrient quality of the commodity, although detection of subtle changes in nutrient quality requires more careful and long-term feeding studies.

A major concern is that residues of fumigants may have long-term toxicological implications and may, in some subtle way, affect processes that regulate cell division. Methods of analysis based on inorganic bromide are no longer satisfactory as a basis for setting tolerances for brominated fumigants, and sophisticated analytical methods are important to ensure that residues of unchanged fumigant or other toxicologically significant molecules can be quantitatively determined.

9.3. PROTECTANTS

The use of protectants to limit the occurrence of insects in stored products is a widespread practice. Malathion, which will be discussed in some detail, has been used for a long time to control a variety of insect pests; however, the problem of resistance to malathion makes it necessary to continue the search for alternatives that provide residual activity without hazardous effects. Other compounds that have been examined include fenitrothion, primiphos-methyl, bioresmethrin, and chlorpyrifos-methyl, alone or in combination. All of these except bioresmethrin are organophosphate insecticides. Currently malathion, methoxychlor, and pyrethrins are among the chemicals used in the U.S. for application to storage bins as residual sprays. The only readily available insecticide approved in the U.S. for direct application to grain is malathion. Pirimiphos-methyl has been approved for this purpose in Great Britain and France.

Malathion.   Malathion (O,O-dimethyl phosphorodithioate of diethyl mercaptosuccinate) may be formulated as a 57% emulsifiable liquid (0.6 kg A.I./ liter), 25% wettable powder, or 4% dust. In the U.S. it has been registered for use on stored grains (including wheat, oats, rice, corn, barley, grain sorghum, and field or garden seeds) against the confused flour beetle (*Tribolium confusum* Jacquelin duVal), rice weevil [*Sitophilus oryzae* (L.)], granary weevil [*Sitophilus granarius* (L.)], sawtoothed grain beetle [*Oryzaephilus surinamensis* (L.)], flat grain beetle [*Cryptolestes pusillus* (Schönherr)], red flour beetle [*Tribolium castaneum* (Herbst)], rusty grain beetle (*Cryptolestes ferrugineus* Stephens)], lesser grain borer [*Rhyzopertha dominica* (F.)], and Indianmeal moth [*Plodia interpunctella* (Hübner)]. The emulsifiable liquid is diluted and sprayed over the surface of the uninfested grain. It may also be used to spray boxcars before they are used for transportation of packaged flour or cereals. Other stored products may also be protected by applications of malathion.

Malathion is one of the least toxic of the currently available insecticides and is extremely versatile. For these reasons, it has been widely used throughout the world. It is used on a large scale by the World Health Organization for control of malaria vectors. The U.S. product volume in 1972 was estimated at about 11 million kg A.I., of a total of 124 million kg of insecticides produced in the U.S. in that year (von Rumker *et al.*, 1974). The other leading insecticides were toxaphene, carbaryl, and methyl parathion, of which 34.5, 24.0, and 23.2 million kg A.I., respectively, were produced in 1972. A further 69,800 kg of malathion was imported into the U.S. in 1972. It is estimated that 3.6 million kg A.I. of the U.S. stock was exported during that year.

Malathion has been widely used in food processing, packaging, and distribution establishments. In the north central U.S., where its major use is for protection of food and feed grains, it is estimated that 0.5 million kg was used in 1972 by industrial and commercial organization.

The U.S. producer of malathion is American Cyanamid. Its manufacture involves reaction of phosphorus pentasulfide with methanol to give *O,O*-dimethyl hydrogen phosphorodithioate. The addition of this intermediate to diethyl maleate yields malathion (Eto, 1974) (Fig. 9.1).

Malathion has very low toxicity to rats, with an acute oral LD_{50} of 1375 mg/kg. In a long-term feeding study, rats fed with 1000 ppm for 92 weeks showed normal growth. It has been synthesized in *d* and *l* forms (toxicities 1014 mg/kg and 2357 mg/kg, respectively). The greater toxicity of the former may be due to increased esterase inhibition shown by *d*-malaoxon, which was four and eight times more effective than the *l* isomer in the inhibitions of acetylcholinesterase and carboxyesterase, respectively. The optical activity is based on the succinic acid moeity. The highly selective toxicity of malathion may be ascribed to the superior ability of mammalian carboxyesterases to hydrolyze the carboxyethyl groups of the succinate portion of the molecule.

Studies of the fate of malathion in the environment indicate that it is rapidly degraded in soil (50–90% in 24 hr) and in water. The half-life at concentrations of 0.5 ppm in water is 0.5–10 days, depending on pH. At pH 8 and 28°C, malathion half-life has been reported as 1 month. In ethanol–buffer (1 : 4; pH 6.0, 70°C), Ruzicka *et al.* (1967) reports its half-life as 7.8 hr. The action of alkali in organic solvent converts it into fumarate and dimethyl phosphorodithioic acid. The latter forms a copper complex used in the quantitative estimation of malathion.

Malathion is not very toxic to mammals, but the detoxication mechanism

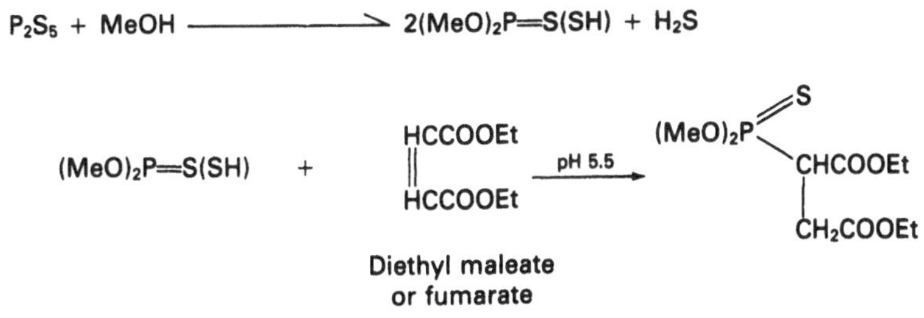

$$P_2S_5 + MeOH \longrightarrow 2(MeO)_2P{=}S(SH) + H_2S$$

Figure 9.1. Manufacture of malathion.

is dependent upon carboxyesterase activity and its action may therefore be potentiated by esterase inhibitors. Some impurities in the technical material such as O,S,S-trimethyl phosphorodithioate may increase its mammalian toxicity. This impurity was detected in one study (Pellegrini and Santi, 1972) at the 1% level, and two related homologs $[(MeO)_2P{=}O(SMe)$ and $(MeO)_2P{=}O(OMe)]$ were detected at the 0.1% and 0.2% levels. Their mammalian toxicities are high (LD_{50} 450, 47, and 96 mg/kg orally in rats) and they have a considerable effect on the toxicity of malathion.

Malathion of 92.2% purity had an LD_{50} of 1580 mg/kg, but 98% malathion had an LD_{50} of 8000 mg/kg; this marked difference indicates the magnitude of the effect of impurities.

A homolog of malathion has been identified as a residue on crops, and this compound, the ethyl butyl analog of malathion, is believed to be a contaminant of the commercial product (Gardner et al., 1969). More recently, the presence of a toxic contaminant, isomalathion, has been implicated in the deaths of workers (Baker et al., 1978).

Malathion is generally decomposed in the environment by hydrolysis and is also degraded by ultraviolet radiation. It does not appear to accumulate in the environment or to build up in food chains. Its biological transformations have been investigated in many species; since it is susceptible to degradation by phosphatases and carboxyesterases, the products are species-dependent. For example, Krueger and O'Brien (1959) found seven metabolites in mice that were fed malathion. The dose was 70–80% detoxified in 0.5 hr, and the major metabolites were the monoester (68%) and phosphatase hydrolysis products (20.5%).

It has been stated that malathion is one of the most benign pesticides available today (von Rumker et al., 1974). However, the onset of insect resistance associated with continued intensive use has been reported for a number of species. A recent FAO report of a global survey of pesticide susceptibility of stored-grain pests (Champ and Dyte, 1976) summarizes the position throughout the world. Resistance was found in 78 of 86 countries surveyed. It was present in all species tested but was most prevalent in *Tribolium* spp. and in *Rhyzopertha dominica*. The implications of the report are profound and extend beyond the future of malathion: there is evidence of resistance to fumigants as well as to insecticides. In its conclusion, the report stresses the need to maintain high standards of hygiene, because the ease with which control could be obtained in the past with insecticides, even with poor standards of hygiene, led to complacency and inadequate concern with the basic principles of food storage. It was recommended that chemical methods be used to give as complete a kill as possible to delay onset of reinfestation. Fumigants should be used for initial control of established infestations and insecticides should be applied when needed to prevent reinfestations.

9.4. ALTERNATIVE CHEMICAL CONTROL TECHNIQUES

Up to this point, I have discussed the use of insecticidal compounds—the fumigants and grain protectants. These conventional techniques may be supplemented by good hygiene and physical methods of insect control (e.g., inert atmospheres, specially designed storage facilities, infrasound treatment, gamma radiation, microwaves) or by newer chemical methods.

Insecticidal residues and the onset of insect resistance are two major problems associated with excessive reliance upon a limited number of chemical insecticides. In all aspects of insect control, it is important to use pesticides wisely, and any decision to use a pesticide should be based on a knowledge of the type and extent of infestation and the economic or other benefit to be expected from the treatment. Many more alternatives must be provided for the user, who is at present limited to a very restricted range of approved treatments. It is the obligation of the research scientist to explore the whole range of possible strategies that might be used in the control of insect pests.

Consideration of the physiology and biochemistry of the insect provides us with many potential sites at which chemical intervention might initiate a chain of events that could result in death or in failure to develop or reproduce. In an excellent review, Levinson (1975) discusses the potential application of insectistatics and pheromones in insect pest control, particularly with regard to the problem of stored-product insects. It is worthwhile to summarize its conclusions, because the author's approach is based on the physiology of the insect and explores the possibilities of utilizing agents that interfere with the normal function of physiologically active compounds. Some of these compounds are now in experimental use, others represent only hypothetical possibilities for utilization. Levinson uses the term *insectistatics* because most such agents affect growth and reproduction rather than having a direct insecticidal effect. He suggests that sublethal levels may be sufficient to exert control, which means we could avoid the problem of the rapid development of resistant species. The following approaches are suggested:

1. Compounds that affect the integument. Inhibition of the pathway of chitin biosynthesis is a promising method of reducing the survival rate of developing insects. A number of antagonists of chitin biosynthesis, of several structural types, are known. One of the most effective of these is the recently introduced compound diflubenzuron, N-([[(4-chlorophenyl)amino]-carbonyl)2,6-difluorobenzamide, an insecticide which may have wide application. Such compounds might be effectively utilized against stored-product insects by formulation in baits.

2. Compounds that affect hormone balance. Applications of compounds that have hormonelike activity are being explored. Such compounds are

often specific as to the species and functions that are affected. Affected functions include larval development, molting ability, egg mortality, and female sterility. (Neurohormones are currently a subject of interest; however, when Levinson's review was published, little was known of their structure, and the topic was not discussed.)

3. Nutrients and regulators of metabolism. Pests of stored products require a number of essential nutrients, including amino acids, carbohydrates, B vitamins, sterols, carotenoids, inorganic salts, and water. Antagonists of these nutrients can suppress growth or affect development, and overdoses of some may have similar adverse affects. Insect steroid metabolism presents an opportunity for design of molecules that may interfere with normal metabolic routes, and azasterols and other cholesterol derivatives may block normal biosynthetic routes. For example, the biosynthesis of ecdysone is important for the regulation of insect molt: the biological precursor of ecdysone is cholesterol, which must be derived from dietary sources, e.g., through degradation of phytosterols.

The utilization of energy resources may be affected by a number of substances termed *hypolipidemic compounds*. These cause rapid depletion of insect lipid content and may increase larval mortality or cause other insectistatic effects.

The absence of nutrients produced by symbiotic microorganisms may be lethal to insect species. Vitamin-producing symbionts such as yeast organisms may be inhibited by low concentrations of chemical antagonists.

4. Sex attractants and mating inhibitors. Sex and aggregation pheromones may be used for: (a) detection of sites of infestation; (b) estimation of population density; (c) luring of insects into traps where they may be killed, sterilized, or infected with pathogens; and (d) air permeation to disrupt mating (Stockel, 1975).

In this brief summary it is impossible to do full justice to Levinson's comprehensive review, which outlines many possible strategies for control based on consideration of insect physiology and biochemistry. The value of such an approach becomes more apparent as we recognize the continued appearance of insecticide resistance among major insect pests. This is not surprising when we consider many of the insecticides in current use and realize that they are designed to act on a limited number of target sites. For example, organophosphates, carbamates, pyrethroids, and organochlorine compounds act by affecting neural transmission. Cholinesterase inhibitors predominate among insecticides frequently used; it does not seem unreasonable that the onset of resistance in an insect species is often also accompanied by the appearance of cross-resistance to other insecticides that have similar modes of action. To avoid this situation, it may be desirable to increase the availability of new insecticides that act by different modes of action. However, even this approach may be more optimistic than can be justified by experience. An insecticide-resistant strain of *Tribolium castaneum* showed greater resistance to a mixture of methyl (*Z*)- and (*E*)-10,11-epoxy-7-ethyl-3,11-dimethyl-2,6-tridecadienoates than normal strains of the species (Levinson, 1975; Dyte, 1972). Brown (1977) has given an account of the problem and points out that multiresistant strains also show cross-tolerance to juvenile hormone mimics and other insect growth regulators. He predicts that resistance to insecticides will accumulate and spread in proportion to our use of chemicals, and he recommends that standard tests for resistance be used systematically at regular intervals. Thus in our continued reliance on insecticides we must be certain that they are used only when needed, and we must be aware of the need to constantly seek alternatives.

Several such alternative approaches have been developed. Considerable research experience has been gained in the potential applications of insect growth regulators and pheromones. Both classes of chemicals are generally rapidly degraded in the environment and are biologically metabolized to innocuous compounds. In fact, maintaining their biological effectiveness over a prolonged period often presents a problem, and special formulation techniques may be required to protect them against oxidation or photochemical breakdown in sunlight.

9.4.1. Compounds That Affect Insect Development

Insect growth regulators (IGRs) include a variety of compounds. Some, like diflubenzuron, affect molt by interfering with the synthesis of chitin; others mimic hormones, particularly the insect juvenile hormones. Siddall (1976) has defined IGRs as "substances which act within an insect to accelerate or inhibit a physiological regulatory process essential to normal development of an insect or its progeny in such a way that the action of the substance is necessarily dependent on the life stage of the insect." The use of IGRs would be insectistatic rather than insecticidal. It has been suggested that the rapid rate of development of stored-product pests renders them particularly suitable for control by IGRs (Levinson, 1975). Some IGRs are very effective against Coleoptera, acting at nanogram levels; sterility of emerging female khapra beetles (*Trogoderma granarium* Everts) is induced by application of 10^{-6} μg of 3,4-methylenedioxyphenyl 6,7-epoxygeranyl ether to single pupae (Metwally *et al.*, 1972). However, IGRs are usually rapidly degraded in the environment and may need to be formulated to provide controlled release. Methoprene [isopropyl (*E,E*)-11-methoxy-3,7,11-trimethyl-2,4-dodecadienoate] provides an example. Metabolism in rice or alfalfa plants gave 7-methoxycitronellal, an unexpected product, formed by oxidative rupture of the 4-ene double bond (Quistad *et al.*, 1974). In soil, breakdown was extensive and rapid, and there was substantial conversion of methoprene to carbon dioxide. The only metabolite that could be identified was the demethylated ester (0.7% of the total applied compound) (Schooley *et al.*, 1975). Mammalian metabolism studies indicate that at practical-use levels no toxic effects would be expected to occur in domestic animals. The most important photochemical reaction of methoprene was isomerization to the biologically inactive 2-*Z* isomer (Quistad *et al.*, 1975*a*). This mode of detoxication is found to occur in mosquitoes and house flies, neither of which can rapidly effect the reverse reaction (Quistad *et al.*, 1975*b*).

The juvenile hormone analogues are promising for control of some insects, but they are often specific for particular species. One problem associated with their use was noted by Brieger (1973), who observed that larvae of *Galleria mellonella* (L.) fed on methyl geranylgeranate grew excessively and remained in this state without pupation for 5 months; the inhibitory effect was reversed when a diet free from juvenoid was fed, whereas the results of topical application of juvenoids are irreversible. The expected appearance of resistant strains has already been mentioned. These difficulties must be considered before utilizing the juvenoids as pest control agents in food storage.

9.4.2. Compounds That Affect Insect Behavior

There is a rapidly increasing amount of literature on insect pheromones and their application to insect pest management. Pheromones and analogous compounds may cause intraspecific, short-term behavioral responses that cease rapidly after perception of the signal (releasers) or may effect more fundamental long-term physiological changes (primers). The chemicals utilized by the insects are often blends of more or less complex organic compounds of relatively low volatility that are secreted by specialized glands and may be detected by olfactory or chemotactic sensilla. Sex pheromones of the Lepidoptera are often secreted by the adult female and detected by the male, which is equipped with elaborate antennae. Detection is followed by orientation toward the odor source and by a complex series of behaviors that results in mating. The use of pheromones in trapping for survey or detection has been mentioned. Attempts to utilize pheromones for suppression of insect populations have usually relied upon the use of pheromone components or closely related analogues to interfere with the behavioral sequences involved in mating. Some success has been achieved by permeating the air with pheromones or related chemicals during the normal period of mating. The successful use of the permeation technique depends on many factors. The chemistry of the pheromone system and the behavioral responses of the insect toward chemical stimuli must be first established and the life cycle, habitat, and population dynamics of the insect must be thoroughly investigated. Finally, there is the matter of effective formulation of pheromones for application in pest management techniques, an area of specialization in which wide experience has not yet been gained.

The biological activity of pheromones is extremely high, and only a few molecules are required to induce behavioral responses. Because the quantities needed are infinitesimally small, as well as because of their extremely low mammalian toxicity and their lack of persistence, pheromones possess great potential for use in pest management systems without causing environmental contamination. However, without an effective delivery system and a careful study of the reproductive biology of the insect, it is just as easy to misuse this potentially powerful technique as it is to misuse conventional pesticides.

The complexity of pheromone systems has become increasingly clear as improved analytical techniques are applied to their study. Formerly many insects were required for conventional chemical techniques of extraction, isolation, and identification. Now it is sometimes possible to identify pheromonal components from a single insect. The sex pheromones of many Lepidoptera and other insects appear to be multicomponent mixtures that differ in component ratio as well as in chemical composition. This knowledge is particularly important in trapping insects, as well as in other behavioral studies, because the precise pheromonal blend must be reproduced for best results.

Other chemicals that affect behavior might also be used in management of stored-product pests. For example, the use of repellents for treating areas or packaging might be useful (DeLong, 1962). Indeed, in one test cockroaches did not enter food-containing cartons for over a week when the cartons were treated with substituted sulfonamides (McGovern *et al.*, 1975).

9.4.2.1. Trapping

Burkholder (1976, 1977) and others have shown the value of trapping techniques for management of stored-product insects. Barak and Burkholder (1976) studied the seasonal patterns of emergence of *Attagenus* and *Trogoderma* in warehouses in Milwaukee, Wisconsin, by using corrugated paper traps baited with pheromones. They were able to detect new infestations and to demonstrate that high populations of *A. megatoma* (F.) and *T. variabile* (Ballion) existed.

Levinson and Levinson (1979) have reported their success in mass-trapping of insects in grain stores. They used contact traps that release the sex pheromone system of the female khapra beetle, (Z)- and (E)-trogodermal [(Z)- and (E)-14-methyl-8-hexadecenal], in the ratio 10 : 1. Both components are capable of stimulating males of five dermestid species [*T. granarium, T. variabile, T. inclusum* (LeConte), *T. simplex* Jayne, and *T. glabrum* Herbst]. In other tests, sticky traps containing a source that releases (Z,E)-9,12-tetradecadien-1-ol acetate (ZETA) or (Z,E)-7,11-hexadecadien-1-ol acetate were used for phyticid and gelechiid species in flour mills and granaries. The species involved were *Ephestia elutella* (Hübner), *Anagasta kuehniella* (Zeller), *E. cautella* (Walker), *P. interpunctella*, and *Sitotroga cerealella* (Olivier).

Pheromones have also been used as lures to attract insects to pathogen-inoculating devices. Male *T. glabrum* beetles in simulated warehouse conditions were attracted by the pheromone to a corrugated cardboard inoculation device that dusted them with spores of a protozoan, *Mattesia trogodermae* Canning, diluted with cellulose powder. The disease was subsequently spread by contamination of females who transferred it to eggs and larvae. The result was substantial reduction of *T. glabrum* populations (Shapas *et al.*, 1977; Schwalbe *et al.*, 1974).

9.4.2.2. Mating Disruption

If pheromones are to be used for population suppression, it is essential to understand the subtleties and underlying complexity of the air permeation technique, because its effects will not resemble those of conventional pesticide application and its effectiveness must be monitored by very different criteria. Promising results have been obtained in attempts to reduce populations of stored-product insects by disruption of mating. However, the method may have disadvantages in certain circumstances. Although a single treatment of pheromone reduced the mating activity of *A. megatoma* in a sealed 208-liter fiber drum (Brukholder, 1973), Burkholder pointed out that such containers might be attractive to insects when they were shipped and opened, and that the warehouses themselves might draw insects from untreated areas. The experiments of Brady *et al.* (1975) were less encouraging. *P. interpunctella* and *E. cautella* were exposed to high pheromone levels for up to 99 days in commercial storage facilities, but the mating activity of the females was not reduced, compared with that of the control.

Greater success in disrupting mating of *E. cautella* was reported by Wheatley (1974). Experiments by Sower and Whitmer (1977) showed that the release of the synthetic pheromone reduced mating frequency of *P. interpunctella* and *E. cautella*. The degree of mating reduction was dependent upon pheromone dose and population density. Reproduction and population were greatly reduced in the presence of ZETA.

9.5. CONCLUSION

In this summary, I have outlined problems associated with the use of conventional fumigants and have indicated a number of alternative approaches to the chemical control of stored-product pests. The newer methods are based on chemicals that are readily degraded and present little threat to the environment.

However, they cannot be applied simply and effectively as can volatile fumigants. When their action is well understood, simple methods of application will be devised, but at present the use of these materials is not yet a practical alternative for insect control. This is unfortunate, since the problems of potentially harmful residues and developing insect resistance limit the time available to us for discovery of substitutes for many conventional fumigants.

REFERENCES

Alumot, E., Nachtomi, E., Bielorai, R., and Harduf, Z., 1974, Significance of fumigant residues in animal feed, in: *Isotope Tracer Studies of Chemical Residues in Food and the Agricultural Environment*, pp. 3–10, International Atomic Energy Agency, Vienna.

Amir, D., and Volcani, R., 1965, Effect of dietary ethylene dibromide on bull semen, *Nature (London)* **206**:99.

Baker, E. L., Jr., Zack, M., Miles, J. W., Alderman, L., Warren, M., Dobbin, R. D., Miller, S., and Teeters, W. R., 1978, Epidemic malathion poisoning in Pakistan malaria workers, *Lancet* **1978-I**:31.

Barak, A. V., and Burkholder, W. E., 1976, Trapping studies with dermestid sex pheromones, *Environ. Entomol.* **5**:111.

Bierer, B. W., and Vickers, C. L., 1959, The effect on egg size and production of fungicide-treated and fumigated grains fed to hens, *J. Am. Vet. Med. Assoc.* **134**:452.

Brady, U. E., Jay, E. G., Redlinger, L. M., and Pearman, G., 1975, Mating activity of *Plodia interpunctella* and *Cadra cautella* during exposure to synthetic sex pheromone in the field, *Environ. Entomol.* **4**:441.

Bridges, R. G., 1955, The fate of labelled insecticide residues in food products. III. *N*-Methylation as a result of fumigating wheat with methyl bromide, *J. Sci. Food Agric.* **6**:261.

Brieger, G., 1973, Juvenile hormone analogue in diet of the waxmoth *Galleria mellonella*, *Naturwissenschaften* **60**:261.

Brown, A. W. A., 1977, The progression of resistance mechanisms developed against insecticides, in: *Pesticide Chemistry in the 20th Century* (J. R. Plimmer, ed.), pp. 21–38. ACS Symposium Series No. 37, American Chemical Society, Washington, D.C.

Burkholder, W. E., 1973, Black carpet beetle: Reduction of mating by megatomoic acid, the sex pheromone, *J. Econ. Entomol.* **66**:1327.

Burkholder, W. E., 1976, Applications of pheromones for manipulating insect pests of stored products, in: *Insect Pheromones and Their Applications* (T. Kono and S. Ishii, eds.), pp. 111–122, Proceedings of a Symposium, Nagaoka and Tokyo, Japan, December 8–11, 1976, Japan Plant Protection Association, Tokyo.

Burkholder, W. E., 1977, Manipulation of insect pests of stored products, in: *Chemical Control of Insect Behavior* (H. H. Shorey and J. J. McKelvey, Jr., eds.), pp. 345–351, Wiley, New York.

Champ, B. R., and Dyte, C. E., 1976, *Report of the FAO Global Survey of Pesticide Susceptibility of Stored Grain Pests*, FAO Plant Production and Protection Series No. 5, Rome.

Cotton, R. T., and Ashby, W., 1952, Insect pests of stored grains and seed, in: *Insects*, pp. 620–639, 1952 Yearbook of Agriculture, U.S. Department of Agriculture, Washington, D.C.

DeLong, D. M., 1962, Beer cases and soft drink cartons as insect distributors, *Pest Control* **30**(7):14.

Dyte, C. E., 1972, Resistance to synthetic juvenile hormone in a strain of the flour beetle, *Tribolium castaneum*, *Nature (London)* **238**:48.

Eto, M., 1974, *Organophosphorus Pesticides: Organic and Biological Chemistry*, CRC Press, Cleveland, Ohio.

Fishbein, L., 1976, Potential hazards of fumigant residues, *Environ. Health Perspect.* **14**:39.

Fowler, D. L., and Mahan, J. N., 1976, *The Pesticide Review 1975*, U.S. Department of Agriculture Agricultural Stabilization Conservation Service, Washington, D.C.

Gardner, A. M., Damico, J. N., Hansen, E. A., Lustig, E., and Storherr, R. W. 1969, Previously unreported homolog of malathion found as residue on crops, *J. Agric. Food Chem.* **17**:1181.

Krueger, H. R., and O'Brien, R. D., 1959, Relationship between metabolism and differential toxicity of malathion in insects and mice, *J. Econ. Entomol.* **52**:1063.

Levinson, H. Z., 1975, Possibilities of using insectistatics and pheromones in pest control, *Naturwissenschaften* **62**:272.

Levinson, H. Z., and Levinson, A. R., 1979, Trapping of storage insects by sex and food attractants as a tool of integrated control, in: *Chemical Ecology: Odour Communication in Animals* (F. J. Ritter, ed.), pp. 327–341, Elsevier/North-Holland Biomedical Press, Amsterdam.

McGovern, T. P., Burden, G. S., and Beroza, M., 1975, *n*-Alkanesulfonamides as repellents for the German cockroach [Orthoptera (Dictyoptera):Blatellidae], *J. Med. Entomol.* **12**:387.

Metwally, M. M., Sehnal, F., and Landa, V., 1972, Reduction of fecundity and control of the khapra beetle by juvenile hormone mimics, *J. Econ. Entomol.* **65**:1603.

Nachtomi, E., 1970, The metabolism of ethylene dibromide in the rat: The enzymic reaction with glutathione *in vitro* and *in vivo*, *Biochem. Pharmacol.* **19**:2853.

Olson, W. A., Habermann, R. T., Weisburger, E. K., Ward, I. M., and Weisburger, J. H., 1973, Induction of stomach cancer in rats and mice by halogenated aliphatic fumigants, *J. Natl. Cancer Inst.* **51**:1993.

Pellegrini, G., and Santi, R., 1972, Potentiation of toxicity of organophosphorus compounds containing carboxylic ester functions toward warm-blooded animals by some organophosphorus impurities, *J. Agric. Food Chem.* **20**:944.

Quistad, G. B., Staiger, L. E., and Schooley, D. A., 1974, Environmental degradation of the insect growth regulator methoprene (isopropyl (2*E*, 4*E*)-11-methoxy-3,7,11-trimethyl-2,4-dodecadienoate). I. Metabolism by alfalfa and rice, *J. Agric. Food Chem.* **22**:582.

Quistad, G. B., Staiger, L. E., and Schooley, D. A., 1975*a*, Environmental degradation of the insect growth regulator methoprene (isopropyl (2*E*, 4*E*)-11-methoxy-3,7,11-trimethyl-2,4-dodecadienoate. III. Photodecomposition, *J. Agric. Food Chem.* **23**:299.

Quistad, G. B., Staiger, L. E., and Schooley, D. A., 1975*b*, Environmental degradation of the insect growth regulator methoprene. V. Metabolism by houseflies and mosquitoes, *Pestic. Biochem. Physiol.* **5**:233.

Ruzicka, J. H., Thomson, J., and Wheals, B. B., 1967, The gas chromatographic determination of organophosphorus pesticides. Part II. A comparative study of hydrolysis rates, *J. Chromatogr.* **31**:37.

Schooley, D. A., Creswell, K. M., Staiger, L. E., and Quistad, G. B., 1975, Environmental degradation of the insect growth regulator isopropyl (2*E*, 4*E*)-11-methoxy-3,7,11-trimethyl-2,4-dodecadienoate (methoprene). IV. Soil metabolism, *J. Agric. Food Chem.* **23**:369.

Schwalbe, C. P., Burkholder, W. E., and Boush, G. M., 1974, *Mattesia trogodermae* infection rates as influenced by mode of transmission, dosage, and host species, *J. Stored Prod. Res.* **10**:161.

Shapas, T. J., Burkholder, W. E., and Boush, G. M., 1977, Population suppression of *Trogoderma glabrum* by using pheromone luring for protozoan pathogen dissemination, *J. Econ. Entomol.* **70**:469.

Siddall, J. B., 1976, Insect growth regulators and insect control: A critical appraisal, *Environ. Health Perspect.* **14**:119.

Sower, L. L., and Whitmer, G. P., 1977, Population growth and mating success of Indian meal moths and almond moths in the presence of synthetic sex pheromone, *Environ. Entomol.* **6**:17.

Stockel, J., 1975, Les phéromones sexuelles chez les insectes de denrées: Possibilités d'applications practiques, *Rev. Zool. Agric. Pathol. Veg.* **74**:158.

von Rumker, R., Lawless, E. W., Meiners, A. F., Lawrence, K. A., Kelso, G. L., and Horay, F., 1974, *Production, Distribution, Use and Environmental Impact Potential of Selected Pesticides*, EPA 540/1-74-001, Environmental Protection Agency, Washington, D.C.

Wheatley, P. E., 1974, Research being undertaken by the Tropical Stored Products Centre in the United Kingdom and overseas, *Bull. OEPP* **4**:495.

Winteringham, F. P. W., 1955, The fate of labelled insecticide residues in food products. IV. The possible toxicological and nutritional significance of fumigating wheat with methyl bromide, *J. Sci. Food Agric.* **6**:269.

Winteringham, F. P. W., Harrison, A., Bridges, R. G., and Bridges, P. M., 1955, The fate of labelled insecticide residues in food products, II. The nature of methyl bromide residues in fumigated wheat, *J. Sci. Food Agric.* **6**:251.

10

Application of Biodegradable Pesticides in India

C. R. Krishna Murti and T. S. S. Dikshith

10.1. INTRODUCTION

Ever since man organized agriculture as a profession, pesticides in some form or another have been in use in plant protection. The rapid strides of the last four decades resulting from the synthesis, manufacture, and application of new man-made chemical compounds in pest control have, however, brought about the dramatic changes in agriculture. By keeping in check many species of unwanted pests and weeds, pesticides have made a great impact on the production and preservation of food, fiber, and other cash crops. The introduction of pesticides has initiated revolutionary changes in farm practice, leading to the incredible possibility that hunger can be banished forever from the earth. So much for the credits of pesticides.

The debits of pesticides have given rise to many serious health and environmental problems. Most of the chlorinated nondegradable pesticides tend to leave residues in living organisms. These residues are retained by the organisms for prolonged periods of their life span and are presumably responsible for a variety of known toxic symptoms. Even when pesticides are present in trace amounts, their chemical diversity, potential toxicity, and persistence adversely affect birds, fish, and trees. Furthermore, under tropical conditions, the chemical transformation of pesticides can be expected to be relatively fast due to heat,

C. R. Krishna Murti and T. S. S. Dikshith ● Industrial Toxicology Research Center, Lucknow 226001, India.

light, humidity, and diverse microbial activity. The food habits of people living in the tropic and subtropic regions are also quite different from those in temperate regions. When considering the impact of toxic chemicals on human health, it becomes imperative to take into account the climatic, socioeconomic, ethnic, and health backgrounds (e.g., nutritional status, coexistent parasitic diseases) of the people exposed to the chemicals.

The per-hectare use of pesticides in India is at present about 330 g as opposed to 1490 g in Japan. The use of pesticides in India is certain to register an upward trend in order to meet the increasing food needs of a growing population and to contain vector-borne human and cattle diseases. The use of pesticides has thus become an essential part of the Indian strategy of crop protection, particularly under an intensive agriculture program envisaging high-yielding and short-duration varieities of cereals and pulses. The toxicological implications of the extensive use of pesticides in agriculture are consequently of great relevance to problems of health planning.

Pesticides came into wide use in agriculture and public health around 1944. The benefits, manifested as enhanced farm productivity and inexpensive control of insect-borne diseases, were so overwhelming that the problem of their toxicity was ignored until 1960.

Pesticides, microorganisms, soil, water, and air interact with one another in a closed network system. Various factors are involved (Venkataraman and Rajya Lakshmi, 1971) in the bioactivation/detoxification of pesticides in the above network. The problem of contamination of grain, pesticides, dairy products, vegetables, and fruits and of the living environment can be visualized from Fig. 10.1. DDT levels in some food products are listed in Table 10.1. Elucidation of the factors controlling the interaction of pesticides with environmental factors has posed a challenge to scientists. The symptoms of poisoning due to accidental or occupational exposure to pesticides have been recognized in India. Episodes of poisoning in 1955 in Cochin and Kerala (Karunakaran, 1958), in the Sitapur–Hardoi area, and in Uttar Pradesh in 1977 and the "Handigodu syndrome" of Karnataka (Report of National Institute of Nutrition, Hyderabad, 1977) have been documented.

Pesticidal chemicals in use today cover hundreds of organic molecules. Among these, the "insecticides" are regarded as the ones which cause the maximum health hazards. The persistent types, such as DDT, BHC, endosulfan, aldrin, dieldrin, endrin, heptachlor, toxaphene, and chlordane, are all varieties of organochlorine insecticides. Being readily soluble in lipids, they accumulate in fat deposits of man and animals. In addition, they are not metabolized fast enough to facilitate their rapid elimination from the body.

Two other important types of insecticides are the organophosphorus compounds [exemplified by parathion, malathion, diazinon, dichlorvos, methyl demeton, phosphamidon, fenitrothion (Sumithion), dimethoate, and quinalphos]

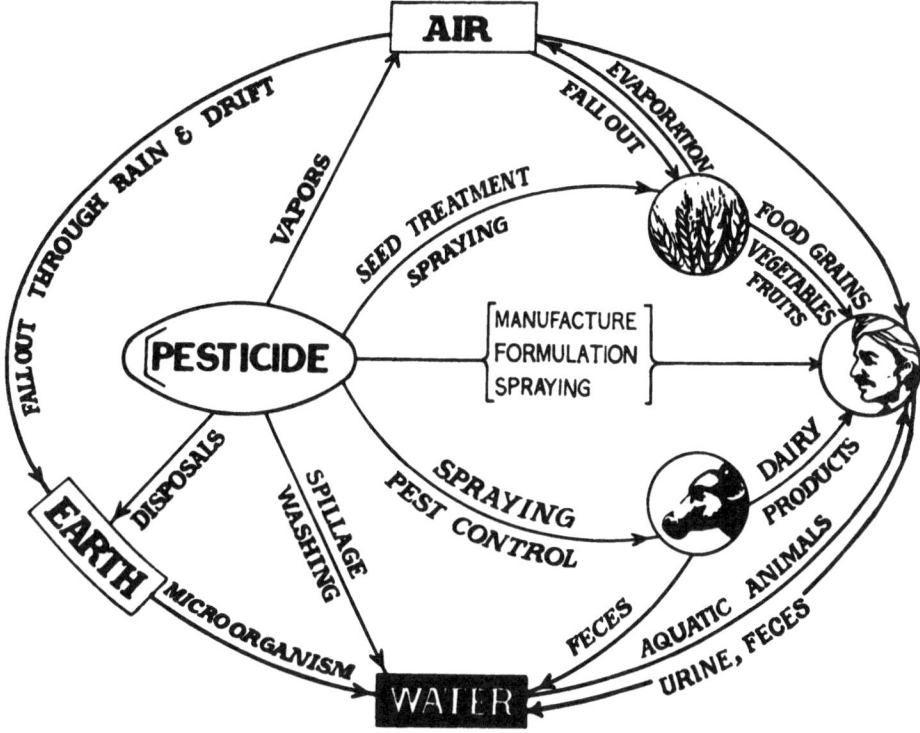

Figure 10.1. Schematic diagram depicting pesticide cycle in the environment.

and the carbamates [such as carbaryl, carbofuran, and aldicarb]. Fortunately, these are slightly more soluble in water and in biological fluids. They are also easily biotransformed and are thus rapidly excreted and consequently do not accumulate in biological tissues to a great extent. A suggestion has been made, therefore, that the persistent organochlorine pesticides should be replaced by the latter two types of biodegradable pesticides. The organophosphates have, in general, quick effects. One has to remember all the same that many organophosphorus insecticides show high acute toxicity to man and animals. Some of them are also implicated in certain types of delayed neural toxicity.

It is a matter of concern that no suitable substitute for DDT/BHC has been found to this point. The properties of persistence and relative resistance to biodegradation make DDT and BHC ideal insecticides for public health and agriculture. An average Indian farmer has to spray his crop once or twice with persistent pesticides to get the same benefit that he derives from 6 to 8 sprays of nonpersistent pesticides.

Table 10.1.   DDT Levels in Food Products in India

Food articles	DDT levels (ppm)	Sampling period	Place of sampling
Butter	0.04 ± 0.14	1965	Pantnagar
	1.1–8.0	1974	Delhi
Milk	0.0032 ± 0.0026	1965	Pantnagar
	Traces–0.2	1969–1971	Hyderabad
Toned milk	Not detectable	1972	Delhi
Eggs	USFDA tolerance	1969–1971	Hyderabad
Eggs (shell-free)	Not detectable–0.24	1973	Delhi
Fat of buffaloes, goats, and cows	0.538	1965	Pantnagar
Fish	Traces	1969–1971	Hyderabad
Mutton and beef	USFDA tolerance	1969–1971	Hyderabad
Wheat flour	12–15	1958	—
Wheat grains	0.41 ± 0.23	1965	Pantnagar
	0.05	1965	Delhi
	4–6	1970	Ludhiana
Cereals	Traces–0.8	1970–1971	Hyderabad
Rice	9–16	1958	—
Pulses	5–35	1958	—
	Traces–0.5	1970–1971	Hyderabad
Groundnut seeds	3.2–4.1	1969	Delhi
Mustard seeds	1.1–2.4	1969	Delhi
Sesame seeds	2.3–3.1	1969	Delhi
Linseed	1.7–2.4	1969	Delhi
Groundnut oil	5.0–7.1	1969	Delhi
Mustard oil	22.1–25.7	1969	Delhi
Sesame oil	10.0–12.1	1969	Delhi
Coconut oil	9.3–10.6	1969	Delhi

Until DDT was banned in the U.S., the average American was exposed to 30 times the amount of environmental levels of DDT as compared to the exposure in India. Yet the blood levels of DDT and its metabolites in Indian subjects are somewhat higher than those of the inhabitants of North America and other parts of the world (Dikshith, 1978). Numerous experimental studies with diverse groups of animals have not produced convincing evidence demonstrating harmful effects caused by DDT administered at doses general populations are expected to receive. BHC has been shown to induce carcinoma in selected species of animals at high doses. Although p,p'-DDD has been shown to modulate microsomal enzyme activity, evidence adduced by scientists in the National Institute of Occupational Health in Ahmedabad, India, indicates a progressive decline in the power of p,p'-DDE to elicit microsomal activity by the process of induction. Fish and birds are more susceptible than humans. Lethal concentrations required to bring about such ill effects can be produced in bird and fish tissues by even a single environmental exposure.

Aldrin, BHC, and heptachlor are very effective soil insecticides because of their relatively high vapor pressure. Toxaphene was once widely used to control external parasites on cattle, sheep, and other domestic animals, the advantage being its ready excretion and hence negligible tissue storage. The use of toxaphene for veterinary purposes is, however, now banned in the United States. Combination products of toxaphene and DDT have also been phased out in India. In many countries, the use of DDT has also been banned in view of its residual effects and suspected carcinogenic potential based on experiments in mice. In India, it is still permitted along with BHC in the campaign against malaria and other insect vector-borne diseases.

Keeping in mind the vast area to be covered in India and the compelling necessity to control malaria, efforts have been made to meet the country's requirements by indigenous production. The current production is around 5000 metric tons, although the installed capacity is 14,000 metric tons. DDT–toxaphene was also sprayed until recently in the form of Heliotox for the control of cotton pests. Residues of DDT were analyzed in the seed and lint of cotton and found to be below the tolerance level of 7 ppm after 4 days. However, when DDT was applied combined with toxaphene the residues were always higher than when DDT was applied alone. The rate of disappearance of DDT from sprays of DDT–toxaphene was much slower than that of DDT from DDT sprays (Anonymous, 1977).

The mechanism of bio- or physicochemical degradation from soil and plants is poorly understood. The need for intensive research in this area must be emphasized. Considering its magnitude, the problem of persistence of residues in plants and in fat deposits of man and animals has not yet attracted the attention of many scientists in India.

The present overview of the situation is prompted by a desire to identify areas of research out of which remedial action can, it is to be hoped, be devised to protect plants, soil, animals, and above all humans from the potential hazards of pesticides and their derivatives and degradation products (Anonymous, 1979*b*).

10.2. THE PESTICIDE INDUSTRY IN INDIA

The manufacture of pesticides began in India in 1952 with the construction of a plant for producing BHC. This was followed by a plant for DDT. Among the South Asian and African countries, excluding Japan, India is the largest manufacturer of basic pesticidal chemicals. In all, 122 pesticides have been

Table 10.2.   List of Insecticides Approved for Registration
under the Insecticides Act, 1968

1. BHC	62. Triallate
2. DDT	63. Alachlor
3. Malathion	64. Alpha napthyl acetic acid
4. Copper oxychloride	65. Chlormaquate chloride
5. Cuprous oxide	66. Nitrofen
6. Copper sulfate	67. Butachlor
7. Lindane (Gamma-BHC)	68. Phorate
8. Carbaryl	69. Monocropotophos
9. Dimethoate	70. Phenthoate
10. Zineb	71. Phosalone
11. Ziram	72. Ethion
12. Thiram	73. Fluchloralin (Basalin)
13. Aldrin	74. Carbendazim (Bavistin)
14. Chlordane	75. Benomyl
15. Heptachlor	76. Dicofol
16. Toxaphene	77. Mancozeb
17. PMA	78. Paraquat dischloride
18. EMC	79. Difonphos
19. MEMC	80. Propoxur
20. Sulfur	81. Carbofuran
21. Lime sulfur	82. Carboxin
22. Diazinon	83. Siramate
23. Oxydemeton	84. Simazine
24. Zinc phosphide	85. Atrazine
25. Captan	86. Linuron
26. 2,4-D	87. Ediphenphos (Hinesan)
27. Dalapon	88. Gibberellic acid
28. Nicotine sulfate	89. Chlorfenvinphos
29. Thiometon	90. Aureofungin
30. Aluminum phosphide	91. Formothion
31. Dichlorvos (DDVP)	92. Chlorpyriphos
32. Methyl bromide	93. DSMA
33. Ethylene dibromide	94. MSMA
34. EDCT	95. Propanil
35. Pyrethrum	96. Calixin
36. Warfarin	97. Difolaton
37. Ferbam	98. Dinocap
38. MCPA	99. Copper aceto arsenite (Paris
39. Trichlorophon (Dipterex)	Green)
40. PCNB	100. Dibromochloropropane
41. Tetradifon	101. Methyl parathion
42. Fenthion	102. Nickel chloride
43. Allathrin	103. Methabenzthiazuron (Tribunil)
44. Carbon tetrachloride	104. Aldicarb
45. DD mixture	105. Streptocycline
46. Sodium cyanide	106. Ethepon
47. Calcium cyanide	107. Barium carbonate

(Continued)

Table 10.2. *(Continued)*

48.	Paradichlorobenzene	108.	Paraquat dimethyl sulfate
49.	Maleic hydrazide	109.	Metoxuron
50.	Pentachorophenol (PCP)	110.	Menazon
51.	Trichloroacetic acid (TCA)	111.	Glyphosate (roundup)
52.	Chlorebenzilate	112.	Amitraz
53.	Metaldehyde	113.	Bendiocarb (Ficam)
54.	Maneb	114.	Benzoylpropethyl (Suffix)
55.	Coumachlor	115.	Cyanazine (Bladex)
56.	Thanite (isobarnyl thiocyanoacetate)	116.	Etrimfoe (Satisfar)
		117.	Glyodin
57.	Endosulfan	118.	Oxadiazon (Ronstar)
58.	Fenitrothion	119.	Oxyfluorfen (Coal)
59.	Phosphamidon	120.	Propetamphos (Safrotin)
60.	Quinalphos	121.	Scilliroside (Silmurin)
61.	Diruon	122.	Thiocyclam hydrogenoxalate

approved for registration and use in agriculture so far (Anonymous, 1980) (Table 10.2). The government has licensed the production of 82,135 tons of various pesticides; out of which a capacity for 67,474 tons has already been installed. At present 23 units are engaged in manufacturing technical-grade pesticides and about 50 units are preparing formulations based on technical-grade pesticides produced indigenously or imported. The quantity and value of pesticides produced in the organized sector during the year 1976–1977 is given in Table 10.3. The production of technical material in 1977 was 40,685 tons. The actual installed capacity of important technical pesticides in 1977 is shown in Fig. 10.2. In addition, about 350 units in the small-scale sector undertake the manufacture of conventional formulations, mainly dust powder (360,000 metric tons) and, to a limited extent, wettable powder (90,000 metric tons), emulsifiable concentrates (45,000 metric tons), and granules (3750 metric tons). A few sophisticated pesticides are also allowed to be imported to cope with the qualitative changes in the cropping pattern inherent to the program of intensive cultivation of cereals, legumes, cotton, tobacco, coffee, and tea. Total imports during 1976–1977 were approximately 6106.2 tons (Anonymous, 1978*a*, 1979*a*).

Table 10.3. Production of Pesticides, 1976–1977

Quantity (tons)	1976	Value (millions of rupees)	1977
Technical material	34,703	4.19	40,685
Formulations			
Solid	70,739	3.32	—
Liquid	11,045	3.50	—

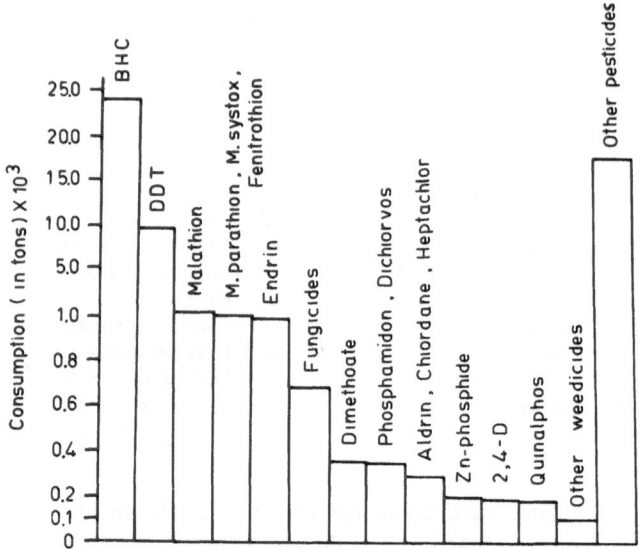

Figure 10.2. Quantity and value of pesticide produced in the country during 1976.

10.2.1. Consumption of Pesticides in India

Estimated requirements and consumption of technical-grade pesticides for agriculture and public health were officially estimated as 58,540 tons during 1976. Other requirements of pesticides are closely related to the plant protection coverage programs. According to the Ministry of Agriculture, the covered area in hectares of plant protection was expected to be around 70 million during 1977–1978, 75 million during 1978–1979, and 100 million by 1982–1983. Based on the anticipated coverage of plant protection measures, the requirements of technical-grade pesticides have been estimated at 62,607 tons in 1977–1978, 66,871 tons during 1978–1979, and approximately 80,000 tons by 1982–1983 (Table 10.4).

Consumption of pesticides for protection of public health in the past and the future estimates are shown in Fig. 10.3.

10.2.2. Development of Process Technology within the Country

An official report reveals that the technology for the production of new pesticides like phenthoates and endosulfan has been generated and that manufacture is expected to commence shortly. During the next 5 years, such pesticides

Table 10.4. Requirements of Pesticides, 1977–1982 (in Metric Tons)

Pesticides	1977–1978	1978–1979	1982–1983
Insecticides			
1. BHC	27,000	28,000	33,000
2. DDT	5,400	5,400	5,600
3. Malathion	2,600	2,800	3,500
4. Methyl demeton			
5. Fenitrothion	1,000	1,700	2,000
6. Parathion			
7. Endosulfan	1,100	1,200	1,600
8. Carbaryl	5,000	6,500	7,500
9. Dimethoate	800	850	1,000
10. Phosphamidon	650	650	650
11. Quinalphos	300	500	1,000
12. Chlordane ⎫			
13. Heptachlor ⎬	860	900	1,000
14. Aldrin ⎭			
15. Phenthoate	300	300	600
16. Monocrotophos ⎫	450	450	600
17. Chlorfenvinphos ⎭			
18. DDVP (dichlorovos)	250	280	300
19. Carbofuran	150	200	250
Acaricides			
1. Dicofol ⎫			
2. Ethion ⎬	80	100	150
3. Tetradifon ⎭			
Fungicides			
1. Dithiocarbamates (Zineb, Ziram, Thiram, and Mancozeb)	2,500	2,700	3,000
2. Sulfur (wettable and dusting powder)	4,000	4,500	5,000
3. Copper sulfate	4,000	4,400	5,000
4. PCNB	75	100	150
5. Captafol	75	80	100
6. Organomercurials	12	13	15
7. Kerathane ⎫			
8. Hinosan ⎪			
9. Carboxin ⎬	155	220	390
10. Carbondazinn ⎪			
11. Benomyl ⎭			
12. Calixin			
13. Nickel chloride	70	80	90
Rodenticides			
1. Zinc phosphide ⎫			
2. Warfarin ⎬	600	650	750
3. Coumeryl ⎭			

(Continued)

Table 10.4. *(Continued)*

Pesticides	1977–1978	1978–1979	1982–1983
Weedicides/herbicides			
1. Dalapon	200	230	250
2. 2,4-D	500	650	1,000
3. Nitrofen ⎱			
4. Propanil ⎰	175	275	500
5. Alachlor			
6. Dutachlor	100	150	300
7. Paraquat	100	200	300
8. Diuran	40	60	100
9. MSMA and DSMA	150	150	300
10. Triazine	10	12	25
11. Fluchlorin	10	12	20
12. MCPA ⎱	15	10	25
13. MCPD ⎰			
14. Sirmate	20	25	40
Nomaticides			
1. DD	10	15	25
2. Fensulfothion	25	30	50
3. Aldicarb	25	30	50
Plant growth regulators			
1. CCS and NAA ⎱			
2. Ethopon	50	60	100
3. Maleic hydrazide			
4. Gibberallic ⎰			
Fumigants			
1. EDD ⎱			
2. M. Dr.	100	125	200
3. EDCT ⎰			
4. All phosphide	100	125	200

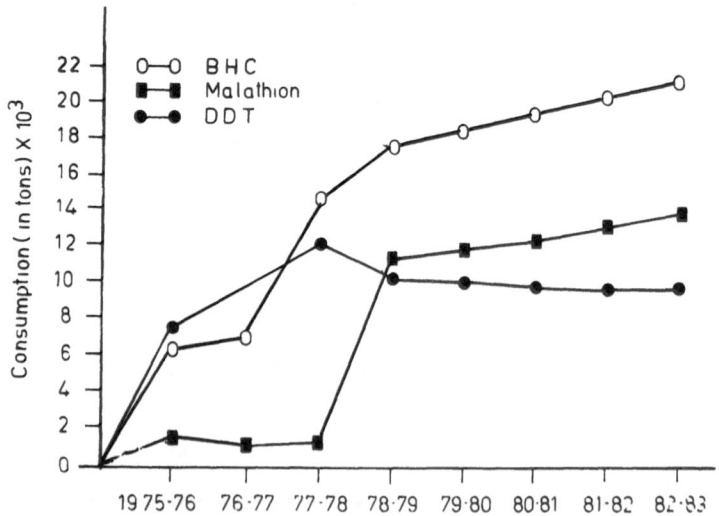

Figure 10.3. Consumption of pesticides for public health program.

as carbaryl, monocrotophos, paraquat, and bavistin are expected to be produced indigenously.

The Indian Council of Scientific and Industrial Research has also supported R&D activities in national laboratories for the development of technology. As a result, process packages for the manufacture of several known pesticides such as endosulfan, MBC, nitrofen, atrazine, simazine, dalapon, monocrotophos, diazinon, quinalphos, phosphamidon, DDVP, methoxychlor, and carboxin have been developed. Works on the following pesticides are at various stages of development: carbaryl, metasystox, methyl parathion, phosalone, thiometon, carbofuran, propanil, divron, paraquat, and diazinon.

10.3. BIODEGRADATION OF PESTICIDES BY MICROORGANISMS

Pesticides are acted upon by a variety of interrelated physical and chemical factors and microbial organisms. Physicochemical reactions could lead to incomplete degradation with the formation of products that continue to persist. More complete transformation of pesticides is mediated essentially by microorganisms, the role of some of which is now well established in soil and water. That many pesticides are biotransformed by microorganisms is now well recognized (Alexander, 1965; Kearney and Kaufman, 1969; Kaufman and Kearney, 1970; Kandaswamy *et al.*, 1977; Sheela and Vasantharajan, 1978*a,b*; Griffiths and Walker, 1970; Patil *et al.*, 1972; Sethunathan, 1973; Balasubramanya and Patil, 1976; Chahal *et al.*, 1977). Factors such as moisture, temperature, organic matter, fertilizers, and surfactants can affect the degradation of pesticides in soil. In general, moisture, high temperature, and high organic matter in soil enhance the rate of degradation. Fertilizers and surfactants, on the other hand, could suppress the rate of degradation significantly, the effect being modulated by the action of soil microflora (Anonymous, 1978*b*).

A major quantity of orthane, ingested by the body, is excreted within 24 hr. Buildup in soil does not occur, nor does it accumulate in the natural food chain (Anonymous, 1973). It kills a wide range of pests, especially those which have developed resistance to chlorinated hydrocarbons. However, it is not as effective as chlorinated hydrocarbons against soil pests. Methomyl, a carbamate insecticide, has been known to undergo biodegradation very rapidly in soil, presumably mediated by soil microorganisms (Harvey and Pease, 1973). Methomyl has no residual effect in tobacco, cotton, and cabbage, since it has a half-life of only 3–6 days (Harvey and Reiser, 1973).

Unlike organochloride insecticides, the organophosphorus compounds are readily degraded on the surface of plants, inside their tissues, and in soil and water and hence may pose less serious problems of environmental pollution than those caused by organochlorine pesticides. The fate of parathion in certain rice-growing fields of India under flooded conditions and the role of microorganisms in its degradation have been investigated. After the first application to a flooded soil, parathion degradation proceeded via nitro group reduction to aminoparathion. But after the second application, substantial hydrolysis occurred in addition to reduction. After the third application, the pathway was essentially one of hydrolysis. Thus, the metabolism of parathion shifted from reduction to hydrolysis after repeated applications (Sethunathan et al., 1975).

Three-day-old larvae of the silk worm Bombyx mori L. were used to monitor the persistance of fensulfothion in soil under laboratory conditions (Sheela and Vasantharajan, 1978a). Paper chromatographic and TLC analysis revealed that fensulfothion and its oxygen analogue were the predominant breakdown products. Compatibility of fensulfothion, chlorfenvinphos, and chloropyriphos was studied with NPK fertilizers. The degradation of fensulfothion was 6–10% in the first 100 days. Chloropyriphos degraded anywhere from 8.9–34.8%, whereas chlorfenvinphos showed the highest degradation rate, 37.5–94.6% (Anonymous, 1978b).

In general, monocrotophos and dicrotophos, when mixed with fertilizers, degraded faster than did phorate and disulfoton mixed with fertilizers. Thus in 120 days at 30°C the rate of degradation of the former was 10–40% as compared to 8–30% of the latter. An increase in temperature from 30° to 50°C was found to enhance the amount of insecticide degraded in all cases. The effect of temperature was, however, more pronounced (1- to 1.5-fold increase) on monocrotophos and dicrotophos than on phorate and disulfoton. Addition of moisture at the 5% level increased the rate of degradation by 1.5- to 3.5-fold at 30°C and 1.5- to 5-fold at 50°C (Anonymous, 1978b).

Fruits of tomato sprayed with carbaryl contained very little residue, suggesting a quick degradation of the insecticide (Singh and Singh, 1970). No residue was detected in the stem, or on cobs of maize and on cauliflower treated with carbaryl (Deshmukh and Saramma, 1971). Abelmoschus esculantus (Bhindi, okra) showed no residues of the insecticide 3 days after spraying, indicating faster dissipation (Raghuraj et al., 1973).

Carbofuran has been used for the control of the sorghum shoot fly in India. Straw as well as grain contained no residues of carbofuran, indicating fast dissipation (Gupta and Dewan, 1974). Baygon (2-isopropoxyphenyl-N-methylcarbamate) was degraded to 2-isopropoxy phenol by Pseudomonas sp. (Gupta et al., 1979).

10.4. INSECTICIDES OF PLANT ORIGIN

Attempts have been made to identify and utilize plant products as insecticides. About 2000 species of plants have been known to offer products possessing insecticidal defense against insect pests. In contrast to organic insecticides, the insecticides of plant origin are relatively less toxic to man, animals, and other plants, but are highly effective with species of insects.

Of the pesticides originating from plants, nicotine sulfate and pyrethrum extract have wide-range use. The bulk of about 15,300 tons of pyrethrum comes from Kenya and Tanzania. A limited amount of about 10 tons is the contribution from India. There is a great potential for the expansion of cultivation of pyrethum in India along the Himalayan foothills—all the way from Assam to Kashmir. Programs are also being developed for producing synthetic pyrethrums, particularly Permethrin. This product is presently undergoing bioefficacy tests.

Various formulations of pyrethrum have been used for household sprays. In Indian the production of different formulations of pyrethrum have gradually increased over the years. During 1976–1977 the total production was about 2000 kiloliters; in 1977–1978 it was about 2700 kiloliters. Further, India imported about 11,500 kg of pyrethrum during the last 2 years.

Production of nicotine sulfate from tobacco waste is steadily increasing in India. During 1966–1967 the total production was about 23,200 kg; presently the total quantity is about 90,000 kg.

Plants and Insecticides. Plants come in contact with insecticides either through direct application or through soil. Direct application of sprays, dusts, or granules to soils often leads to a low but detectable level of residues at the time of harvest. Insecticides have been recovered from fruits, vegetables, mushrooms, grains, spices, forage crops, feeds, tobacco, and trees. Moreover, products processed from such contaminated plants also contain residues of insecticides.

Cyclodiene insecticides have been found to undergo extensive rearrangement and metabolism in living organisms and as a result of exposure to ultraviolet light. The metabolites formed possess significant toxicity, comparable to that of the parent compounds. Organophosphorus compounds undergo oxidative desulfuration in plants, and the reaction is mediated by the mixed-function oxidases in the presence of NADPH and oxygen (O'Brien, 1967).

The thio ether oxidation of certain organophosphorus compounds has been demonstrated *in vivo* in plants. This reaction involves the conversion of the thio ether moiety to the respective sulfoxide and sulfone; it has been shown with demeton, phorate, and fensulfothion.

In plants, carbaryl is metabolized to 4- and 5-hydroxy carbaryl, *N*-hydroxymethylcarbaryl, and 1-naphthol conjugated with glucose and other sugars. In cotton plants hydrolytic and nonhydrolytic pathways contributes almost equally to the metabolism of carbaryl. Plants grown in carbofuran-treated soil metabolize the insecticide to 3-hydroxycarbofuran, 2,3-dihydro-7-hydroxy-2,2-dimethyl benzofuran, and 2,3-dihydro-3,7-dihydroxy-2,2-dimethyl benzofuran. These products are largely stored as glycosides in plants (Knaak *et al.*, 1970).

Endosulfan (10 ppm) temporarily inhibits the growth of root and shoot in germinating gram seeds in lower concentrations, the meristematic tissues recovering from the toxic effects after 10 days of treatment. Germinating seeds implanted in agar slants mixed with different concentrations of endosulfan pick up relative amounts of the insecticide within 24 hr. Accumulation of the insecticide in the seed suggests a dose dependency.

Field experiments are, however, open to the criticism that under natural conditions or a change of weather plant surfaces may become contaminated with the soil which has earlier received treatment with the insecticide and is later translocated in the plant (Lichtenstein and Schulz, 1965; Saha and McDonald, 1967). Furthermore, the reaction between pesticide residues which penetrate plant tissues and the constituents of plants are not fully known. Plant microsomes have been investigated in connection with protein biosynthesis, but in general the interaction of these organelles with the cyclodiene group and other types of insecticides remains unexplored (Whaley *et al.*, 1960).

Studies have been made on the uptake, translocation, and accumulation of phosphamidon residues in mustard plants (*Brassica compestris* var. Sarsonprain). Analysis of top, middle, and bottom portions of the plant sprayed with 0.03 and 0.06% of phosphamidon suggested that more residues were found on the top portion of the plant. Accumulation of residue was maximum in the inflorescence as compared to leaves sampled from the middle and bottom parts of the plant, suggesting the translocation of the insecticide through cell sap (Yadav and Gupta, 1975).

De novo synthesis of acetylcholinesterase in roots of *Pisum sativum* and the inhibition of the enzyme have been reported (Kasturi, 1978; Kasturi and Vasantharajan, 1976). Fensulphothion did not inhibit the *de novo* synthesis of acetylcholinesterase in *P. sativum* but inhibited its activity (Kasturi, 1978).

Ideally, the ultimate evaluation of a pesticide should be made under conditions comparable to those occurring in actual use. Valuable information on the metabolism of pesticides can also be obtained from comparative studies on insects and other animals and on plants that are maintained and tested in a controlled environment. It is of utmost importance that all the products formed during the metabolism of pesticides be detected, identified, and evaluated individually and in combination. The metabolism of different pesticides in plants has been reviewed extensively (Casida and Lykken, 1969; Kuhr, 1970; Menzer and Dautermann, 1970).

The persistence of pesticides has been the subject of research on a limited scale by some institutes under the umbrella of the Indian Council of Agriculture Research, mainly in the agricultural universities. Thus, work on residues has been conducted on crops, such as sorghum, maize, cotton, sugar cane, and a variety of vegetables (e.g., cabbage, cauliflower, tomato, brinjal). Organophosphorus compounds, carbamates, and chlorinated hydrocarbons have been used most often, and proper dosages have been worked out (Agnihothrudu and Mithyantha, 1978).

10.5. FARM MANAGEMENT AND METABOLISM

10.5.1. Organophosphorus Compounds

A majority of the organophosphorus insecticides in use are basically of a single chemical nature and are the derivatives of phosphoric acid. They also have a uniform mode of action. Organophosphorus compounds have the characteristic feature of persistence only for short periods of time.

Organophosphorus insecticides have a brief half-life ranging from 1 to 3 weeks. Phosphamidon, for example, has a half-life of 1–3 weeks in soil and water. Phosphamidon leaches out from many soils, and as such it does not accumulate in the top layer of soil. Samples of air taken in orchards 1–24 hr after spraying show less than 0.01 mg of phosphamidon/m^2 (Voss and Geiss-bühler, 1971).

The rates of degradation of phosphamidon, diethylphosphamidon and gamma chlorophosphamidon have been assessed under laboratory and greenhouse conditions. These compounds are degraded rapidly in green leaves. Fruits degraded them at a much lower rate. Phosphamidon is degraded in sea water, its half-life in sea water being approximately 2 weeks. The rate of degradation in soil depends upon the type of soil and the initial residue level.

Dicrotophos persisted in soil up to 75 days. Degradation slowed down in the presence of fertilizers (Pandey and Agnihotri, 1975). While diazinon was found in harvested paddy plants even 50 days after application, no residues could be detected in soil (Gupta, 1974). There was quick degradation of chlorfenvinphos in soil, and no residue was found in the potato plant and its tubers (Misra *et al.*, 1977). Disulfoton degraded in soil 30 days after application (Rajukkannu *et al.*, 1973). There is, however, a need to estimate the level of pesticide residues in potatoes *(Solanum tuberosam)* and onions *(Allium cepa)*, which are kept in cold storage and released periodically into the market. Phorate and disulfoton dissipated quickly from the rape seed (Jain *et al.*, 1974). Dimethoate (0.03% spray) degraded quickly, and no residue was seen after 48 hr of treatment of tobacco plants (Joshi and Ramaprasad, 1969). Dimethoate was not found on peach and guava *(Psidium guajava)*. Approximately 50% of the initial deposit was degraded within 3–5 days. Grapes treated with fenthion four times at 15-day intervals showed very low residues (Rajukkannu *et al.*, 1977a). Rapid degradation, however, was noticed, and in 8 days no residue could be detected.

Persistence of malathion residues in the cow pea *(Vigna sinensis)* has been studied (Dewan *et al.*, 1969). Degradation of malathion and its formulations WDP, granules, E.C., and dusts was faster under higher temperatures, low humidity, and bright sunshine (Hameed and Rattan Lal, 1971). In winter, E.C. formulation took 12 days, WDP 14 days, and dusts 5 days for residues to reach levels below the tolerance limit of 8 ppm. Malathion applied (0.05–0.15%) on paddies degraded rapidly, reaching undetectable levels within 3 days (Srivastava *et al.*, 1975). The half-life ranged from 1.3 to 2.1 days. The level was below the EPA tolerance limit of 8 ppm in 48 hr after a single spray. However, the half-life of malathion on green grass is 2.46 months (Murthy and Srivastava, 1977).

Malathion spray (0.5 and 1.0%) left an initial residue of 11.67–16.72 ppm on small fruits, 3.2–10.39 ppm on medium-sized fruits, and 2.58–4.68 ppm on normal-sized fruits of okra *(A. esculantus)*. However, the level of residue dropped to below 3 ppm after 48 hr. Also, washing of the fruits removed more than 80% of the malathion residue (Jat and Srivastava, 1973). Folin application of dicrotophos (0.05%) left a residue of 7.5 ppm on Bengal gram *(Cicer arietinum)* pods at harvest. A spray of endosulfan (0.07%) at the time of pod formation in Bengal gram left a high residue of the insecticide both on the whole plant and in the grain even 25 days after treatment, suggesting that care be taken during the spray schedule and in the pattern of use (Pandey *et al.*, 1977).

In cow pea pods treated with monocrotophos (0.75–1.25 kg A.I./ha) the half-life of the pesticide ranged between 2.7 and 3.1 days (Awasthi *et al.*, 1977*a*). Monocrotophos applied to soil is quickly degraded and no residue was seen in sugar cane juice (Awasthi *et al.*, 1977*b*). Soybeans sprayed with carbaryl (0.1% showed no detectable levels of residues in grains, straw, and husks at harvest (Awasthi *et al.*, 1979).

Parathion dissipated and degraded rapidly in cabbage (Singh *et al.*, 1971). Residues were reduced to less than 1.0 ppm in 1 day and were undetectable after 21 days. The half-life of parathion on cabbage varied from 1.67 to 1.81 days, and no residue could be detected in random samples of cabbage collected from the market. Phorate applied to puddled paddy soils degraded completely within 30 days (Rajukkannu *et al.*, 1977).

When Bengal gram was sprayed with 0.04–0.05% solutions of tetrachlorovinphos, carbophenothion, and trichlorfon, residues were found to be excessive in the grains at harvest. Examination of the harvest grains showed 6.0 ppm of tetrachlorvinphos, 3.5 ppm of carbophenothion, and 13.5 ppm of trichlorofon (Pandley *et al.*, 1977).

10.5.2. Organochlorine Insecticides

Residue levels of DDT and BHC on spinach *(Spinacia olearacea)* leaves were estimated after spraying them with 0.1% solutions. While the residue levels of DDT decreased from 53.4% to 32.8% between 3 and 7 days, the corresponding decrease of BHC was 30.6 to 18.8 for the same duration (Jagalan and Chopra, 1971). In groundnut plants, the residue of BHC decreased rapidly between 15 and 75 days to levels below the tolerance limit (Chopra *et al.*, 1973).

DDT degraded faster on *A. esculantus* L. (Singh and Deshmukh, 1974). Residues of DDT in Bengal gram (*C. arietinum* L.) were much below the tolerance limits (Singh *et al.*, 1973). Dusting of BHC (5%) on *B. compestris* L. var. Sarsonprain showed 0.20 ppm residue after 10 days, suggesting rapid dissipation of the compound (Misra *et al.*, 1971).

Analysis of milk, butter, eggs, and different vegetable oils collected from the market indicated that DDT and BHC were invariably present at high concentrations and above tolerance limits. Some of the samples showed more than 50 ppm of BHC. In comparison to the earlier studies of 1965 and 1972 the survey conducted during 1974 showed an increase in DDT of about 3.3 times. Concentration of DDT ranged from 1.1 to 8.0 ppm in butter and 5.01 to 25.7 ppm in vegetable oils. In contrast to butter and oil, eggs were contaminated with low residues of DDT (Agnihotri *et al.*, 1974*a,b*; Dikshith, 1978). BHC dust (5%) translocated faster in cow peas (*Vigna catjang* walh) than in green gram (*Phaseolus aureus* Roxb).

Brinjal (*Solanum melongena* L.) sprayed with 0.01% of lindane contained only traces of lindane after 5 days, showing a quick dissipation from the plant (Jain and Gupta, 1976). A comparative study with carrots (*Daucus carotae* L.), radishes, (*Raphanus sativus* L.), and beet roots (*Beta vulgare* L.) suggested that the maximum amount of insecticide is absorbed by carrots, followed by radish and beet root (Yadav, 1976; Yadav *et al.*, 1977; Srivastava and Kavadia, 1976). Residues of BHC disappeared by about 88% in chili (*Capsicum annum* L.) within a period of 150 days under the climatic conditions of Jodhpur (Pal and Kushwah, 1977).

Endrin (0.02%) sprayed on rice plants did not leave any residues in the grain, straw, and bran, but at higher concentrations the residues were detected on both grain and straw (Rajukkannu *et al.*, 1976).

Endosulfan sprayed on *A. esculantus* dissipated rapidly, and the plants showed very little residue (Singh, 1972). The insecticide did not leave any residues on cauliflower (*Brassica oleracea* L. var. *botrytis*). The initial deposit of endosulfan was 29.8 ppm on leaves and 18.6 ppm on curds, which declined to 0.9 and 0.6 ppm, respectively, after 32 days (Awasthi *et al.*, 1974; Verma and Rattan Lal, 1976; Kavadia *et al.*, 1974). Similar were the observations of Nath *et al.* (1974) on *A. esculantus*. The residues dissipated quickly in the first 48 hr and were 6 ppm on the sixth day after treatment. Endosulfan residues on the fig *(Ficus carica)* and tomato disappeared faster within 5–7 days (Joia and Kalra, 1974; Singh and Deshmuth, 1974; Dixit *et al.*, 1975; Shankar and Kavadia, 1976; Srivastava *et al.*, 1976). *P. aureus* (Roxb) and *Cajanus cajian*

(Sprengl) crops sprayed with endosulfan for the control of jassids *(Empeasia devastanus)* showed very few residues after 14 days of treatment. Endosulfan was reduced to 0.21 ppm from an initial deposit of 4.20 ppm after 50 days of treatment in mustard *(Brassica juncea* Coss.). A rapid decline was found in the residual content of endosulfan in *C. arietinum* L. (Bengal gram) and also Chick pea (Dixit *et al.,* 1977; Pandey *et al.,* 1977). Berries of *Zizyphus zujuba* Lamk (Ber) showed no residues of endosulfan after 5 days of treatment (Kathpal *et al.,* 1977).

At harvest, maize did not show any residues of endosulfan. The initial residue levels of 20.23 ppm dissipated quickly, and the insecticide could not be detected within 4 days (Kavadia *et al.,* 1977).

Aldrin, endrin, dieldrin, chlordane, endosulfan, and heptachlor have a wide spectrum of activity, and many members of the cyclodiene group also have a high mammalian toxicity. Like other chlorinated hydrocarbons, they too are known to be persistent. Aldrin was found to be converted to dieldrin after application to green gram at 5% concentration (Agnihotri *et al.,* 1977*b*). A maximum concentration of dieldrin was found on the thirtieth day after treatment, and 80.8% of this was degraded during the subsequent 70-day period. In 180 days, 96.4% of aldrin, 96.4% of dieldrin, and 86.4% of heptachlor were lost from Delhi soils (Agnihotri *et al.,* 1977*a,b*). The conversion of both aldrin and heptachlor into their epoxides was indeed rapid.

Repeated sprays of 0.07% endosulfan on okra, tomato, and brinjal *(Solanum brinjal* L.) once in 15 days left initial deposits of 2.74, 4.35, and 3.50 ppm, respectively, which were reduced to 0.32, 0.0, and 0.20 ppm in 10 days (Rajukkannu *et al.,* 1976). The initial deposit of endosulfan on mustard leaves was 4.20 ppm, which was reduced to 0.21 in 50 days (Dixit *et al.,* 1977). From an average initial deposit on fruits of 2.14 ppm after the first spray, endosulfan levels rose to 5.14 ppm after the second spray (Kathpal *et al.,* 1977). The residues had a half-life of 10.8 days for the first and 8.13 days for the second spray. BHC and DDT sprayed on spinach showed interesting behavior (Jagalan and Chopra, 1971).

10.5.3. Carbamate Compounds

In tobacco plants, aldicarb applied to soil in the form of 10% granules at 15 kg/ha persisted for 36 days (Ramaprasad and Joshi, 1974). Investigations on the dissipation of aldicarb in soil and pea plants revealed that the initial residue of aldicarb was 13.70 ppm and that its degradation followed first-order kinetics with a half-life of 17 days (Dixit *et al.,* 1976). In peas, residues persisted for 110 days and were concentrated in the top portions of the plant. Absorption and metabolism of carbofuran in Sorghum was very rapid (Baskaran and Jothwani, 1976).

10.5.4. Fungicides, Herbicides, and Fumigants

Reports on the residues of fungicides in India are very sketchy. Since most of the organic fungicides have low mammalian toxicity, problems of excessive residues of the parent compound are not generally serious. Soil organic matter is a potential absorber of PCNB. The half-life of the fungicide in the soils varied from 15.4 to 53 days. Carboxin was rapidly absorbed by sugarcane and was degraded in the plant within 7 days (Agnihotri *et al.*, 1973). Absorption and translocation of carboxin and oxycarboxin in pearl millet showed a time-dependent loss of the fungicides (Bhaktavatsalam and Tripathi, 1974; Tripathy *et al.*, 1976). Two of the degraded products of benomyl, one methyl-2-benzimidazole carbamate and the other unidentified (Rf, 0:30) were found up to 45 and 15 days, respectively (Kannaiyan *et al.*, 1975). Tridemorph was degraded rapidly on tea leaves to levels of less than 0.1 ppm in 14 days (Venkataraman, 1977).

Work conducted in India on residue levels of herbicides on crop, soil, and water has also been meagre. The half-life period in soils for 2,4-D ranged from 14.53 to 32.2 days, for atrazine from 20.3 to 52.58 days, and for monuron from 50.75 to 115.50 days. Based on the study, it was found that atrazine and monuron were better herbicides for soil application than 2,4-D and paraquat (Mithyantha, 1973). Spraying of dodine on citrus plants left no residue (Ray and Addy, 1976). Tomato plants showed little residue after treatment with fungicides (Jhooty and Munshi, 1976).

Aureofungin, benomyl, carbondaxins, ceresan, ferbam, mancozeb, and MBC were applied to control rotting on ginger rhizomes. The effects of carbondazim persisted up to 90 days, while the effects of others disappeared much more quickly (Arora *et al.*, 1977a). The residue of benzimidazole on sugar beets during harvest was between 3.15 and 6.2 ppm, much below the tolerance level, indicating rapid dissipation (Bandopadhyay and Mukhopadhyay, 1977). Degradation of 2,4-D, atrazine, and monuron was fast when moisture was high, and the degradation followed first-order kinetics (Mithyantha, 1973). Grains and plant of maize contained no simazine and atrazine residue (Kulshrestha *et al.*, 1976). Fumigation of wheat with iodofenphos for the control of *Tribolium* sp. indicated no evidence of residue (Girish *et al.*, 1971; Chawla *et al.*, 1976).

Treatment of groundnut *(Arachis hypogeae)* seeds, pulses, food grains, almonds, walnuts, coffee beans, and seeds of coriander with methyl bromide, methyl iodine, and phosphine showed little residue in the food material (Muthu *et al.*, 1976; Sinha *et al.*, 1976). The pattern of dissipation and the residue level

Table 10.5. Common and Botanical Names of Plants
Cited in the Text

Common name	Botanical name
1. Arhar; red gram	*Cajanus cajan* Sprengl
2. Barley	*Hordeum vulgare* L.
3. Beet root	*Beta vulgare* L.
4. Bengal gram; chickpea	*Cicer arietinum* L.
5. Ber	*Zizyphus zujuba* Lamk
6. Bhindi; okra	*Abelmoschus esculantus* Moench
7. Black gram; mung	*Phaseolus mungo* var. *radiatus* L.
8. Brinjal	*Solanum brinjal* L.
9. Cabbage	*Brassica oleracea* var. *capitata*
10. Carrot	*Daucus carotae* L.
11. Cauliflower	*Brassica oleracea* L. var. *botrytis*
12. Chili	*Capsicum annum* L.
13. Cotton	*Gossypium* sp.
14. Cow pea	*Vigna catjang walh*
15. Eggplant	*Solanun melongena* L.
16. Fig	*Ficus carica*
17. Finger millet; Ragi	*Eleusinea corocana* Gaertn
18. Green gram	*Phaseolus aureus* Roxb
19. Groundnut	*Arachis hypogeae*
20. Jawar	*Sorghum vulgare pers*
21. Knol khol	*Brassica oleracea* var. *colocarpa* L.
22. Maize	*Zea mays* kinn.
23. Mustard	*Brassica juncea* *Brassica compestris.* L.
24. Oat	*Avena sativa*
25. Onion	*Allium cepa*
26. Paddy; rice	*Oryza sativa*
27. Pea	*Pisum sativum* L.
28. Guava	*Psidium guajava*
29. Potato	*Solanum tuberosam*
30. Radish	*Raphanus sativus* L.
31. Soybean	*Glycine max.* Merr.
32. Spinach	*Spinacia olearacea*
33. Tobacco	*Nicotina tabacum* L.
34. Wheat	*Tritum vulgare* *Tritium aestivum* L.
35. Coriander	*Coriandrum sativum*
36. Ginger	*Zingibar* sp.

of different pesticides in a variety of Indian crops (Table 10.5) have been compiled by Bindra and Kalra (1971) and Agnihothrudu and Mithyantha (1978).

10.6. POSTHARVEST STORAGE

With the advent of modern organic insecticides for storage, pest control has opened a new chapter in applied storage entomology. Some work on the efficacy of some of these organic insecticides has been in progress in India for nearly two decades. The Ministry of Agriculture has suggested various programs to increase agricultural production and productivity through increased use of pesticides. Some of the schemes for supply of pesticides for the protection of stored grains in the model villages are the "Save Grain" campaign of the Agriculture Ministry; the national program of rodent control, weed control and pest management; and centrally sponsored schemes for control and eradication of pests and diseases in endemic areas. Aerial application to about 1,555,000 acres and ground spraying of 667,000 acres with different pesticides took place during the year 1977–1978 (Anonymous, 1977*a*).

Over two-thirds of the population in India depends upon agriculture as a main occupation. This accounts for about 50% of the national increase. The cultivators and farmers in India store food grains and other agricultural commodities produced in their fields to meet their annual household requirements. Reports indicate that as much as 60–70% of the total production is retained by the farmer and that only 30–40% is released to marketing channels as surplus. During 1977–1978, about 75–88 out of 126 million tons of food grain were retained by farmers. It was kept in storage that was far from satisfactory. The faulty storage conditions often account for the huge quantitative and qualitative losses of the food grains. It has been indicated that 9.3% of food grains are lost during post harvest and 6.68% during storage. In terms of money, this is tantamount to an annual loss of over 6360 million rupees.

Farmers usually store the food grains in bulk in different kinds of storage structures. These structures are normally constructed from the material available locally in the villages. The farmers use mud and split bamboo as materials. The stores are either inside the house or outside in an open area, with the latter constructed either above or below the ground. Structures built above ground are called *Kothis,* those built underground, *Khattis*. Since the walls of the storages are not waterproof, loss of grain due to absorption of moisture is a regular occurrence. The high moisture content of the stored grain leads to fungal infection and caking of grains on all the exposed walls.

The structures made from split bamboo and mud give no protection from moisture during the rainy seasons or protection from insects and rodents. Since the structures are not air-tight, chemical fumigation will not be possible or effective. Jute bags and polyethylene-lined jute bags are also used in rural areas to store grains. However, it is now established that bulk storage is preferable to bag storage.

In recent years, efforts have been made by different organizations in the country to design good storage structures to save the food grains. The Indian Grain Storage Institute at Hapur developed various designs for outdoor structures to store many kinds of commodities; these are identical to elevator storage. These structures have been constructed with facilities to load and unload the bulk grains, to fumigate them periodically, and to keep them free from insects, moisture, and rodents. The insects that attack the stored grains include a variety of species. Some of the insects destroy all kinds of stored grains, and others damage broken or milled food grains. The high temperature and humidity inside the storage structure greatly facilitate the growth and movement of the stored-grain pests. To a certain extent, the infestation of different insects increases with higher moisture content above the 10% level. By controlling the moisture content and the temperature of the stored grains, it is possible to minimize pest activity. The most common insect pests that attack different food products are shown in Table 10.6 (Agarwal, 1979; Pingale, 1964).

Presently, different insecticides are used to control the insect pests and to protect the food grains. Malathion spray, ethylene dibromide mixed with EDCT, and phosphine are the most common.

Apart from insects and rodents, microorganisms also damage most of the food grain in postharvest storage conditions. Climatic conditions in India are very favorable for the growth and sustenance of microorganisms in the grain storages. Microorganisms impart different effects on the food grains and lead to loss of grains. The infected grain develops an odd color and a bad odor and tastes different. The kernel discoloration, loss of nutritional value, and production of mycotoxins and other toxins are examples of harmful effects to the user.

Proper drying, aeration, and control of humidity and temperature are a few factors that would minimize the spoilage of grain by microorganisms (Agarwal, 1979).

DDT and BHC were tested with encouraging results against *Sitophilus oryzae, Tribolium castaneum,* and *Silvanus surinamensis.* The toxicity of free and sorbed vapor of BHC and DDT has also been tested. The question of hazardous residue and contamination in food grains has also received the attention of several investigators (Mookherjee, 1964).

Bioassay tests of insecticides have been made using *Trogoderma granarium, Latheticus oryzae, Oryzaephilus surinamensis. Laemophloeus minutus, Tribolium castaneum, Lasioderma serricorne,* and *Sitophilus oryzae.* These studies help as guiding factors for the choice of a suitable insecticide for the control of insect pests.

The use of fumigants for the control of insect pests in storage is the most

Table 10.6.   Insect Pests Which Infest Stored
Products

Insect	Food product
Araecerus fasciculatus	Coffee beans
Bruchus analis	Pulses
Bruchus pisorium Linn	Pulses
Callosobruchus chinensis L.	Pulses
Callosobruchus maculatus Fobr.	Pulses
Carpophilus sp.	
Corcyra cephalonica Staint.	Cereals
Coryoborus Sp.	Tamarind
Ephestia cautella	Cashew nuts
	Groundnuts
	Linseed
Gnorimoschema operculella	Potatoes
Laemophloeus minutus	
Lasioderma serricorne	Black pepper
	Chilis
	Dry ginger
	Turmeric
Latheticus oryzae	Cereals
Necrobia rufipes (F.)	Cashew nuts
Orzaephilus surinamensis	Cashew nuts
	Groundnuts
Oryzaephilus sp.	Black pepper
Plodia interpunctella H.	Cashew nuts
Rizopertha dominica Fab.	Cereals
Silvanus surinamensis	
Sitotroga cerealella Oliv	Cereals
Sitophilus oryzae	Cereals
Sitophilus sp.	
Stegobium paniceum	
Stegobium sp.	Black pepper
	Chilis
	Coriander
	Dry ginger
	Turmeric
Tenebroides mauritanicus L.	Cashew nuts
Tribolium castaneum Hbst.	Cereals
	Cashew nuts
Tribolium sp.	Cereals
	Black pepper
	Pulses
	Groundnut
Trogoderma granarium Everts	Cereals
	Pulses

commonly adopted measure. Fumigation with cyanide is made for the control of infestation of grains. Correlations have been made between the susceptibility of insects to fumigation with HCN gas and the amount of HCN recoverable from them immediately after fumigation. Ethylene dibromide is used as a fumigant for the control of insect and fungal infestation in grain and root crops such as tapioca. The extent of variation caused by certain factors in the toxicity of ethylene dichloride–carbon tetrachloride mixture has also been studied (Muthu and Pingale, 1955). One of the very important factors involved in the fumigation of infested grains is temperature, but little work has been done in India to correlate temperature with fumigation practices. Tests have been conducted with two fumigants, CS_2 and ethylene dichloride, using *T. castaneum* as the test insect, and the effect of temperatures before, during, and after fumigation on the toxicity of the compounds has been studied. Temperature and initial moisture content of grains are two very important factors in the overall effectiveness of the fumigants, but our knowledge in this area is also very inadequate (Bhatnagar and Srivastava, 1974).

The use of chemically inert dusts, though reported to be effective by several workers, has failed in recent studies, and hence does not offer much scope in the control of pests. Preharvest prophylaxis for infestation control in stored food grains by using malathion has been suggested. More work, however, seems to be necessary in this direction before the method can be recommended for general use. In India, insecticides of plant origin have been safely used on food grains. The sweet flag powder (*Acorus calamus*) and pyrethrum have often been suggested for the control of stored-product insect pests. The future of pyrethrum, however, lies in making less expensive formulations with longer-lasting effects (Mookherjee, 1964).

The important means of pest control undoubtedly lies in fumigation. The use of HCN, CS_2, and even naphthalene has been known and recommended for grain fumigation from early times. Although the most commonly used fumigant in India is a mixture of ethylene dibromide and carbon tetrachloride (EDCT), chemicals like ethylene dibromide and a mixture of methyl bromide and ethylene dibromide or methyl bromide have also been recommended and used. Although methyl bromide has been used in India for grain fumigation for a long time, there is a void in our knowledge regarding its use in different commodities, including the oil seeds. The way it is absorbed in these commodities and ultimately is reacted upon by them to produce harmful residues has not been investigated. The role of the temperature and moisture content of grains on the overall effectiveness of fumigants commonly used is also still unknown. Phosphine, a well-known fumigant, has been used for the protection of wheat in India with encouraging results both in stacks and in flat storage as well (Mookherjee, 1964; Muthu *et al.*, 1971). However, much remains to be done regarding its effective use in other commodities under varying conditions and in countering the problem of hazardous residues, if any exist.

While chemical control of storage pests is being actively practiced for the safe storage of grains in India, biological methods of control using insects and microbes *(Bacillus thuringiensis)* are mostly of theoretical interest at this time. Some records have been made of the occurrence of chalcid and other parasites on different species of grain pests (Mookherjee, 1964).

The properties of common fumigants used in India have been described by a number of workers (Dhaliwal and Rattan Lal, 1973). Effects of temperature during prefumigation, fumigation, and postfumigation periods have been studied. The actions of hydrocyanic acid gas, methyl bromide, and ED/CT against *Lasioderma serricorne* Fab.; of EDCT, MB, and HCN for fumigation of ginger; and of ethylene dibromide as a general fumigant are on record. Carbon disulfide has been reported to be a suitable fumigant for potatoes. Relative toxicities of fumigants and fumigant mixtures have also been studied. Monro (1963, 1964) has reviewed behavior and residual effects of several fumigants with reference to storage of food grains and fumigation techniques.

Records of commercial fumigation under Indian conditions are few. Studies have been made to analyze the permeability of liquid fumigants through polyethylene sheets (Muthu and Narasimhan, 1964). ED/CT was the main fumigant used until recently. Practical experience with this chemical mixture suggests that it is not very useful in grain meant for long storage. In short-term storage, surviving insects do not get an opportunity to create a problem, and therefore it may be satisfactory. A recirculatory technique to increase its efficacy under gas-tight covers has been attempted (unpublished records). This device provides for better mortality and reduction in the dosage. The lack of ovicidal action by the fumigant, however, limits the scope of its use.

10.7. BIOEFFICACY AND RESIDUE EFFECTS OF PESTICIDES

The efficacy of various pesticides, such as lindane, aldrin, and heptachlor, against white grubs of groundnut has been reported (Pradhan *et al.*, 1964; Beri and Dewan, 1964; Bhatnagar, 1975). The comparative efficacy of organochlorine and organophosphorus insecticides has been studied by different workers (Shetty and Nayar, 1964; Bhatnagar *et al.*, 1964).

The relative efficacy of fenitrothion, malathion, gardona, and idofenphos used as grain protectants has been determined (Krishnaiah *et al.*, 1976). Studies show fenitrothion to be the most effective grain protectant. Malathion and gardona proved almost equally effective. Idofenphos was found to be least effective.

The effects of pesticides on the metabolic processes of plants and other chemical constituents in addition to their utility in insect control have been investigated. Application of dicrotophos, monocrotophos, endosulfan, and chlor-fenvinphos altered the biochemical constituents of brinjal plants (Uttamaswamy et al., 1976). It was reported that changes brought about by these in phenolics, sugars, and minerals appeared to influence the population of the red spider mite.

Investigations on the effect of parathion on the pea crop have revealed that residues could lead to a marginal increase in the protein content, whereas sulfur and phosphorus contents remained unaffected (Jagirdar et al., 1974). The contents of reducing and total sugars decreased significantly at the time of harvest, while nonreducing sugars were maximum at this period. Carbaryl and cytrolane also brought about changes in phenolics and sugars in brinjal plants (Kumaresan and Bhaskaran, 1975). In contrast to cytrolane, the carbaryl-treated plant showed a lesser increase in phenolics, and correspondingly the insect infestation was more than that in cytrolane-treated and control plants. Contents of reducing and nonreducing sugars were found likely to be enhanced in the treated plants.

Effects of the treatment of insecticides on the crop yield have also been investigated (Chakraborty et al., 1973; Chatterjee, 1972). A significant difference in the grain yield was obtained in insecticide-treated (phosphamidon, fenitro-thion, and lindane) plots over controls. A high dose of lindane mixed with urea registered the highest yield, closely followed by phosphamidon when applied singly. The maximum yield was obtained in the plots that received fenitrothion, followed by lindane and phosphamidon, respectively (Chakraborty et al., 1973). Malathion, sumithion, sevin, and thiodan lead to an increase in yield over control on paddies (Chatterjee, 1972).

A single administration of endrin (3 μg) to the adult male grasshopper Poecilocerus pictus reduced the activity of alkaline and acid phosphatases in hemolymph and testicular tissue, but not in alimentary tissues of the insects (Vasuki and Dikshith, 1968). The pattern of the two enzymes after endrin treatment in vitro using a coccid, Dactylopous confusus, as the test system suggested a gradual inhibition of alkaline phosphatase activity and indicated a dose dependency (Dikshith and Vasuki, 1970).

Isolation of active compounds from a variety of plants and their identification for insecticidal activity has been pursued with some positive results. Several species of plants grown in India were examined for the insecticidal property. The insecticidal activity of the active material isolated through solvent extraction and steam evaporation of plants suggested that they do possess insecticidal properties and could control insect pests without causing deleterious effects to higher animals and man. Extracts of A. calamus L. (sweet flag) were found to be toxic to flies and mosquitoes, and a significant knockdown effect was noticed in them in comparison to DDT. The active compound showed a synergistic effect with DDT. Woolen fabrics treated with the extract were not affected by the woolly bear. Seed oil of Anona squamosa L. (custard apple) was found to be poor in comparison to pyrethrin when it was tested against mosquitoes, house-flies, flour beetles, and woolly bears. The seed oil failed to control mosquitoes and flour beetles as a contact insecticide.

The seed oil and leaf extract of *Azadirachta indica* L. (Indian neem) also did not kill flies, mosquitoes, floor beetles, and wool-destroying insects. However, the nonfatty alcohol extract of the neem seed cake showed aphicidal activity (Sinha and Gulati, 1968). Nutmeg leaf oil (*Myristica fragraus* Hout.) was relatively toxic to flies and mosquitoes but was ineffective against woolly bears. Petroleum ether extracts of roots, stem, and leaves of *Abrus precalorius* L. (wild liquorice root), and *Nerium odorum* Soland (sweet scented oleander) were not very toxic to flies and mosquitoes, whereas the extracts of *Curcuma long* L. (turmeric) and *Andropogen citrulus* D.C. (lemon grass oil) were found to be toxic to insects (Anonymous, 1951, 1954, 1964, 1965).

10.8. PESTICIDES IN FORESTRY

Forests constitute one of the most important natural wealths of any country. Besides valuable timber, they yield a variety of products of great economic importance. Forests in India are covered by several very valuable kinds of trees, in addition to a variety of medicinal plants and wild life. Teak *(Tectona grandis)*, shisham *(Dalbergia sisso)*, gamtar *(Gmelina arborea)*, deodar (Cedrus deodar), sal *(Shorea robusta)*, mahogany *(Seietenia macrophylla)*, oak *(Quecrus incana)*, sandal *(Santalum album)*, *Causurina*, neem (*A. indica* L.), and bamboo are some of the forest trees which have helped sustain the forest wealth for ages. Large tracts of forest also have a direct influence on the local rainfall.

Forests play an important role in the national economy. Their destruction or deforestation is a matter of serious concern. The area of forests in India comprises 783,692 km^2 (302,688 square miles) and is unevenly distributed. Insects, in addition to other factors, are one of the greatest agents of destruction of forests. Because of their high rate of reproduction and short life cycles, most forest insects have the ability to multiply to astronomical numbers. In nature, such optimum conditions do not exist because they are offset by destructive influences such as climate, weather, availability of food, prevalence of diseases, and other enemies which destory insects. The importance of various other agencies varies at different times and densities, but all are interdependent to a great extent. Under normal conditions, control is maintained by such natural factors, and a state of equilibrium prevails in the natural forest for all the populations constituting the fauna of the forest. When environmental conditions favor rapid increase of destructive pests, natural control factors are incapable of checking the outbreak and widespread damage often results.

In the widest sense, forest operations with pesticides destory the stable equilibrium of the undisturbed environment and produce a new one, which may be temporarily stable but which often permits multiplication of plant feeders to an injurious degree. This disturbance reaches its extreme degree in large mono-specific plantations in which the population of the pest and its natural enemies are widely out-of-balance. The incidence of the pest is either maintained at a high level or is subject to oscillations in the form of epidemics alternating with scarcity (Mathur, 1964).

To quote Beeson (1941), "Indian forestry is not static . . . it is experimental and progressive and is continually producing new conditions under which well-known pests create fresh ecological problems and unknown insects spring into prominence as pests." The control of forest insects is therefore not a simple problem. The forest is faced continually with insect problems at every stage in the growth of the tree, coniferous or deciduous. Before the seeds are collected, they may be destroyed by certain insects. The insect damage continues even during storage of seeds. The seedlings, saplings, and trees in the forest are injured by defoliators and sapsuckers, girdled by bores, or killed by root-eating insects. This ability of insects to attack the tree in all phases of its growth greatly influences the practice of forestry both directly and indirectly.

The spike diseases of sandal *(S. album)* cause a hugh loss of forest revenue in Karnataka, Tamil Nadu, and parts of the Kerala States. The disease is caused by a virus and four species of insects. *Jassus indicus* Walker, *Moonia varlabilis* Distent, *Petalocephala uniformin* Distant, and *Sarima nigro clypeata* Meliacher are the vectors of the viral disease. It is a matter of great concern that no chemical control has thus far been found to combat this deadly disease.

A variety of insect pests cause damage and loss of the forest trees. It has not been possible to control the attack of insects with any one kind of insecticide. However, several workers have suggested treating the infected parts of the trees with DDT, endrin, BHC, dieldrin dusts and sprays, injections of a mixture of creosote and fuel oil, and pentachlorophenol as prophylactic measures before the onset of the monsoon or rainy season.

Chemical control methods should be supplemented with appropriate silvicultural practices like mixed plantations of trees to minimize the pest population in forests.

10.9. SAFETY EVALUATION STUDIES

10.9.1. Toxicity to Fish

The indiscriminate use of pesticides in agriculture and public health operations has widened the scope of disruption of the ecological balance as many of the nontarget and beneficial organisms, which include important members of the food chain, perish in the process, thus adversely affecting the secondary and tertiary productivity of freshwater ecosystems. Aerial spraying of pesticides reaches the streams through runoff and causes heavy mortality of nontarget aquatic insect predators, which in turn increases the vector and pest populations. The tragic incidence of Handigodu syndrome in Karnatka State (India) was probably due to the consumption of pesticide-poisoned crabs and fish by the local population (Report of National Institute of Nutrition, 1977; Koundinya, 1978). According to a rough estimate, 25% of the pesticides used on land may ultimately find their sink in the sea, and their cumulative effect on coastal water can be expected to be considerable. India, a major subcontinent, is a major producer of inland estuarine and marine fish. The impact of pesticides on the fish population has therefore attracted some attention (Joshi and Rege, 1980; Ahmed *et al.*, 1978).

In vitro studies by O'Brien (1967) have revealed that fish are highly susceptible to organochlorine compounds in general and to endrin in particular. This is in accordance with the indication that fish lack the mixed-function oxidases responsible for drug oxidation (O'Brien, 1967; Brodie and Maicke, 1962). Presumably, fish dispose of foreign lipid-soluble compounds directly by diffusion through gills or skin into the surrounding water without prior conversion to more polar derivatives (Brodie and Maike, 1962). However, Potter and O'Brien (1964) showed that trout liver slices converted parathion into paraoxon, and since then several trout microsomal enzymes affecting drug oxidation, all requiring NADPH and oxygen, have been described (Creaven *et al.*, 1965, 1967; Chan *et al.*, 1967; Lotlikar *et al.*, 1967; Buhler and Rasmusson, 1968). The oxidizing system was different in one or more components of the electron transport chain as compared to the mammalian liver, and possibly the level of aldrin epoxidase was also low. A lethal dose of fenitrothion had an inhibitory effect on the cholinesterase activity in nervous and other tissues of fish, with a concomitant increase of acetylcholine content and decreased SDH and increased LDH activities. These observations indicated that anaerobic metabolism is favored in fenitrothion-treated fish (Koundinya, 1978; Koundinya and Ramamurthi, 1978a,b, 1979a).

Toxicity studies in fish reported from India have revealed significant accumulation of organochlorines in tissues (Verma and Gupta, 1976). Among various chlorinated insecticides examined for their toxicity (namely, DDT, lindane, dieldrin, aldrin, endrin, endosulfan, and chlordane) endrin was extremely toxic to fish and endosulfan was least toxic (Santha Ram *et al.*, 1976; Basak and Konar, 1976, 1977; Joshi *et al.*, 1975; Rao, 1975; Saxena and Agarwal, 1970; Amminikutty and Rege, 1977; Reddy and Gomathy, 1977; Sastry and Sharma, 1978; Banerjee, 1970; Verma *et al.*, 1975). In catfish, endrin was reported to be 70,000 times more toxic than carbaryl (Saxena and Agarwal, 1970). Biochemical studies carried out with endrin in fish revealed that α-amylase activity was inhibited by more than 50%; this could be regained in the presence of a sodium ion concentration of 1 ppm (Bhattacharya *et al.*, 1975; Kumar and Bhattacharya, 1977). During a study on the uptake and metabolism of DDT in *Gambusia affinis*, two metabolites of DDT, namely, p,p'-DDE and p,p'-DDT, were detected (Pillai *et al.*, 1977) and DDE was the major metabolite. Unlike chlorinated hydrocarbon insecticides, very little accumulation of organophosphorus insecticides occurs in tissues (Verma and Gupta, 1976). Effects of these insecticides on the metabolic fate and activities of various lysosomal enzymes in different tissues have also been studied (Srivastava *et al.*, 1977; Mukhopadhyay *et al.*, 1977). Several deformities were observed in fertilized eggs of *C. carpiocommunis* exposed to different concentrations of diazinon, malathion, fenitrothion, and phosphamidon (Kaur and Toor, 1977). Parathion was reported to be highly toxic and dimethoate least toxic to fish. Sumithion (fenitrothion) inhibited the activity of acetylcholinesterase in the nervous and nonnervous tissues of the fish. The insecticide inhibited the activity of succinic dehydrogenase and tissue respiration, but lactic dehydrogenase was raised, suggesting the operation of an anaerobic glycolytic pathway (Koundinya and Ramamurthi, 1978*a,b*). The activity of GDH, GPT, GOT, and total ninhydrin positive substance (TNPS) in different tissues of fish was increased by sumithion. GDH has been linked with increased oxidation of glutamate. The rise of TNPS suggested protein catabolism and increased synthesis of amino acids in the insecticide-treated fish. A rise in blood glucose level supported the observation (Koundinya and Ramamurthi, 1979*a,b*, 1980).

10.9.2. Toxicity to Wildlife

Poultry are often exposed to a variety of pesticides either by ingestion of contaminated feed or through pesticide in henhouses. Pesticides are lethal to poultry if ingested in high concentrations. However, the lethal dose of a pesticide is governed by the species of the bird and the nature of the compound. Contamination of poultry with nonlethal levels may impair one or more of a number of production characteristics such as growth, egg production, egg size, shell thickness, fertility, and hatchability.

Toxicological studies carried out on poultry with a few organophosphorus and chlorinated pesticides in India are of interest while considering the action of biodegradable pesticides. Thiometon, when sprayed aerially for the protection of crops, did not induce any toxic effects in poultry (Ranade *et al.*, 1978). Residues of rabon, an organophosphorus insecticide, were found in the fat of a treated hen (Yadav and Shaw, 1970). In the egg yolk, residues appeared 2 days after initiation of treatment and disappeared 5 days after the last treatment. Fenitrothion was found to be more toxic than malathion to chick embryos (Paul and Vadamudi, 1976). The effect of fenitrothion on the growth rate was correlated with the growth-promoting endocrine gland. The reduced utilization of several metabolites such as nicotinamide, nicotinic acid, and tryptophan during embryonic development could also be responsible for the toxic manifestation. Inadvertent use of malathion for the control of ectoparasites in poultry has resulted in their large-scale killing (Chawla *et al.*, 1977). Malathion inhibited brain cholinesterase activity in house sparrows (Mehrotra *et al.*, 1967). A correlation has been found with the aging of house sparrows and inhibition of rat brain esterase by different organophosphorus compounds (Mehrotra and Singh, 1972). Telodrin produced varying degrees of degenerative hemorrhagic changes in the liver and kidney of cockerels (Verma *et al.*, 1967). Metabolic effects of DDT in earthworms and snails, toxic effects of various insecticides in bees and the effect of malathion on enzyme activities of acetylcholinesterase, asparatate, and alanine aminotransferase in snails have also been reported (Yadav *et al.*, 1976; Agarwal *et al.*, 1978; Dale, 1975; Kapil and Lamba, 1974; Singh *et al.*, 1974; Yadav *et al.*, 1978; Ahmed *et al.*, 1978). Carbaryl, phosphamidon, and endosulfan significantly inhibit the activity of gut amylase, acetylcholinesterase of cerebral ganglion, and coelomic fluid of earthworms both *in vivo* and *in vitro* (Dikshith *et al.*, unpublished data).

10.9.3. Toxicity to Animals

Ingestion of insecticide-contaminated forage crops by animals leads to buildup of residues in the body fat of such animals. Chlorinated hydrocarbons are by far the most common residues found in milk, since they are concentrated and stored in the fat in animals and translocated to the milk fat. It was reported as early as 1947 that DDT residues appeared in the milk of cows that ingested feed treated with the insecticide (Carter, 1947). Since that time, DDT, dieldrin, BHC, lindane, chlordane, heptachlor, aldrin, endrin, and toxaphene have all been detected in milk when the feed of the cow has been treated with these compounds at levels necessary to control the insect pests. In contrast, organophosphorus compounds have not shown such residual effects. The work of Cook (1957) indicates that the absence of residues in the milk of cows fed with organophosphorus compounds is due to the inactivation of the compound by the rumen fluid of the cow.

Insecticides can be detected in blood after exposure. DDT, dieldrin, and lindane have been identified in the blood of most of the examined animals (Schafer, 1968). Toxicological effects, metabolism, and persistence of lindane have been explored in laboratory animals and domestic goats (Anonymous, 1964; Gopalaswamy and Aiyar, 1977; Datta, 1978; Datta and Dikshith, unpublished data). The stimulatory effects of organochlorine insecticides on protein biosynthesis altered the general metabolism and mixed-function oxidases (Bhatia *et al.*, 1971, 1972; Bhatia and Subramanian, 1972*a,b;* Bhatia *et al.*, 1973; Kohli *et al.*, 1977; Krishnamurthy *et al.*, 1965; Somasundaram *et al.*, 1978; Rao, 1975).

Various concentrations of BHC, dieldrin, DDVP, lindane, diazinon, and parathion solution, when coated on the skin of rats, guinea pigs, monkeys, and dogs, produced loss in body weight and histopathological changes in the skin (Dikshith *et al.*, 1971; Dikshith and Datta, 1972*a*; Dikshith *et al.*, 1974, 1976, 1978*b*; Sundaram *et al.*, 1978). BHC (0.2%) exposure led to an increase in the weight of the liver and altered the microsomal protein content and the level of cytochrome P-450 (Rajamanickam and Padmanabhan, 1974). Acute exposure to chlordane produced a significant change in the serum alkaline phosphatase activity, and chronic exposure produced hyperproteinemia, hyperglycemia, and a significant increase in serum acid and alkaline phosphatase activities in Indian desert gerbils (Karel, 1976; Karel and Saxena, 1976). Biochemical effects of DDT and also its carcinogenic potential have been reported (Aravindakshan *et al.*, 1977; Nageshwar Rao and Subrahmanyam, 1974; Gupta and Agarwal, 1977; Kashyap and Gupta, 1971; Dikshith *et al.*, 1975*b*; Kar and Dikshith, 1970). A significant increase in the levels of liver and kidney enzymes by the beta isomer of BHC has been observed. γ-BHC produced significant alterations in hepatic asparate amonotransferase and the hepatic alkaline and acid phosphatase (Srinivasan and Radhakrishnamurthy, 1977).

Among the organophosphorus insecticides, toxicity of malathion in rats has been studied in detail (Chauhan *et al.*, 1973, 1974; Krishnamurthy *et al.*, 1965; Pawar and Makhija, 1975; Bhagavat and Ramachandran, 1973, 1975). It has been shown that inhibition of acetylcholine esterase activity due to malathion administration in the brain and heart was dose related, while such a relationship was not observed in other tissues. In another study conducted to investigate the effects of malathion on hepatic drug metabolism and lipid peroxidation in young rats, the protein content was found to increase significantly in males but to decrease significantly in females. There was an appreciable increase in aminopyrine-*N*-demethylase activity and in acetanilide hydroxylase activity in both male and female rats. Other insecticides studied included metasystox, phorate, pyrethrum, dichlorovos, and baygon (Mitra *et al.*, 1978; Thontadarya *et al.*, 1974; Saxena and Karel, 1975; Pawar and Makhija, 1975; Fatehyab and Mahdi Hasan, 1977). Effects of pesticides on reproduction in mammals have been investigated (Agarwal and Ahmed, 1978). Carbaryl (200 mg/kg, 3 days/week) did not alter the fertility of male rats (Dikshith *et al.*, 1975*a*). Endosulfan (2.0 mg/kg) did not suggest any reproductive effects in male and female rats (Dikshith *et al.*, unpublished data).

Toxicological studies on DDT, BHC, lindane, endrin, endosulfan, parathion, fenitrothion, diazinon, malathion, phenthoate, dichlorovos, phosphamidon, quinalphos, and carbaryl using different species of laboratory animals have also been carried out at the Industrial Toxicology Research Center, Lucknow. The objectives included exploration of the *in vivo* cytogenetic, morphological, pharmacological, biochemical, and reproductive alterations induced by pesticides in the experimental animals. Repeated oral, dermal, intraperitoneal, intravenous, and intratesticular administration, alone or in combination with other insecticides, produced varied toxicological effects (Datta, 1978; Datta and Dikshith, 1973, 1980; Dikshith, 1973, unpublished data; Dikshith *et al.*, 1971; Dikshith and Datta, 1972*a,b*, 1973).

Repeated oral feeding of endosulfan produced significant depletion of hepatic glycogen in male albino rats. The high activity of phosphorylase, hexokinase, aldolase, and succinate dehydrogenase suggested a rapid cycling of glycogenolysis, glycolysis, and Krebs cycle, respectively. There was no change in the activity of fructose-1,6-diphosphatase, but glucose-6-phosphatase showed a significant increase which indicated a partial disturbance in gluconeogenesis. Endosulfan also produced significant inhibition of glucose-6-phosphate dehydrogenase and lactate dehydrogenase, which in turn would block the HMP and anaerobic glycolysis. The significant increase in the activity of ATPase suggested the energy requirement for the metabolism of endosulfan-poisoned animals (Kushwah and Dikshith, 1980; Dikshith *et al.*, 1974, 1975*a,b*, 1976, 1978*a–c*, 1979, 1980*a*, unpublished; Gupta, 1976*a,b;* Gupta and Paul, 1974; Gupta and Chandra, 1975; Kohli *et al.*, 1974*a,b;* Kohli and Khanna, 1974; Anand *et al.*, 1977; Khanna *et al.*, 1975; Matin, 1974; Matin and Kar, 1972, 1973, 1974; Matin *et al.*, 1976, 1977; Kar and Dikshith, 1970; Kar and Matin, 1971, 1972, 1974; Nath *et al.*, 1978; Raizada *et al.*, 1979, 1980; Kushwah and Dikshith, 1980).

Storage of endosulfan after repeated oral feeding for 30 days did not differ significantly in the presence of metepa or otherwise. The highest level of residue was observed in the kidney (6.5 ppm), while the lowest was in the blood (0.96 ppm). The observation did not suggest any kind of additive, antagonistic, or potentiation effects of metepa and endosulfan in male rats (Nath *et al.*, 1978). Male and female rats, however, behaved in a different manner in the induction of a toxic response (Dikshith *et al.*, 1980*a*).

Skin painting rats with fenitrothion (0.1 ml of 95% purity) showed that the insecticide is absorbed quickly through the skin, and a significant level was seen in the blood within 2 hr after treatment. Insecticide level in the blood was maximum after 8 hr and later showed a decrease. Inhibition of acetylcholinesterase after a single application of fenitrothion was 19.6% after three applications it was 64.1%, and five applications produced total inhibition (Kohli *et al.*, 1974*a*). Fenitrothion also caused loss of water from vital organs like the kidney, brain, and heart. The spleen and brain also demonstrated maximum mobilization of metals (Khanna *et al.*, 1975).

Malathion (500 mg/kg) administered through intraperitoneal injections produced a significant increase of blood glucose and plasma sodium and glycogen of the liver, kidney, heart, and spleen of rats. There was a change in plasma potassium and brain glycogen levels of treated rats (Gupta and Paul, 1974). Rats treated with a single dose of fenitrothion (750 mg/kg) through skin painting did not suggest any relationship between the RBC Mg^{2+} level and inhibition of cholinesterase activity, but the latter showed a continuous decrease in plasma up to 8 hr after treatment (Khanna et al., 1977; Anand et al., 1977).

Rats treated with a single dose of phenthoate orally or dermally exhibited typical symptoms of organophosphorus poisoning and inhibition of acetylcholinesterase activity in the blood and brain (Gupta, 1976a). Dermal painting of endosulfan in chloroform produced clinical symptoms of toxicity and mild to severe histopathological changes in some of the vital organs of the animal (Gupta, 1976a).

Exposure of male rats to parathion (2.6 mg/kg), lindane (17.6 mg/kg), or their combination through oral intubation daily for a period of 90 days produced histological and biochemical alterations in the liver and testis. The focal necrosis of the liver, although observed in all the treatments, was very prominent in the animals exposed to lindane alone. The kidney and epididymis, however, did not show any significant histological lesions. The activity of acetylcholinesterase in the blood and brain decreased markedly, whereas that of succinic dehydrogenase, adenosine triphosphatase, and the alkaline and acid phosphatases in the liver and testis showed significant alterations for all three treatments (Dikshith et al., 1978a).

Dermal application of benzene hexachloride in daily doses of 100,200 and 500 mg/kg for a total period of 30 days caused significant changes in male guinea pigs. The animals exposed to high doses of BHC died within 5–12 days. There was no mortality in 100 mg/kg per day, but significant pathologic and biochemical changes were observed in the vital organs of the experimental animals. Massive congestion and thickened blood vessels were seen in the liver of the BHC-treated animals in comparison to the controls. Similarly, testicular changes included mild to severe pathologic lesions. There was no change in the epididymis, kidney, spleen, brain, and lungs. The changes in the skin were mild and no signs of dermatitis were observed in the BHC-painted areas. The activity of glutamic oxaloacetic transaminase (GOT), glutamic pyruvic transaminase (GPT), and alkaline phosphatase in the liver and serum revealed significant changes from that of the controls (Dikshith et al., 1978b).

Daily oral administration of paraquat, a well-known herbicide, at a dose of 11 mg/kg for 30 days induced no toxic symptoms in rabbits. There were no deaths due to paraquat feeding. The morphological changes in the liver, kidney, testis, epididymis, and adrenal were not significant. Of the 12 animals, only one showed marked emphysema, interstitial and interalveolar fibrosis of the lung. The lumen of the smaller bronchioles was filled with edematous fluid. In contrast to mild morphological changes the activity of GOT and GPT in the lungs and serum of treated animals indicated a significant decrease and increase respectively. Serum alkaline and acid phosphatase also presented a significant depletion or mild elevation of the respective enzymes (Dikshith et al., 1979). Prolonged feeding of zineb (1.0 g/kg per day) has produced marked hyperplasia of thyroid in male rats, suggesting the blockade of iodide–iodine conversion. It also produced testicular damage in rats (Raizada *et al.*, 1979).

Repeated administration of organophosphorus insecticides such as quinalphos, methyl demeton, and phosphamidon in low doses inhibited acetylcholinesterase activity and induced no ill effects in animals. Rest and immediate cessation from further exposure to insecticides normalized the level of acetylcholinesterase activity. The behavior of different species of test animals, like rats, rabbits, guinea pigs, and domestic goats, toward low levels of organophosphorus compounds was comparable (Dikshith *et al.*, 1980*a–c*, unpublished data).

10.9.4. Toxicity to Man

Pesticides have exerted highly neurotoxic effects in animals and humans. Studies have hitherto stressed the convulsive properties of several pesticidal compounds that are used in pest and vector control operations (Joy, 1976). These potentially toxic chemicals are also known to mimic neurologic syndromes such as headaches, peripheral neuropathy, ataxia, seizures, status epilepticus, and clinical entities resembling pulmonary edema, myocardial infarction, diabetic comas, encephalitis, and asthma (Holmes, 1965). While assessing the health hazards of pesticide residues, two types of injury have to be considered: first, the possibility of an acute illness resulting from ingesting residues for a short period of time, and second, the long-term effects that may accrue after ingesting small quantities of residues daily for many years. Exposure to residues appears to cause only a mild disease manifested as gastrointestinal symptoms. Epidemiologically, the symptoms noticed due to residues are quite distinguishable from the acute effects produced by direct exposure. The majority of individuals with high amounts of body residues frequently become sick. In contrast, in poisoning episodes due to direct exposure to technical grade or formulations of pesticides, it is unusual to have more than one or two cases among any group of workers. Accidental poisoning in Kerala due to parathion-contaminated flour and in Karnataka and the involvement of members of the food chain like fish and crabs in the Handigodu syndrome have focused attention on exercising greater caution and control in the spread of pesticides to villages. With regard to organophosphorus pesticides, cases of acute poisoning were reported in individuals exposed to these in their occupations. Over 100 deaths in India during the spring of 1958 resulted from eating food accidently contaminated with parathion during shipment (Mutalik *et al.*, 1966; Karunakaran, 1958; Report of the National Institute of Nutrition, 1977).

Periodic surveys have indicated that humans in India show significantly higher storage levels than their counterparts in the USA. Signs of intoxication due to aldrin and dieldrin involve the central nervous system and may include electroencephalographic changes, muscle tremors, and convulsions. Levels of SGOT, SGPT, and serum LDH were greatly enhanced in the group occupationally exposed to pentachlorophenol. Very high levels of alkaline phosphatase have also been found in exposure to common organochlorines. Levels of albumin and beta and gamma globulins are also found to vary significantly with different types of occupational exposures, suggesting, primarily, involvement of the liver.

Cases of poisoning of men due to ingestion or exposure to organophosphorus and chlorinated hydrocarbon insecticides have been frequently reported in India. Organophosphorus and carbamate pesticides have been known to cause depression in the cholinesterase activity of the blood and brain. Studies have suggested that inhibition of acetylcholinesterase activity in RBC and the brains of pesticide-intoxicated animals would return to near-normal values when the animals are not further exposed and given a period of rest (Dikshith *et al.*, 1976, 1980a–c, unpublished data). This information could be used for controlling cases of organophosphorus poisoning under field conditions. The work conducted in India with special reference to toxic effects of these cases in human beings is briefly summarized as follows.

Thirty-four patients with cases of diazinon poisoning were admitted to the Ruby Hall Hospital in Pune, India, between January 1967 and May 1969. Diazinon was shown to cause rapid and severe depression of serum cholinesterase activity in 17 patients. Similar studies were undertaken in 158 males from Delhi and Punjab including 84 occupationally exposed to organophosphorus pesticides (Karnik *et al.*, 1970; Kashyap and Gupta, 1971a,b). The exposed group of individuals showed a significant depression in cholinesterase level. Blood cholinesterase activity was found to reflect the length of duration of exposure. Electrocardiographic changes were observed in 12% of the 86 cases of diazinon poisoning (Shah and Undavia, 1972). Impairment of consciousness (10%), fasciculation (27%), convulsion (1%), toxic delirium (50%), and paralysis (26%) were observed in poisoned people. A field study on the toxicological hazards to workers engaged in ultra-low-volume aerial spraying of phosphamidon revealed significant alterations in the plasma acetylcholinesterase activity of the sprayers. The maximum percentages of plasma cholinesterase inhibition, which occurred 1–3 days postspray, were 0–25% in 11 subjects, 26–50% in 19 subjects, and over 50% in 2 subjects. The distribution of parathion, malathion, dimethoate, sumithion, and phosphamidon in the human stomach, intestine, lungs, spleen, and heart in five different cases of suspected poisoning has been reported (Kashyap and Gupta, 1976; Tewari and Harpalani, 1977).

Studies with human volunteers have suggested that 2,4-D is quickly absorbed and above 75% of the compound is excreted unchanged in the urine 96 hr after administration (Kohli *et al.*, 1974a). A similar study with 2,4,5-T has also shown that this compound is absorbed readily from the gastrointestinal tract and is excreted in the urine without undergoing any metabolic alteration in the system (Kohli *et al.*, 1974b).

Residues of DDT and its metabolites in blood samples from 182 people in Delhi have been reported (Agarwal *et al.*, 1976). The average total DDT concentration in the whole blood ranged from 0.177 to 0.683 mg/liter in males and from 0.166 to 0.32 mg/liter in females, and p,p'-DDE, p,p'-DDD, and p,p'-DDT were detected as metabolites. DDE accounted for most of the total DDT. Eleven members of a village community and five domestic animals developed symptoms of neurotoxicity in the form of myoclonic jerks and major motor seizures on being exposed to chlorinated (aldrin and gammaxene) insecticides for a period of 6–12 months (Gupta, 1975). Eight cases with grand mal epilepsy in a village of Uttar Pradesh, secondary to accidental contamination of food grain by BHC, were also reported (Nag *et al.*, 1977). The distribution of endrin in different tissues from five different victims after autopsy was assayed by TLC. It was found that the largest amounts of the insecticide remained in the stomach and intestine (Tewari and Sharma, 1977). Deaths occurred within 1–2 hr of the ingestion of the insecticide. Small amounts of organophosphorus, organochlorine, and carbamate insecticides in human biological material were detected by TLC (Ganguly and Bhattacharya, 1973).

Toxicological experiments on occupational exposure to pesticides in pest control operators have been conducted by the National Institute of Occupational Health (NIOH) in Ahmedabad, India, in collaboration with the Industrial Toxicology Research Center in Lucknow. In a study conducted by the NIOH involving 120 exposed workers in a warehouse, 60 each of warehouses and godowns were found to be exposed to celphos, DDVP, and malathion, while the PCA workers were mostly exposed to chlordane, aldrin, malathion, and heptachlor. A significant reduction in plasma and RBC cholinesterase levels was found. Liver function tests, namely, SGPT and alkaline phosphatase, showed no significant difference between the control and both of the exposed groups.

10.10. FUTURE PERSPECTIVES

Pesticide research is an unending process. Identification and isolation of newer molecules and compounds and preparation of newer formulations are the only ways to control the increasing menace of pests and to reduce the ill effects of pesticides to man. Areas for further investigations can be categorized tentatively as follows:

1. Identification and isolation of biologically active molecules which could easily be biodegraded and synthesized. Documentation of phytochemicals already isolated and exploring the possibility of chemically transforming them. This would take care of the soil, water, and air even with the projected high levels of consumption of chemical pesticides.

2. Exploration of the possibility of screening microorganisms which can actively mediate the process of biodegradation, particularly in soil and water, by enrichment culture, genetic engineering, and other microbiological techniques. Studies on bacteria, fungi, and actinomycetes which have the potential of producing antifungal and antinematodal reagents.

3. Utilization of pesticides, biodegradable or otherwise, in large quantities during the coming years. It would be prudent to arrive at realistic methods for their safety evaluation and to frame the protocols to suit our local requirements. Standardization of reliable analytical (*in vitro* and *in vivo*) techniques for quantitating residues and assessing their biological effects.

4. Detailed studies on the versatile biochemical activity, for example, of plants, algae, and lichens to uptake and biotransform pesticides presently considered nonbiodegradable.

5. Development of simple field tests for the identification of residues and their toxicity.

6. Studies on photochemical mechanisms of the degradation of pesticides, especially in the presence of environmental pollutants, and the nature of the products thereof.

7. Determination of the health effects of pesticides on agricultural communities, farm animals, domestic pests, and on other nontarget organisms.

REFERENCES

Agarwal, N. S., 1979, Controlling stored grain pests in rural areas, *Pestic. Inf.* 4:83.

Agarwal, S. P., and Ahmad, A., 1978, Effect of pesticides on reproduction in mammals, *Pesticides* 12:15.

Agarwal, H. C., Pillai, M. K. K., Yadav, D. V., Menon, K. B., and Gupta, R. K., 1976, Residues of DDT: its metabolites in human blood samples in Delhi, India, *Bull. WHO* 54:349.

Agarwal, H. C., Yadav, D. V., and Pillai, M. K. K., 1978, Metabolism of 14C-DDT in *Pheritima posthuma* and effects of pretreatment with DDT, lindane and dieldrin, *Bull. Environ. Contam. Toxicol.* 19:295.

Agnihothrudu, V., and Mithyantha, M. S., 1978, Pesticide Residues, A Review of Indian Work, Pallis India Limited R.D. Laboratories, Fertilizers and Pesticides Division, Bangalore, India.

Agnihotri, V. P., Singh, K., and Budhraja, T. R., 1973, Persistence and degradation of Vitavax in soil and sugarcane setts and its effect on soil fungi proc., *Indian Natl. Sci. Acad.* 39B:561.

Agnihotri, N. P., Dewan, R. S., and Dixit, A. K., 1974a, Residues of insecticides in food commodities from Delhi. I. Vegetables, *Indian J. Entomol.* 36:160.

Agnihotri, N. P., Dewan, R. S., Jain, H. K., and Pandey, S. Y., 1974b, Residues of insecticides in food commodities from Delhi. II. High fat content food materials, *Indian J. Entomol.* 36:203.

Agnihotri, N. P., Pandey, S. Y., and Jain, H. H., 1977a, Persistence of BHC and Aldrin in soil and translocation in Mung (*Phaseolus aureus* L.) and Lobia (*Vigna sinensis* Siva), *Indian J. Entomol.* 36:261.

Agnihotri, N. P., Pandey, S. Y., Jain, H. A., and Srivastava, K. P., 1977b, Persistence of aldrin, dieldrin, lindane, heptachlor, and p,p'-DDT in soil, *J. Entomol. Res.* 1:89.

Ahmed, T. K., Ramama Rao, K. V., and Swami, K. S., 1978, Effect of malathion on enzyme activity in foot mantle and hepatopancreas of snail, *Indian J. Exp. Biol.* 16:258.

Alexander, M., 1965, Biodegradation: Problems of molecular recalcitrance and microbial fallibility, *Adv. Appl. Microbiology* 7:35.

Amminikutty, C. K., and Rege, M. S., 1977, Effects of acute and chronic exposure to pesticides, Thiodon Ec35 and Agallol'3' on the liver of widow *Tetra gymnocorymbus ternetzi* (Boulenger), *Indian J. Exp. Biol.* 15:197.

Anand, M., Khanna, R. N., Misra, D., and Sharma, H. K., 1977, Changes in brain acetylcholine of rats after dermal application of fenitrothion (Sumithion), *Indian J. Physiol. Pharmacol.* 21:121.

Anonymous, 1951, Study of insecticidal properties of *Acorus calamus* Linn, *Def. Res. Lab Rep.* Bio/51/76, Kanpur, India.

Anonymous, 1954, Insecticidal properties of nutmeg leaf oil, *Def. Res. Lab. Rep.* Ento/l/46, Kampur, India.

Anonymous, 1964, Use of pesticides, *Residue Rev.* 6:1.

Anonymous, 1965, Studies on insecticidal properties of Haldi, *Curcuma longa* Linn, *Def. Res. Lab. Rep.* 51/64, Kanpur, India.

Anonymous, 1973, The dependable way to knock out budworm in cotton, *Ortho News*, U.S.A.

Anonymous, 1977, Research report, Rallis India Limited, R & D Chemicals, Bangalore, India.

Anonymous, 1978*a*, Status of pesticides industry in India, *Pesticides* 12:15.

Anonymous, 1978*b*, A decade of service 1967–77, Publication from Division of Agricultural Chemistry, IARI, New Delhi.

Anonymous, 1979*a*, Report of the working group on pesticides Industry for the Plan (1978–79 to 1983–84), Ministry of Petroleum, Chemicals and Fertilizers, Government of India, India.

Anonymous, 1979*b*, Status report of research and development work done in India, Indo-US Workshop on Biodegradable Pesticides, Industrial Toxicology Research Centre, Lucknow, India.

Anonymous, 1980, Report of Pesticide Registration Committee, Ministry of Agriculture and Irrigation, Government of India.

Aravindakshan, A., Bikram Chand, Ramachandran, M., and Hussain, Q. Z., 1977, Effect of dietary DDT on certain biochemical changes in albino rats, *Indian J. Exp. Biol.* 15:578.

Arora, A., Vyas, S. C., and Jain, A. C., 1977*a*, Persistence of systemic fungicides carbendazim and benomyl on plants, *PANS (U.K.)* 23:430.

Awasthi, M. D., Dixit, A. K., Verma, S., Handa, S. K., and Dewan, R. S., 1974, Dissipation of endosulfan residues from cauliflower crop, *Indian J. Plant Protect.* 2:24.

Awasthi, M. D., Dixit, A. K., Verma, S., Handa, S. R., and Dewan, R. S., 1977*a*, Fate of monocrotophos and carbaryl on the cowpea, *Indian J. Plant Protect.* 5:55.

Awasthi, M. D., Kalara, A. N., and Dewan, R. S., 1977*b*, Residues of insecticides in sugarcane juice and gur following chemical protection of crop from insects, *Pesticides* 11:33.

Awasthi, M. D., Handa, S. K., Dixit, A. K., and Chatterjee, N. S., 1979, Dissipation of carbaryl residues in/on soybean crop, *Indian J. Entomol.* 41:181.

Balasubramanya, R. H., and Patil, R. B., 1976, Degradation of carboxin and oxy-carboxin by a species of *Pseudomonas* isolated from soil, *Madras. Agric. J.* 63:505.

Bandopadhyay, R., and Mukhopadhyay, A. N., 1977, Control of cerospora leaf spot of sugar beet with systemic fungicides, *Pantnagar J. Res.* 2:258.

Banerjee, S. C., 1970, Detoxification of pond water treated with endrin, *Indian J. Appl. Chem.* 33:185.

Basak, P. K., and Konar, S. K., 1976, Toxicity of six insecticides to fish, *Geobios (Jodhpur)* 3:209.

Basak, P. K., and Konar, S. K., 1977, A method for the determination of safe concentration of insecticides to protect fishes, *Indian J. Environ. Health* 19:283.

Baskaran, P., and Jothwani, M. G., 1976, Persistence of carbofuran and its principal metabolite, 3-OH carbofuron in grain sorghum, *Indian J. Plant Protect.* 4:186.

Beeson, C. F. C., 1941, *The Ecology and Control of the Forest Insects of India and the Neighboring Countries*, Vasant Press, Dehradun, India.

Beri, Y. P., and Dewan, R. S., 1964, Relative efficiency of different types of jute cloth bags against penetrating of stored grain pests and insecticides, in: *Pesticides*, pp. 144–147, Symposium on Pesticides, Central Food Technology Research Institute, Mysore, India.

Bhagavat, V. M., and Ramachandran, B. V., 1973, Determination of malathion in enzymatic digests by ferric hydroxamate method, *J. Assoc. Off. Anal. Chem.* **56**:1339.

Bhagavat, V. M., and Ramachandran, B. V., 1975, Enzymic hydrolysis of malaoxon by mouse liver homogenates, *Biochem. Pharmacol.* **24**:2002.

Bhaktavatsalam, G., and Tripathi, K. K., 1974, Uptake and translocation of carboxin and oxy-carboxin in pearl millet, *Indian J. Mycol. Plant Pathol.* **4**:21.

Bhatia, S. C., and Subramanian, T. A. V., 1972a, Effect of dieldrin on certain enzyme systems of rat liver, *Br. J. Exp. Pathol.* **53**:419.

Bhatia, S. C., and Subramanian, T. A. V., 1972b, Mechanism of dieldrin induced fat accumulation in rat liver, *J. Agric. Food Chem.* **20**:993.

Bhatia, S. C., Sharma, S. C., Damodaran, V. N., and Subramanian, T. A. V., 1971, Changes in rat ascorbic acid status and adrenocortieal activity during acute dieldrin toxicity, *Indian J. Biochem. Biophys.* **8**:57.

Bhatia, S. C., Sharma, S. C., and Subramanian, T. A. V., 1972, Acute dieldrin toxicity, biochemical changes in blood, *Arch. Environ. Health* **24**:369.

Bhatia, S. C., Sharma, S. C., and Subramanian, T. A. V., 1973, Effect of dieldrin on hepatic carbohydrate metabolism and protein biosynthesis *in vivo*, *Toxicol. Appl. Pharmacol.* **24**:216.

Bhatnagar, O. K., 1975, Efficacy of various pesticides against white grubs of groundnut, *Pesticides* **9**:22.

Bhatnagar, S. P., Yadava, C. P. S., Bhatnagar, K. N., and Srivastava, B. P., 1964, Comparative efficacy of some chlorinated and phosphatic insecticides against *Chrotogonus trachyptenus* Blance., Symposium on Pesticides, Central Food Technology Research Institute, Mysore, India.

Bhatnagar, V. S., and Srivastava, B. P., 1974, Effect of temperature on the toxicity of some insecticides to *Tribolium castaneum* (Herbst) (Tenebrionidae: coleoptera), *Bull. Grain Technol.* **12**:211.

Bhattacharya, S., Mukherjee, S., and Bhattacharya, S., 1975, Toxic effects of endrin on hepato-pancreas of teleost fish, *Indian J. Exp. Biol.* **13**:185.

Bindra, O. S., and Kalra, K. L., 1971, A review of work done in India on pesticide residues, Symposium on Progress and Problems in Pesticide Residue Analysis, Ludhiana, India.

Brodie, B. B., and Maicke, R. P., 1962, *Proceedings of the First International Pharmacological Meeting*, Vol. 6, *Comparative Biochemistry of Drug Metabolism*, p. 299, Pergamon Press, New York.

Buhler, D. R., and Rasmusson, M. E., 1968, The oxidation of drug by fishes, *Comp. Biochem. Physiol.* **25**:223.

Carter, R. H., 1947, Estimation of DDT in milk by determination of organic chlorine, *Anal. Chem.* **19**:54.

Casida, J. E., and Lykken, L., 1969, Metabolism of organic pesticide chemicals in higher plants, *Annu. Rev. Plant Physiol.* **20**:607.

Chahal, D. S., Bans, I. S., and Chopra, S. L., 1977, Degradation alcchor (2-chloro-*N*(methoxy methyl)-2′, 6′-diethyl acetanilide) by soil fungi, *Plant Soil* **45**:689.

Chakraborty, D. P., Mauti, R. K., and Dhua, S. P., 1973, Studies on the efficacy of some insecticides and their compatibility with urea against major pests of paddy under field condition, *Pesticides* **7**:15.

Chan, T. M., Gillett, J. W., and Terriare, L. C., 1967, Interactions between microsomal electron transport system of trout and male rat in cyclodiene epoxidation, *Comp. Biochem. Physiol.* **20**:731.

Chatterjee, D. K., 1972, Effects of a few moderate to slightly toxic insecticides on some rice pests and on crop yield, *Pesticides* **6**:19.

Chauhan, U. P. S., Rastogi, V. K., Jaggi, C. B., and Ray Sarkar, B. C., 1973, Effect of acute malathion poisoning on acetylcholinesterase in various tissues of rats, *Indian J. Exp. Biol.* **11**:576.

Chauhan, U. P. S., Jaggi, C. B., and Rastogi, V. K., 1974, Hypertrophy of adrenals and ascarbic acid status in various tissues on malathion treated rats, *Indian J. Med. Res.* **62**:987.

Chawla, R. P., Joia, B. S., Udean, A. S., Kalra, R. L., and Bindra, O. S., 1976, Toxicity and residues of idofenphos as influenced by its distribution in the stored wheat, Proceedings of the All India Symposium on Modern Concepts of Plant Protection, Udaipur, p. 81.

Chawla, R. S., Hothi, D. S., Singh Bulwant, and Grewal, G. S., 1977, Malathion poisoning in poultry, *Pesticides* **11**:30.

Chopra, S. L., Nandra, K. S., and Kumari, S., 1973, Persistence of some pesticides in groundnut plant (*Arachis hypogoea* L.), *J. Res. (Punjab)* **10**:199.

Cook, J. W., 1957, Action of rumen fluid on pesticides: *In vitro* destruction of some organophosphate pesticides by bovine rumen fluid, *J. Agric. Food Chem.* **5**:859.

Creaven, P. J., Parke, D. V., and Williams, R. J., 1965, A fluorometric study of the hydroxylalation of bipheyl *in vitro* by liver preparations of various species, *Biochem. J.* **96**:870.

Creaven, P. J., Davies, W. H., and Williams, R. T., 1967, Dealkylation of alkoxybiphenyls by trout and frog liver preparations, *Life Sci.* **6**:105.

Dale, D., 1975, Studies on the inhibition of cholinesterase from Indian Honey bee, *Pesticides* **9**:25.

Datta, K. K., 1978, Studies on the cytopathological effects of lindane in experimental animals and goat, Ph.D. dissertation, Agra University, Agra, India.

Datta, K. K., and Dikshith, T. S. S., 1973, Histopathologic changes in the testis and liver of rats repeatedly exposed to pesticides, *Exp. Pathol.* **8**:363.

Deshmukh, S. N., and Saramma, P. V., 1971, Estimation of carbaryl residues in maize and cauliflower, *Indian J. Entomol.* **33**:338.

Dewan, R. S., Misra, S. S., Handa, S. K., and Lal, R., 1969, Persistence of malathion residues on cowpea, *Vigna sinensis* fruits and grain, *Indian J. Entomol.* **31**:93.

Dhaliwal, G. S., and Lal, R., 1973, Relative toxicity of some fumigants to the larvae of *T. grananiun* and *Cada cautella* and the susceptibility of different stages of these insects to phosphamidon, *Indian J. Entomol.* **35**:134.

Dikshith, T. S. S., 1973, *In vivo* effects of parathion on guinea pig chromosomes, *Environ. Physiol. Biochem.* **3**:161.

Dikshith, T. S. S., 1978, DDT-Residue and hazards, *J. Sci. Ind. Res.* **37**:316.

Dikshith, T. S. S., and Datta, K. K., 1972*a*, Effect of parathion on the skin of guinea pigs, *Experientia* **28**:169.

Dikshith, T. S. S., and Datta, K. K., 1972*b*, Pathologic changes induced by pesticides in the testis and liver of rats, *Exp. Pathol.* **7**:309.

Dikshith, T. S. S., and Datta, K. K., 1973, Endrin induced cytological changes in albino rats, *Bull. Environ. Contam. Toxicol.* **9**:65.

Dikshith, T. S. S., and Datta, K. K., 1978, Endosulfan: Lack of cytogenetic effects in male rats, *Bull. Environ. Contam. Toxicol.* **20**:826.

Dikshith, T. S. S., and Vasuki, K., 1970, Alkaline and acid phosphatases and the effect of endrin on *Dactylopius confusus* (Dactylopiidae: coccoidea), *Enzymologia* **39**:77.

Dikshith, T. S. S., Chandra, P., and Datta, K. K., 1971, Effect of lindane on the skin of albino rats, *Experientia* **29**:684.

Dikshith, T. S. S., and Datta, K. K., and Chandra, P., 1974, Interaction of lindane and diazinon on the skin of rats, *Exp. Pathol.* **9**:219.

Dikshith, T. S. S., Behari, J. R., Datta, K. K., and Mathur, A. K., 1975*a*, Effect of diazinon in male rats. Histopathological and Biochemical studies, *Environ. Physiol. Biochem.* **5**:293.

Dikshith, T. S. S., Datta, K. K., and Pandya, K. P., 1975b, Effect of DDT on the free amino acid pool of brain and kidney in guinea pigs, *Environ. Physiol. Biochem.* **5**:404.

Dikshith, T. S. S., Datta, K. K., and Chandra, P., 1976, 90 days dermal toxicity of DDVP in male rats, *Bull. Environ. Contam. Toxicol.* **5**:574.

Dikshith, T. S. S., Tandon, S. K., Datta, K. K., Gupta, P. K., and Behari, J. R., 1978a, Comparative response of male rats to parathion and lindane: Histopathological and biochemical studies, *Environ. Res.* **17**:1.

Dikshith, T. S. S., Datta, K. K., Kushwah, H. S., and Raizada, R. B., 1978b, Histopathological and biochemical changes in guinea pigs after repeated dermal exposure to benzene hexachloride (BHC), *Toxicology* **10**:55.

Dikshith, T. S. S., Nath, G., and Datta, K. K., 1978c, Combined cytogenetic effects of endosulfan and metepa in male rats, *Indian J. Exp. Biol.* **16**:1000.

Dikshith, T. S. S., Datta, K. K., Raizada, R. B., and Kushwah, H. S., 1979, Effect of paraquat dichloride in male rabbits, *Indian J. Exp. Biol.* **17**:926.

Dikshith, T. S. S., Datta, K. K., and Raizada, R. B., 1980a, Response of carbon tetrachloride treated male rats to benzene hexachloride and quinalphos, *Indian J. Exp. Biol.* **18**:1267.

Dikshith, T. S. S., Raizada, R. B., and Datta, K. K., 1980b, Interaction of phosphamidon and benzene in female rabbits, *Indian J. Exp. Biol.* **18**:1273.

Dikshith, T. S. S., Raizada, R. B., and Datta, K. K., 1980c, Response of female guinea pigs to repeated oral administration of quinolphos, *Bull. Environ. Contam. Toxicol.* **24**:739.

Dixit, A. K., Awasthi, M. D., Handa, S. K., Verma, S., and Dewan, R. S., 1975, Residues and residual toxicity of malathion and endosulfan on okra fruits, *Indian J. Entomol.* **37**:251.

Dixit, A. K., Agnihotri, N. P., Dewan, R. S., and Saxena, H. P., 1976, Dissipation of aldicarb in soil and pea plant, *Indian J. Agric. Sci.* **46**:117.

Dixit, A. K., Bhattacharjee, N. S., Handa, S. K., Awasthi, M. D., and Dewan, R. S., 1977, Dissipation of phorate, disulfoton and endosulfan in/on soybean crop, *Indian J. Plant Protect.* **5**:70.

Fatehyab, S., and Mahdi Hasan, 1977, Effect of organophosphate insecticide dichlorvos on the amino acid content of different regions of the rat brain and spinal cord, *Indian J. Exp. Biol.* **15**:759.

Ganguly, S. K., and Bhattacharya, J., 1973, Detection of small amounts of pesticides in human biological material by TLC, *Forensic Sci.* **2**:333.

Girish, G. K., Goyal, R. K., and Krishnamurthy, K., 1971, Efficacy and residual toxicity of iodofenphos and malathion (5% dust) against stored grain pests. II, *Pesticides* **5**:18.

Gopalaswamy, U. V., and Aiyar, A. S., 1977, Mammalian toxicity and metabolism of lindane, *Indian J. Biochem. Biophys.* **14**:36.

Dixit, A. K., Agnihotri, N. P., Dewan, R. S., and Saxena, H. P., 1976, Dissipation of aldicarb in soil and pea plant, *Indian J. Agric. Sci.* **46**:117.

Dixit, A. K., Bhattacharjee, N. S., Handa, S. K., Awasthi, M. D., and Dewan, R. S., 1977, Dissipation of phorate, disulfoton and endosulfan in/on soybean crop. *Indian J. Plant Protect.* **5**:70.

Griffiths, D. C., and Walker, N., 1970, Microbiological degradation of parathion, *Meded. Rijks. Landbouwwet. Gent.* **35**:807.

Gupta, B., and Agarwal, A. C., 1977, Metabolism and distribution of DDT in mouse in relation to poisoning symptoms, *Indian J. Exp. Biol.* **15**:402.

Gupta, M., 1974, Determination of diazinon residues by bioassay and thin-layer chromatography *Indian J. Plant Protect.* **2**:103.

Gupta, K. G., Sud, R. K., Aggarwal, P. K., and Aggarwal, J. C., 1979, Effect of Baygon on some soil biological processes and its degradation of *Pseudomonas* ssp., *Plant Soil* **42**:317.

Gupta, P. C., 1975, Neurotoxicity of chronic chlorinated hydrocarbon insecticide poisoning: A clinical study in man, *Indian J. Med. Res.* **63**:901.

Gupta, P. K., 1976*a*, Duration of phenthoate induced changes in blood and brain cholinesterase and toxicity of phenthoate in rats, *Chemosphere* **5**:201.

Gupta, P. K., 1976*b*, Endosulfan induced neurotoxicity in rats and mice, *Bull. Environ. Contam. Toxicol.* **15**:708.

Gupta, P. K., and Chandra, S. V., 1975, The toxicity of endosulfan in rabbits, *Bull. Environ. Contam. Toxicol.* **14**:513.

Gupta, P. K., and Paul, B. S., 1974, Effect of malathion on oxygen consumption and blood cholinesterase of the hen, *Arch. Environ. Health.* **29**:167.

Gupta, R. C., and Dewan, R. S., 1974, Residues and metabolism of carbofuran in soil, *Pesticides* **8**:36.

Hameed, S. F., and Lal, R., 1971, Residues of malathion on cabbage, cauliflower knolkhol estimated by bioassay and chemical assay methods, *Indian J. Entomol.* **33**:326.

Harvey, J., Jr., and Pease, H. L., 1973, Decomposition of methomyl in soil, *J. Agric. Food Chem.* **27**:784.

Harvey, J., Jr., and Reiser, R. W., 1973, Methomyl in tobacco, corn and cabbage, *J. Agric. Food Chem.* **21**:775.

Holmes, J. H., 1965, *Research in Pesticides*, Academic Press, New York.

Jagalan, P. S., and Chopra, S. L., 1971, Degradation and persistence behavior of BHC and DDT on spinach, *Pesticides* **5**:15.

Jagirdar, H. S., Sethi, R. K., and Chopra, S. L., 1974, On some metabolic activity of peas, *Pesticides* **8**:32.

Jain, H. K., Pandey, S. Y., Agnihothri, N. P., Dewan, R. S., Saxena, A. N., and Peshwani, K. M., 1974, Dissipation of phorate and disulfoton in rape seed crop, *Indian J. Plant Protect.* **1**:37.

Jain, P. C., and Gupta, H. L., 1976, Persistence of lindane, malathion and parathion residues in brinjal fruits, *Ann. Arid. Zone* **15**:37.

Jat, N. R., and Srivastava, B. P., 1973, Extent of malathion residue in and on okar (*Aelmonscho esculantus* Moench) fruits, *Indian J. Entomol.* **35**:143.

Jhooty, J. S., and Munshi, G. D., 1976, Persistence of fungicides on tomato leaves, *Indian Phytopathol.* **29**:80.

Joia, B. S., and Kalra, R. L., 1974, A note on the dissipation of ultra low volume formulations of endosulfan, fenitrothion, fenthion and malathion on okra, *Indian J. Agric. Sci.* **44**:897.

Joshi, A. G., and Rege, M. S., 1980, Acute toxicity of some pesticides and a few inorganic salts to the mosquito fish, *Gambusia affinis* (Baird and Girad), *Indian J. Exp. Biol.* **18**:435.

Joshi, B. G., and Ramaprasad, G., 1969, Residues of some common insecticides in fluecured tobacco, *Pesticides* **3**:17.

Joshi, H. C., Kapoor, D., Parwan, R. S., and Gupta, R. A., 1975, Toxicity of some insecticides to Chironomid larvae, *Indian J. Environ. Health* **17**:238.

Joy, R. M., 1976, Convulsive properties of chlorinated hydrocarbon insecticides in the cat central nervous system, *Toxicol. Appl. Pharmacol.* **35**:95.

Kandaswamy, D., Chendrayan, K., Rajukkannu, K. M., and Balasubramanian, M., 1977, On the variation in the degradation of carbofuran by three soil fungi, *Curr. Sci.* **46**:280.

Kannaiyan, J., Tripathi, R. K., and Hene, Y. L., 1975, Degradation and persistence of benomyl in lentil, *Indian Phytopathol.* **28**:305.

Kapil, R. P., and Lamba, D. P. S., 1974, Toxicity of some important insecticides to *Apis cerane* Fab, *Indian J. Entomol.* **36**:6.

Kar, P. P., and Dikshith, T. S. S., 1970, Dermal toxicity of DDT, *Experientia* **26**:634.

Kar, P. P., and Matin, M. A., 1971, Duration of diazinon induced changes in the brain acetylcholine of rats, *Pharmacol. Res. Commun.* **3**:351.

Kar, P. P., and Matin, M. A., 1972, Possible role of aminobytyric acid in paraoxon induced convulsions, *J. Pharm. Pharmacol.* **24**:996.

Kar, P. P., and Matin, M. A., 1974, Possible role of cerebral amino acids in acute neurotoxic effects of DDT in mice, *Eur. J. Pharmacol.* **25**:36.

Karel, A. K., 1976, Acute chlordane toxicity on the serum alkaline phosphate activity of merines hurrina jerdou gerbil, *Arch. Int. Physiol. Biochem.* **84**:63.

Karel, A. K., and Saxena, S. C., 1976, Chronic chlordane toxicity effect on blood biochemistry of Indian desert gerbil, *Pestic. Biochem. Physiol.* **6**:11.

Karnik, V. M., Jchaporia, R. N., and Wadia, R. S., 1970, Cholinesterase levels in diazinon poisoning in relation to severity of poisoning, *J. Assoc. Physiol.* **18**:337.

Karunakaran, C. O., 1958, The Kerala food poisoning, *J. Indian Med. Assoc.* **31**:204.

Kashyap, S. K., and Gupta, S. K., 1971a, Acute and chronic toxicity studies of DDT in albino rats, *Indian J. Med. Res.* **59**:284.

Kashyap, S. K., and Gupta, S. K., 1971b, The effect of occupational exposure to organophosphorus pesticides on blood cholinesterase, *Indian J. Med. Res.* **59**:289.

Kashyap, S. K., Gupta, S. K., 1976, Effect of ULV aerial spray of phosphamidon on human volunteers, *Indian J. Med.* **64**:579.

Kasturi, R., 1978, Alleviation of phytotoxicity of Fensulfothian (Dasanit) on peas, *J. Indian Inst. Sci.* **60**:9.

Kasturi, R., and Vasantharajan, V. N., 1976, Properties of acetylcholinesterase from *Pisum Sativum*, *Phytochemistry* **15**:1345.

Kathpal, T. S., Bhatnagar, V. S., Gupta, H. C. L., and Srivastava, B. P., 1977, Residues of endosulfan in/on ber (*Ziziphus jujuba* Lamk) fruits and leaves, *Pesticides* **11**:37.

Kaufman, D. D., and Kearney, P. C., 1970, Microbial degradation of *S*-triazine herbicides, *Residue Rev.* **32**:235.

Kaur, K., and Toor, M. S., 1977, Toxicity of pesticides to embryonic stages of fish, *Indian J. Exp. Biol.* **15**:193.

Kavadia, V. S., Noor, A., and Saxena, R. C., 1974, Residues and persistence of endosulfan (Thiodan) in head and leaves of cauliflower, *J. Food Sci. Technol.* **11**:63.

Kavadia, V. S., Gupta, H. C. L., Pareek, B. L., and Sharma, K. P., 1977, Residues of endosulfan, carbaryl and malathion in maize, *Entomology* **2**:17.

Kearney, P. C., and Kaufman, D. D. (eds.), 1969, *Degradation of Herbicides*, Marcel Dekker, New York.

Khanna, R. N., and Hasan, M. E., and Kohli, J. D., 1975, Effect of dermal application of fenitrothion on tissue levels of copper, zinc and manganese in rats, *Chemosphere* **5**:259.

Khanna, R. N., Misra, D., and Hasan, M. Z., 1977, Effect of Fenitrothion on mangnesium level and cholinesterase activity in rats, *Indian J. Physiol. Pharmacol.* **21**:209.

Knaak, J. B., Munger, D. M., McCarthy, J. F., and Salter, L. D., 1970, Metabolism of carbofuran, alfalfa residues in the dairy cow, *J. Agric. Food. Chem.* **18**:832.

Kohli, J. D., Hasan, M. Z., and Gupta, B. N., 1974a, Dermal absorption of fenitrothion in the rat, *Bull. Environ. Contam. Toxicol.* **11**:285.

Kohli, J. D., Khanna, R. N., Gupta, B. N., Khan, M. M., Zandon, J. S., and Sirkar, U. P., 1974b, Absorption and excretion of 2,4,5-T in man, *Arch. Int. Pharmacodynam. Ther.* **210**:250.

Kohli, J. D., Khanna, R. N., Gupta, B. N., Dhar, M. M., Tandon, J. S., and Sirkar, K. P., 1974c, Absorption and excretion of 2,4-D dichlorophenoxy acetic acid in man, *Xenobiotica* **4**:97.

Kohli, K. K., Maggon, K. K., Subramanian, T. A. V., 1977, Induction of mixed function oxidases on oral administration of dieldrin, *Chem. Biol. Interact.* **17**:249.

Koundinya, P. R., 1978, Studies on physiological response of the fresh water Telcost *Tilapia mossambica* (Peters) to pesticide impact, Ph.D. dissertation, Sri Venkateswara University, Tirupati, India.

Koundinya, P. R., and Ramamurthi, R., 1978a, *Indian J. Env. Health* **20**:6.

Koundinya, P. R., and Ramamurthi, R., 1978b, Effect of Sumithion (Fenitrothion): Some system in the fish, *Indian J. Exp. Biol.* **16**:809.

Koundinya, P. R., and Ramamurthi, R., 1979*a*, Effect of organophosphate pesticide sumithion (Fenitrothion) on some aspects of carbohydrate metabolism in a fresh water fish, *Sarotherodon (Tilapia) mossambicus* (Peters), *Experientia* **35**:1632.

Koundinya, P. R., and Ramamurthi, R., 1979*b*, Tissue respiration in *Tilapia mossambicus* (Peters) exposed to lethal (LC$_{50}$) concentration of sumithion and sevin, *Indian J. Environ. Health* **20**:426.

Koudinya, P. R., and Ramamurthi, R., 1980, Toxicity of Sumithion and Sevin to the freshwater fish *Sarotherodon mossambicus* (Peters), *Curr. Sci.* **49**:875.

Krishnaiah, N. V., Khare, B. P., and Sharma, V. K., 1976, Relative efficacy of some safer organophosphate insecticides used as grain protectants, *Pesticides* **10**:39.

Krishnamurthy, K., Subramanya, T. S., Urs, R., and Jayaraj, P., 1965, Of insecticide residues in books. Part I. Effects of a poor rice diet on the toxicity of dieldrin to albino rats, *Indian J. Exp. Biol.* **3**:168.

Kuhr, R. J., 1970, Metabolism of carbamate insecticidal chemicals in plants and insects, *J. Agric. Food Chem.* **18**:1023.

Kulshrestha, G., Dewan, R. S., and Mani, V. S., 1976, Dissipation of simuzine and atrazine in soil and their uptake by corn plants, *Pesticides* **10**:21.

Kumar, D., and Bhattacharya, S., 1977, Reversibility of endrin inhibition of alpha-amylase activity from fish liver, *Indian J. Exp. Biol.* **15**:927.

Kumaresan, D., and Baskaran, P., 1975, Biochemical changes in brinjal due to insecticides in relation to insect occurrence, *Indian J. Exp. Biol.* **13**:515.

Kushwah, H. S., and Dikshith, T. S. S., 1980, *In vivo* and *in vitro* response to endosulfan *vis a vis* cholmergic phenomenon, 2nd Congress of the Federation of Asian and Ocean Biochemists and Golden Jubilee Annual Meeting of the Society of Biological Chemists (India), December 14–18, Bangalore, India, abstract, pp. 127–128.

Lichtenstein, E. P., and Schulz, K. R., 1965, Residues of aldrin and heptachlor in soils and their translocation into various crops, *J. Agric. Food Chem.* **13**:57.

Lotlikar, P. D., Miller, E. C., Miller, J. A., and Halver, J. E., 1967, Metabolism of the carcinogen, acetylamino fluorence of rainbow trout, *Proc. Soc. Exp. Biol. Med.* **124**:160.

Mathur, R. N., 1964, Forest entomology in: *Entomolology in India*, pp. 437–456, The Entomological Society of India, New Delhi, India.

Matin, M. A., 1974, Effect on paraoxon on cholinesterase activity in certain brain regions of diabetic rats, *Eur. J. Pharmacol.* **29**:168.

Matin, M. A., and Kar, P. P., 1972, Central effect of paraoxon in diabetic rat, *Biochem. Pharmacol.* **21**:2285.

Matin, M. A., and Kar, P. P., 1973, Further studies on the -aminobutyric acid in paraoxon induced convulsions, *Eur. J. Pharmacol.* **21**:217.

Matin, M. A., and Kar, P. P., 1974, Effect of barbiturates and isoniazid on cerebral hemisphere-aminobutyric acid content in *pp'*-DDT treated mice, *Pharmacol. Res. Commun.* **6**:357.

Matin, M. A., Kar, P. P., and Anand, M., 1976, Modification of *pp'*-DDT induced convulsions by changes in the level of cerebral-aminobutyric acid in mice, *J. Neurochem.* **27**:979.

Matin, M. A., Kar, P. P., Hasan, M. Z., and Anand, M., 1977, Comparison of the chronic effect of -chlordane and *pp'*-DDT on the level of cerebral amino acid and free ammonia in mice, *Pharmacol. Res. Commun.* **9**:613.

Mehrotra, K. N., and Singh, V., 1972, Ageing in esterases inhibited by organophosphates, *Indian J. Entomol.* **34**:112.

Mehrotra, K. N., Beri, Y. P., Misra, S. S., and Phokela, A., 1967, Physiological effects of malathion on the house sparrow, *Passer domesticus* L., *Indian J. Exp. Biol.* **5**:219.

Menzer, R. E., and Dauterman, W. C., 1970, Metabolism of some organophosphorus insecticides, *J. Agric. Food Chem.* **18**:1031.

Misra, S. S., Verma, S., Handa, S. K., and Lal, R., 1971, BHC and parathion residues on crop of yellow sarson, *Indian J. Agric. Sci.* **41**:276.

Misra, S. S., Awasthi, M. D., and Dewan, R. S., 1977, Residues of some content insecticides in potatoes, *J. Fed. Sci. Tech.* **14**:11.

Mithyantha, M. S., 1973, Studies on retention and persistence of pesticides in soils, Ph.D. dissertation, University of Agricultural Science, Bangalore, India.

Mitra, P. K., Sud, S. C., and Bahga, H. S., 1978, Acute oral toxicity of metasystox in buffalo calves, *Indian J. Exp. Biol.* **16**:813.

Munro, H. A. U., 1964, *Manual of Fumigation for Insect Control, FAO Agric. Stud.* No. 79.

Mookherjee, P. B., 1964, Stored grain pests, in: *Entomology in India*, pp. 317–330, The Entomological Society of India, New Delhi, India.

Mukhopadhyay, P. K., Guha, P. K., and Banerjee, S. K., 1977, Biochemical effects of organophosphorus insecticides in fishes, *Indian J. Biochem. Biophys.* **14**:57.

Murthy, K. S. R. K., and Srivastava, B. P., 1977, Dissipation of malathion residues from green gram p. aureus Toxb. seeds, *Indian J. Entomol.* **32**:146.

Mutalik, G. S., Wadia, R. C., and Pai, V. R., 1966, *J. Indian Med. Assoc.* **46**:263.

Muthu, M., and Narasimhan, K. S., 1964, Studies on methods for selecting materials as fungation sheets. I. Permeability of liquid fumigants through polyethylene, Symposium on Pesticides, Central Food Technology Research Institute, Mysore, India.

Muthu, M., and Pingale, S. V., 1955, Extent of variations caused by certain factors in the toxicity of ethylene dichloride–carbon tetrachloride mixture to insects, *Indian J. Entomol.* **17**:193.

Muthu, M., Rangaswamy, J. R., and Vijayashankar, Y. N., 1976, Insecticidal doses of methyl iodide in foods and its residues, *J. Food Sci. Technol.* **13**:43.

Muthu, M., Narasimhab, K. S., and Majumdar, S. K., 1971, Symposium on Phosphine Used on a Fumigant on Food Stuffs, Symposium on Program Problems in Pesticide Residue Analysis, Ludhiana, India.

Nag, D., Singh, G. C., and Senon, S., 1977, Epilepsy epidemic due to benzene hexachlorine, *Trop. Geogr. Med.* **29**:229.

Nageshwar Rao, T., and Subrahmanyam, D., 1974, Effect of DDT on rat adipose tissue lipolytic activity, *Indian J. Biochem. Biophys.* **14**:50.

Nath, G., Kathpal, T. S., and Srivastava, B. P., 1974, Persistence of endosulfan residues in/on bhindi fruits, *Indian J. Plant Protect.* **2**:45.

Nath, G., Datta, K. K., and Dikshith, T. S. S., Tandon, S. K., and Panda, K. P., 1978, Interaction of endosulfan and metepa in rats, *Toxicology* **11**:385.

O'Brien, R. D., 1967, *Insecticide Action and Metabolism*, Academic Press, New York.

Pal, S. K., and Kushwah, K. S., 1977, Proceedings of the Symposium on Insects and Environment, the University of Delhi, February, abstracts, p. 43.

Pandey, S. Y., and Agnihothri, N. P., 1975, Effect of fertilization on the degradation of dichlorotophos, disulfoton and phorate in soil, *Fertil. News* **20**:32.

Pandey, S. Y., Jain, H. K., Agnihothri, N. P., Dewan, R. S., and Saxena, H. P., 1977, Residues from foliar application of carbophenothion, tetrachlorvinphos, dicrotophos, trichlorofon and endosulfan on bengal gram *(Cicer arietinum)*, *Indian J. Plant Protect.* **5**:47.

Patil, K. C., Matsumuru, F., and Boush, G. M., 1972, Metabolic transformation of DDT, dieldrin, aldrin, and endrin by marine microorganisms, *Environ. Sci. Technol.* **6**:629.

Paul, B. S., and Vadamudi, V. P., 1976, Teratogenic studies of benitrothion on white leghoon chick embryos, *Bull. Environ. Contam. Toxicol.* **15**:223.

Pawar, S. S., and Makhija, S. J., 1975, Hepatic amonopyrene N. demethylase, acentanilide hydroxylase and lipid peroxidation in young growing rats during the treatment of insecticides, *Bull. Environ. Contam. Toxicol.* **14**:714.

Pillai, M. K. K., Agarwal, H. C., and Yadav, D. V., 1977, Tolerance uptake and metabolism of DDT in *G. effinis*, *Indian J. Exp. Biol.* **15**:40.

Pingale, S. V., 1964, Progress in handling of grain in storage in India, in: *Entomology in India*, pp. 331–351, The Entomological Society of India, New Delhi, India.

Potter, J. L., and O'Brien, R. D., 1964, Parathion activation by livers of aquatic and terrestrial vertebrates, *Science* **4**:55.

Pradhan, S., Jotwani, M. G., and Sarup, P., 1964, Bioassay of different insecticides on the important insect pest and predators of agricultural importance, in: *Pesticides* (S. K. Majumdar, ed.), pp. 92–103, Academy of Pesticide Control, Mysore, India.

Raghuraj, R., Rajukkannu, K., Tirumurthi, S., Asaf Ali, K., Krishnamurthy, K. K., and Subramanian, T. R., 1973, Estimation of carbaryl insecticide residues on bhindi fruits, *Madras Agric. J.* **60**:1083.

Raizada, R. B., Datta, K. K., and Dikshith, T. S. S., 1979, Effect of Zineb on the histology of the rat thyroid, *Bull. Environ. Cont. Toxicol.* **22**:208.

Raizada, R. B., Misra, P., Saxena, I., Datta, K. K., and Dikshith, T. S. S., 1980, Weak estrogenic activity of lindane in rats, *J. Toxicol. Environ. Health.* **6**:471.

Rajamanickam, C., and Padmanabhan, G., 1974, Biochemical effect of Hexachlorobenzene, *Indian J. Biochem. Biophys.* **11**:119.

Rajukkannu, K., Asaf Ali, K., Raghuraj, R., Tirumurthi, S., Subramanian, T. R., and Krishnamurthy, K. K., 1973, Estimation of disulfoton residues on bhindi fruits by chemical and bioassay methods and dissipation of disulfoton in soil, *Madras Agric. J.* **60**:534.

Rajukkannu, K., Raghuraj, R., Asaf Ali, K., and Krishnamurthi, K. K., 1976, Residues of endrin, parathion, carbaryl, and endosulfan in vegetables, *Pesticides* **10**:14.

Rajukkannu, K., Raghuraj, R., Krishnamurthi, K. K., and Subramanian, T. R., 1977, Persistence of phorate and carborfuan in flooded soils, *Pesticides* **11**:14.

Ramaprasad, G., and Joshi, B. G., 1974, Efficacy of gramlar systemic insecticides for the control of Myzus persical on Lanka tobacco, *Indian J. Agric. Sci.* **44**:357.

Ranade, V. V., Jahagirdar, H. V., and Shingatgeri, M. K., 1978, Aerial spray of thiometon on livestock and poultry, *Pesticides* **12**:36.

Rao, T. S., 1975, Median tolerance limits of some chemicals to the freshwater fish, *C. rapio*, *Indian J. Environ. Health* **17**:140.

Ray, S., and Addy, S. K., 1976, Residue levels of Diodine in relation to canker development in citrus trees, *Indian Phytopathol.* **29**:246.

Reddy, T. C., and Gomathy, S., 1977, Toxicity and respiration effects of pesticides, thiodan (endosulfan) on catfish, *Indian J. Environ. Health* **19**:360.

Report of National Institute of Nutrition, 1977, ICMR, Hyderabad, India.

Saha, J. G., and McDonald, H., 1967, Insecticide residues in wheat grown in soil treated with aldrin and dieldrin, *J. Agric. Food Chem.* **15**:205.

Santha Ram, K. R., Thayumanavan, B., and Krishnaswamy, S., 1976, Toxicity of some insecticides to *Daphnia carinate* king, an important link in the food chain in the freshwater ecosystem, *Indian J. Ecol.* **3**:70.

Sastry, K. V., and Sharma, S. K., 1978, Endrin toxicity on liver of *C. punctatus*, *Indian J. Exp. Biol.* **1**:371.

Saxena, P. U., and Agarwal, S., 1970, Toxicity of some insecticides to the Indian catfish *Anat. Anz.* **127**:502.

Saxena, S. C., and Karel, A. K., 1975, A note on the effect of pyrethrum on haemoglobin concentration of Indian desert gerbil, *Pyrethrum Post* **12**:161.

Schafer, M. L., 1968, Pesticides in blood, *Residue Rev.* **24**:19.

Sethunathan, N., 1973, Microbial degradation of insecticides in flooded soil and in anaerobic cultures, *Residue Rev.* **47**:143.

Sethunathan, N., Rajaram, K. P., and Sidaramappa, R., 1975, Persistence and microbial degradation of parathion in Indian rice soils under flooded conditions in origin and fate of chemical residues in food, agriculture and fisheries, IAEA, Vienna, pp. 9–18.

Shah, R. M., and Undavia, S. V., 1972, Diazinon poisoning with special reference to electrocardiograph and autopsy findings, *Med. Surg.* **12**:6.

Shankar, A., and Kavadia, V. S., 1976, Residues of endosulfan in/on tomato fruits, Proceedings of the All India Symposium on Modern Concepts of Plant Protection, Udaipur, India, pp. 75–76.

Sheela, S., and Vasantharajan, V. N., 1978a, Persistence of fensulfothion in soil, *J. Environ. Sci. Health* B12:15.

Sheela, S., and Vasantharajan, V. N., 1978b, Acetylcholine utilization by organophosphorus pesticides metabolizing microorganism, *Indian J. Exp. Biol.* 16:478.

Shetty, K. M., and Nayer, S. V., 1964, A comparative trial of BHC and some organic phosphate insecticides for the control of "Shabt lonse" of fowls, *Menopon* gallinae, Symposium on Pesticides, Central Food Technology Research Institute, Mysore, India.

Singh, H., and Singh, G., 1970, Evaluation of some important pesticides for the control of fruit, borer, *Heliothis armigera* infesting the tomato, *Indian J. Entomol.* 32:205.

Singh, H., Brar, H. S., and Mavi, G. S., 1973, Insecticidal trial for the control of *Helicoverpa armigera* (Hubner) on gram, *Indian J. Entomol.* 35:325.

Singh, J., 1972, Studies on the residues of carbaryl, DDT, endosulfan, malathion in/on okra fruits, M.S. thesis, Punjab Agricultural University, Ludhiana, India.

Singh, J., and Deshmukh, S. N., 1974, Estimation and dissipation of DDT and endosulfan residues in and on the fruits of okra, *Indian J. Agric. Sci.* 44:516.

Singh, J., Krueger, H. R., Desmukh, S. N., and Bindra, O. S., 1971, Dissipation of parathion residues from cabbage, *Indian J. Agric. Sci.* 41:328.

Singh, M., Sharma, P. L., and Dhaliwal, H. S., 1974, Toxicity of insecticides to honeybee workers, *Apis cerana indica F., Pesticides* 8:28.

Sinha, A. K., Nath, G., Kathpal, T. S., and Srivastava, B. P., 1976, Insecticidal efficiency and residues of phosphine in maize, Proceedings of the All India Symposium on Modern Concepts of Plant Protection, Udaipur, India, pp. 81–82.

Sinha, N. P., and Gulati, K. C., 1968, Neem seed cake on a source of pest control chemicals (II) an aphicidal factor, in: *Pesticides* (Sk. Majumdar, ed.), pp. 215–220, Academy of Pest Control Science, Mysore, India.

Somasundaram, K., Damodaran, V. N., and Subramanian, T. A. V., 1978, Biochemical changes following absorption of dieldrin through skin, *Indian J. Exp. Biol.* 16:1003.

Srinivasan, K., and Radhakrishnamurthy, R., 1977, Effects of beta and gamma isomers of BHC on some liver and kidney enzymes in albino rats, *Curr. Sci.* 46:568.

Srivastava, A. S., Prasad, R., Singh, Y. P., and Singh, D. N., 1975, Persistence of malathion in paddy plants *(Oryza sativa), Curr. Sci.* 44:317.

Srivastava, B. P., and Kavadia, V. S., 1976, Uptake and translocation of some insecticides in carrots, radishes and beetroots raised on treated soil, Proceedings of the All India Symposium on Modern Concepts of Plant Protection, Udaipur, India, pp. 76–78.

Srivastava, B. P., Mathur, M. C., Kathpal, T. S., and Nath, G. 1976, Control of fig midge by endosulfan and its residues in and on fig fruits, Proceedings of the All India Symposium on Modern Concepts of Plant Protection, Udaipur, India, p. 80.

Srivastava, G. N., Gupta, R. A., Peer Mohamed, M., and Nath, G., 1977, Effect of sublethal ethyl parathion on the metabolism and activity of the Indian Weed fish, *Indian J. Environ. Health* 19:66.

Sundaram, K. S., Damodaran, V. N., and Venkitasubramanian, T. A., 1978, Absorption of dieldrin through monkey and dog skin, *Indian J. Exp. Biol.* 16:101.

Tewari, S. N., and Harpalani, S. P., 1977, Detection and determination of organophosphorm insecticides in human body tissues in five cases of poisoning, *J. Chromatogr.* 130:229.

Tewari, S. N., and Sharma, T. C., 1977, Isolation and determination of chlorinated organic pesticides by thin layer chromatography and the application of toxicological analysis, *J. Chromatogr.* 131:275.

Thontadarya, T. S., Gowda, H., Prabhuswamy, H. P., and Shetty, S. V. R., 1974, Effect of phorate residue in the treated rice plant and water on buffalo calves, *Mysore J. Agric. Sci.* **8**:228.

Tripathy, R. K., Singh, A., and Singh, S. L., 1976, Residue analysis of wheat grain and straw produced from Vitavax treated seed, *Pesticides* **10**:33.

Uttamaswamy, S., Kumaresan, D., Vasudevan, P. P., Menon and Jairaj, S., 1976, Biochemical changes in egg plant due to insecticidal sprays in relation to the mite incidence, *Indian J. Exp. Biol.* **14**:639.

Vasuki, K., and Dikshith, T. S. S., 1968, Alkaline and acid phosphatases in the grasshopper *poecilocerus pictus* Fab. (Orthoptera:Acrididae) and the effect of endrin, *Enzymologia* **34**:277.

Venkataraman, C. G., 1977, Degradation of calixin in tea shoots harvested at different intervals after treatment, *Plant. Chron.* **72**:143.

Venkataraman, G. S., and Rajya Lakshmi, B., 1971, Interactions between pesticides and soil microorganisms, *Indian J. Exp. Biol.* **9**:521.

Verma, M. P., Bahga, H. S., and Soni, K., 1967, Toxic effects of insecticides telodrin in poultry, *Indian J. Exp. Biol.* **5**:245.

Verma, S., and Lal, R., 1976, Residues and residual toxicity of endosulfan on cauliflower, *Indian J. Agric. Sci.* **46**:125.

Verma, S. R., and Gupta, S. P., 1976, Pesticides in relation to water pollution, accumulation of aldrin and ethyl parathion in the few tissues of *C. fasciatus* and *Motopterus, Indian J. Environ. Health* **18**:10.

Verma, S. R., Gupta, S. P., and Tyagi, M. P., 1975, Studies on the toxicity of lindane in *Colisa fasciatus*, (Part 1: TLM measurements and histopathological changes in certain tissues), *Gegenbaurs Morphol. Jahr.* **121**:39.

Voss, G., and Geissbuhler, 1971, Rate of degradation of phosphamidon and residue levels, *Residue Rev.* **37**:133.

Whaley, W. G., Malenhauer, H. H., and Leech, J. H., 1960, The ultrastructure of the merstematic cells, *Am. J. Bot.* **47**:407.

Yadav, C. P. S., and Gupta, H. P., 1975, Uptake, translocation and accumulation of phosphamidon residue toxins in mustard, Brassica camp estris, *Indian J. Entomol.* **37**:327.

Yadav, C. P. S., and Shaw, F. R., 1970, Residues of rabon in tissues and egg yolks of poultry, *J. Econ. Entomol.* **63**:1097.

Yadav, D. V., Pillai, M. K. K., and Hari, C., Agarwal, 1976, Uptake and metabolism of DDT and lindane by the earthworm, *Bull. Environ. Contam. Toxicol.* **16**:541.

Yadav, D. V., Agarwal, H. C., and Pillai, M. K. K., 1978, Uptake metabolism and excretion of DDT by the fresh water snail, *Vivipara heliformis, Bull. Environ. Contam. Toxicol.* **19**:300.

Yadav, P. R., 1976, Studies on persistence of BHC in soils, its phytotoxicity and residues in some crops, Ph.D. dissertation, University of Udaipur, Udaipur, India.

Yadav, P. R., Srivastava, B. P., and Kavadia, V. S., 1977, Absorption of BHC in some root crops raised on treated soils, *Indian J. Entomol.* **39**:247.

Index